Oncologic Medicine

Oncologic Medicine

Clinical Topics and Practical Management

Edited By

Alton I. Sutnick, M.D., F.A.C.P.
Dean and Professor of Medicine
The Medical College of Pennsylvania

And

Paul F. Engstrom, M.D., F.A.C.P.
Director, Department of Medicine
American Oncologic Hospital,
Fox Chase Cancer Center
and Assistant Professor Of Medicine
The University Of Pennsylvania School of Medicine

University Park Press
Baltimore • London • Tokyo

UNIVERSITY PARK PRESS
International Publishers in Science and Medicine
Chamber of Commerce Building
Baltimore, Maryland 21202

Copyright © 1976 by University Park Press

Typeset by Service Composition Co., Inc., Baltimore, Maryland.

Manufactured in the United States of America by Universal Lithographers, Inc., and The Maple Press Co.

Library of Congress Cataloging in Publication Data
Main entry under title:

Oncologic medicine.

    Includes index.
    1. Cancer. I. Sutnick, Alton I. II. Engstrom,
Paul F. [DNLM: 1. Neoplasms. 2. Neoplasms—
Therapy. QZ266 058]
  RC261.047   616.9'94   76-13489
ISBN 0-8391-0883-4

Contents

Contributors

Richard Axel, M.D.
Assistant Professor of Pathology,
Institute of Cancer Research
Columbia University College of
    Physicians and Surgeons
New York, New York 10032

Claus Bahne Bahnson, Ph.D.
Head, Section of Oncologic
    Psychology and Psychiatry
American Oncologic Hospital
Fox Chase Cancer Center
Philadelphia, Pennsylvania 19111;
Director, Department of Behavioral
    Sciences
Eastern Pennsylvania Psychiatric
    Institute
Philadelphia, Pennsylvania 19129

Robert E. Bellet, M.D.
Research Physician,
American Oncologic Hospital
Fox Chase Cancer Center
Philadelphia, Pennsylvania 19111

Jane Berkelhammer, Ph.D.
Postdoctoral Associate,
The Institute for Cancer Research
Fox Chase Cancer Center
Philadelphia, Pennsylvania 19111

Richard S. Bornstein, M.D.
Assistant Clinical Professor
    of Medicine,
Temple University School
    of Medicine;
Attending Physician,
Albert Einstein Medical Center—
    Northern Division
Temple University School
    of Medicine
Philadelphia, Pennsylvania 19141

Isadore Brodsky, M.D., F.A.C.P.
Professor of Medicine,
Director, Division of Hematology
    and Medical Oncology,
and Director of the Cancer
    Institute,
The Hahnemann Medical College
    and Hospital of Philadelphia
Philadelphia, Pennsylvania 19102

Ronald I. Cantor, M.D.
Clinical Instructor in Medicine,
Jefferson Medical College of
    Thomas Jefferson University
Philadelphia, Pennsylvania 19107

Paul P. Carbone, M.D., F.A.C.P.
Chairman, Eastern Cooperative
    Oncology Group
Silver Spring, Maryland 20910;
and Special Assistant to the
    Director,
Division of Cancer Biology and
    Diagnosis
National Cancer Institute
Bethesda, Maryland 20014

Peter A. Cassileth, M.D.
Assistant Professor of Medicine,
The University of Pennsylvania
School of Medicine
Philadelphia, Pennsylvania 19174

Richard H. Creech, M.D., F.A.C.P.
Associate Physician,
American Oncologic Hospital
Fox Chase Cancer Center
Philadelphia, Pennsylvania 19111;
Assistant Professor of Medicine,
The University of Pennsylvania
School of Medicine
Philadelphia, Pennsylvania 19174

Paul F. Engstrom, M.D., F.A.C.P.
Director, Department of Medicine
American Oncologic Hospital
Fox Chase Cancer Center
Philadelphia, Pennsylvania 19111;
Assistant Professor of Medicine,
The University of Pennsylvania
School of Medicine
Philadelphia, Pennsylvania 19174

Audrey E. Evans, M.D.
Professor of Pediatrics,
The University of Pennsylvania
School of Medicine
Philadelphia, Pennsylvania 19174;
Chief of Pediatric Oncology,
Childrens' Hospital of
Philadelphia
Philadelphia, Pennsylvania 19146

Anthony A. Fuscaldo, Ph.D.
Assistant Professor of Medicine,
The Hahnemann Medical College
and Hospital of Philadelphia
Philadelphia, Pennsylvania 19102

Kathryn E. Fuscaldo, Ph.D.
Associate Professor of Medicine,
and Associate Director of the
Cancer Institute

The Hahnemann Medical College
and Hospital of Philadelphia
Philadelphia, Pennsylvania 19102

James M. Gerson, M.D.
Instructor in Pediatrics,
The University of Pennsylvania
School of Medicine
Philadelphia, Pennsylvania 19174;
Assistant Pediatrician in Oncology,
Childrens' Hospital of
Philadelphia
Philadelphia, Pennsylvania 19146

S. Benham Kahn, M.D., F.A.C.P.
Professor of Medicine,
Associate Director, Division of
Hematology and Medical
Oncology
The Hahnemann Medical College
and Hospital of Philadelphia
Philadelphia, Pennsylvania 19102

Donald Kaye, M.D., F.A.C.P.
Professor and Chairman,
Department of Medicine
The Medical College of
Pennsylvania
Philadelphia, Pennsylvania 19129

B. J. Kennedy, M.D., F.A.C.P.
Masonic Professor of Oncology,
Professor of Medicine and Director,
Section of Medical Oncology
University of Minnesota Medical
School—Minneapolis
Minneapolis, Minnesota 55455

Melvin J. Krant, M.D.
Co-Director, Oncology Department
Lemuel Shattuck Hospital
Boston, Massachusetts 02130

J. Frederick Laucius, M.D.
Instructor in Medicine,
Jefferson Medical College of
Thomas Jefferson University
Philadelphia, Pennsylvania 19107

W. Thomas London, M.D.,
F.A.C.P.
Research Physician,
The Institute for Cancer Research
Fox Chase Cancer Center
Philadelphia, Pennsylvania 19111;
Assistant Professor of Medicine,
The University of Pennsylvania
School of Medicine
Philadelphia, Pennsylvania 19174

Rita M. Lysik, B.A.
Research Assistant,
Veterans' Administration Hospital
Northport, New York 11768

Michael J. Mastrangelo, M.D.,
F.A.C.P.
Research Physician,
The Institute for Cancer Research
Assistant Physician and Director
of Immunotherapy Clinic,
American Oncologic Hospital
Fox Chase Cancer Center
Philadelphia, Pennsylvania 19111;
Clinical Assistant Professor
of Medicine,
Temple University School
of Medicine
Philadelphia, Pennsylvania 19140

Nathaniel H. Mayer, M.D.
Assistant Professor of
Rehabilitation Medicine,
Temple University School
of Medicine
Philadelphia, Pennsylvania 19140;
Director of Rehabilitation,
American Oncologic Hospital
Fox Chase Cancer Center
Philadelphia, Pennsylvania 19111

Daniel G. Miller, M.D., F.A.C.P.
President and Director,
Preventive Medicine Institute—
Strang Clinic
New York, New York 10001

Richmond T. Prehn, M.D.
Senior Member,
The Institute for Cancer Research
Fox Chase Cancer Center
Philadelphia, Pennsylvania 19111;
Professor of Pathology,
The University of Pennsylvania
School of Medicine
Philadelphia, Pennsylvania 19174

Kristen Ries, M.D.
Assistant Professor of Medicine,
The Medical College of
Pennsylvania
Philadelphia, Pennsylvania 19129

Richard K. Root, M.D.
Professor of Medicine and Chief,
Infectious Disease Section
Department of Internal Medicine
Yale University School of Medicine
New Haven, Connecticut 06510

Richard V. Smalley, M.D., F.A.C.P.
Associate Professor of
Medicine and Head,
Section of Medical Oncology
Temple University School
of Medicine
Philadelphia, Pennsylvania 19140

J. Bruce Smith, M.D., F.A.C.P.
Research Physician,
The Institute for Cancer Research
Fox Chase Cancer Center
Philadelphia, Pennsylvania 19111

Sol Spiegelman, Ph.D.
Professor of Human Genetics
and Development,
Director, Institute of Cancer
Research
Columbia University College of
Physicians and Surgeons
New York, New York 10032

Alton I. Sutnick, M.D., F.A.C.P.
Dean and Professor of Medicine,
The Medical College of
    Pennsylvania
Philadelphia, Pennsylvania 19129

Eugene J. Van Scott, M.D.
Professor of Dermatology,
Temple University School
    of Medicine
Philadelphia, Pennsylvania 19140;
Associate Director,
Skin and Cancer Hospital
Philadelphia, Pennsylvania 19140

Arthur J. Weiss, M.D., F.A.C.P.
Assistant Professor of Medicine,
Jefferson Medical College of
    Thomas Jefferson University
Philadelphia, Pennsylvania 19107

Stanley Zucker, M.D., F.A.C.P.
Associate Professor of Medicine,
State University of New York
    at Stony Brook
Stony Brook, New York, 11794;
Acting Chief of Hematology,
Veterans' Administration Hospital
Northport, New York 11768

Preface

Many changes in the practice of medical oncology have developed over the past decade. We have seen remarkable improvements in the treatment of acute lymphocytic leukemia, Hodgkin's disease, neuroblastoma, Wilms' tumor, Burkitt's lymphoma, and choriocarcinoma. With proper diagnosis and staging, and with the best conditions for management, likely cures have occurred in 50 to 80% of these patients, many of them even with disseminated disease. The accomplishments of the past have been great, and we look forward to even more impressive developments in the future.

This volume, which marks the 50th anniversary of The Institute for Cancer Research of The Fox Chase Cancer Center, provides information about developments in a number of areas in medical oncology. Many of these are already in the hands of the practitioner; some are now in active clinical trial; others represent possibilities for the future. In all cases, the emphasis is on the clinician and the practical problems of cancer patient management. Many of these products of clinical and laboratory research programs have proven their value and cover many fields, ranging from molecular biology and cellular immunology to chemotherapy, psychology, and rehabilitation medicine.

The past 10 years have been generous to us in the cancer field. Now, in the 50th year of The Institute for Cancer Research, and as we celebrate the Bicentennial commemoration of the founding of our country, we look forward to another decade in which we expect the yield to be even greater in the prevention of mortality and morbidity due to malignant disease. As we present this volume, this is our conviction. We offer our support and cooperation to all those who provide a reasonable route towards that end.

Oncologic Medicine

Molecular Virology of Human Neoplasia

Richard Axel, M.D.,
and Sol Spiegelman, Ph.D.

A rational approach to the prevention, diagnosis, and therapy of neoplasia will inevitably benefit from an understanding of the etiology of this disease. Although considerable progress has been made in these areas, the molecular events responsible for the conversion of a normal cell to a cancer cell remain obscure. In approaching the problem of the etiology of human cancer, we were unavoidably influenced by our previous experience with RNA viruses and our assessment of the information available on the relationship between viruses and cancer. Both DNA and RNA viruses have been identified as capable of producing tumors in animals in laboratory experiments. Nevertheless, we decided to concentrate our experimental efforts on the RNA oncornaviruses, a choice made for two reasons. One is that the RNA oncogenic agents predominate quantitatively in the animal systems studied. The second reason is that it is the RNA tumor viruses that have been repeatedly demonstrated to cause tumors in their indigenous hosts. Thus, from the viewpoint of the natural history of the disease, the RNA oncogenic viruses appeared to us as the more

This research was supported by the National Institutes of Health, National Cancer Institute, Virus Cancer Program Contract NO1-CP-3-3258, and by the National Cancer Institute Grants CA-02332 and 16346-01A1.

probable "natural" candidates for etiologic agents of cancer in the animal kingdom, including man.

Over the past few years an experimentally consistent model of transformation of animal cells by tumor viruses has been formulated, which postulates the exogenous introduction of new viral sequences through infection with a tumor virus. If the virus involved is of the RNA variety, the insertion of the new information into the host cell genome is presumed to require the synthesis of viral DNA by a DNA polymerase templated by the viral RNA. In this scheme, replication of the oncornavirus would involve successive transfers of information from the viral RNA to proviral DNA to progeny RNA. Replication of the provirus would proceed via information transfer from DNA to DNA (Temin, 1964; Varmus, Vogt, and Bishop, 1973; Evans, Baluda, and Shoyab, 1974; Sweet et al., 1974).

The evolution of such a scheme in animal systems has provided the rationale for experiments designed to detect the presence of oncornavirus particles in human neoplasias. The detection of putative human viral agents, however, requires more sensitive devices than those that sufficed to establish their presence in the inbred animal systems. In searching for such tools, we quite naturally turned to molecular hybridization and the other methodologies developed by molecular biologists in the past several decades.

Our approach, therefore, relied heavily on technology initially developed in model systems and allowed us to answer sequentially the following questions:

1. Do human neoplasias contain base sequences in their RNA that are homologous to the information present in RNA tumor viruses known to cause similar cancers in animals?
2. Does the virus-specific RNA in human tumors possess the size and physical association with reverse transcriptase that characterize the RNA of the animal viruses?
3. If such RNA exists in human tumors, is it encapsulated in a particle possessing the density and size of the RNA tumor viruses?
4. Does a copy of this RNA reside within the DNA genome of the tumor cell and, if so, is it restricted to the DNA of neoplastic cells?

ANIMAL MODELS AS A POINT OF DEPARTURE

To understand better the biologic rationale underlying the experiments described, it is useful to summarize briefly some of the salient features of the animal model systems used as a guide. Table 1 lists a representative group of animal viruses, including those actually employed to generate the molecular probes used (Axel, Schlom, and Spiegelman, 1972a, 1972b; Hehlmann, Kufe, and Spiegelman, 1972a, 1972b; Kufe, Hehlmann, and Spiegelman, 1972). There are two avian viruses, avian myeloblastosis virus (AMV) and Rous sarcoma virus (RSV), that cause leukemias and sarcomas in chickens. In addition, we have the murine leukemia virus (MuLV) and murine sarcoma virus (MuSV) that induce similar diseases in mice, and finally the murine mammary tumor virus (MMTV) that is the unique etiologic agent for mammary tumors.

When these viruses are examined for sequence homologies among their nucleic acids, a rather informative pattern emerges. It will be noted that the two chicken agents (AMV and RVS) have sequences in common but do not show detectable homology with any of the murine agents. Turning to the murine viruses, we find that the nucleic acids of the leukemia, lymphoma, and sarcoma agents show homology to one another but not to either of the two avian agents or to the MMTV. Finally, the MMTV has a singular sequence homologous only to itself.

If analogous virus particles are associated with the corresponding human diseases, certain predictions might be hazarded on the basis of the specificity patterns exhibited in Table 1, and these may be listed as follows:

1. In view of the lack of homology between the avian and murine agents, it is unlikely that human agents (should they exist) would show homology to the avian group.

2. It follows that the murine tumor viruses would represent a more hopeful source of the molecular probes needed to search for similar information in the analogous human cancers.

3. If particles are found to be associated with human leukemias, sarcomas, and lymphomas, their RNAs might show homology to one another and possibly to that of the MuLV.

4. If RNA particles are identified in human breast cancer, they should not exhibit homology to the RNA of the viruses causing the human mesenchymal neoplasias or to RLV RNA, but might exhibit some homology to the RNA of the MMTV.

Table 1. Comparison of some representative oncornaviruses

Virus[a]	Indigenous host	Homology[b]					Disease
		AMV	RSV	MuLV	MSV	MMTV	
AMV	Chicken	+	+	−	−	−	Leukemia
RSV(RAV)	Chicken	+	+	−	−	−	Sarcoma
MuLV	Mouse	−	−	+	+	−	Leukemia, lymphoma
MSV(MuLV)	Mouse	−	−	+	+	−	Sarcoma
MMTV	Mouse	−	−	−	−	+	Breast cancer

[a]AMV, avian myeloblastosis virus; RSV, Rous sarcoma virus; RAV, Rous avian virus; MuLV, murine leukemia virus; MSV, murine sarcoma virus; MMTV, murine mammary tumor virus.

[b]The results of molecular hybridizations between [^{3}H]DNA complementary to the various RNAs and the indicated RNAs. The plus sign indicates the hybridizations were positive and the minus sign indicates none could be detected.

VIRAL-SPECIFIC RNA IN HUMAN NEOPLASIAS

Using the technology developed in the previous experiments, we began to probe human neoplasias for the presence of RNA molecules with information homologous to that of an analogous animal virus of proven oncogenic potential. The experimental design we adopted is depicted in Figure 1. A highly radioactive DNA copy of a viral RNA is synthesized using the endogenous reverse transcriptase and the 70 S RNA of the appropriate animal virion. This DNA is now used as a probe in annealing reactions to test for homologous virus-specific sequences in the RNA of various human neoplasias. The presence of viral sequences is assessed by Cs_2SO_4 equilibrium density gradient centrifugation. The movement of the [³H]DNA to the RNA region of the density gradient is the signal that the probe used has found complementary sequences in the tumor RNA with which it is being challenged.

The murine agents were initially chosen to produce the necessary molecular probes to look for corresponding information in the human disease. The desire to monitor the biologic consistency of our findings

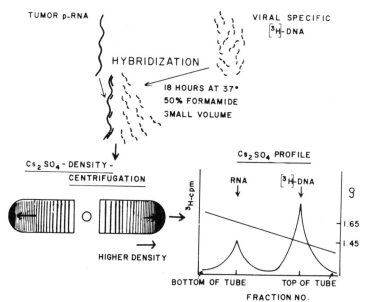

Figure 1. Molecular hybridization and detection with virus-specific [³H]DNA and tumor RNA (see text for further details).

dictated that we examine a number of human neoplasias simultaneously. This would permit us to determine quickly whether our findings in man mirrored biologically what was known from the animal experimental models. For this purpose, from the onset we focused our attention in parallel on the mesenchymal neoplasias and on breast cancer.

In Figure 2*A* we observe the sort of positive response we find when mouse mammary tumor virus (MMTV DNA) is annealed with polysomal RNA (pRNA) from human breast carcinomas (Axel et al., 1972b). This profile is in contrast to the negative outcomes observed when similar reactions were carried out with pRNA from normal breast tissue or from fibrocystic disease tissue (Figure 2*B*), where no MMTV [^{3}H]DNA is observed hybridized in the RNA region. Of the 29 malignant breast tumors examined, 67% gave positive responses with values that can be assigned a better than one chance out of a thousand of being significant. None of the pRNA samples derived from normal breasts or the nonmalignant fibrocystic and gynecomastia tissues and fibroadenomas yielded positive reactions with the MMTV DNA.

Table 2 summarizes in diagrammatic form the outcome of this survey of human neoplasias with the animal virus probes. The plus signs indicate that the corresponding [^{3}H]DNA formed complexes with the indicated tumor RNAs and the minus signs indicate that no such complexes were detected. The proportion of positives among those complexes labeled plus in earlier studies (Axel et al., 1972b; Hehlmann et al., 1972a, 1972b; Kufe et al., 1972) ranged from about 67% for breast cancer to 92% for the leukemias. As our technology improved, so did our percentage of positives among the neoplastic samples.

What is most noteworthy of the pattern exhibited in Table 2 is its concordance with the predictions deducible from the murine system. Thus, human breast cancer contains RNA homologous only to that of the MMTV. Human leukemias, sarcomas, and lymphomas all contain RNA showing sufficient homology to that of the murine Rauscher leukemia virus (RLV) to make a stable duplex. These mesenchymal neoplasias contain no RNA homologous to the MMTV RNA. Finally, none of the human tumors contains RNA detectably related to that of the AMV. Recently, Gallo and his associates (Gallo et al., 1973) have confirmed the homology of leukemic RNA to that of RLV and in the process have shown even more relatedness to the RNA of a simian sarcoma virus. In summary, the specificity pattern of the

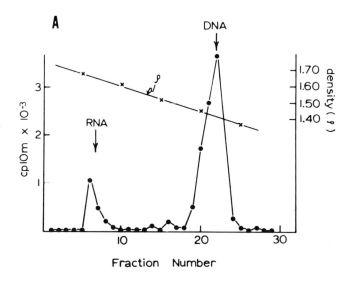

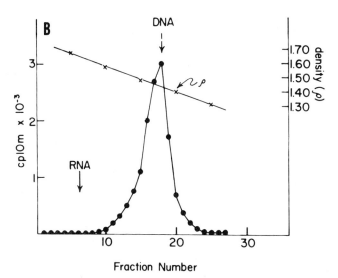

Figure 2. Cesium sulfate equilibrium density gradient centrifugation of MMTV-tritiated DNA. *A*, after annealing to 400 µg of polysomal RNA from human breast tumor (C13791); *B*, after annealing to 400 µg of polysomal RNA from biopsy specimens of fibrocystic disease of breast.

Table 2. Homologies among human neoplastic RNAs and animal tumor viral RNAs

Viral RNAs[a]	Human neoplastic RNAs[b]			
	Breast cancer	Leukemia	Sarcoma	Lymphoma
MMTV	+	−	−	−
RLV	−	+	+	+
AMV	−	−	−	−

[a]MMTV, murine mammary tumor virus; RLV, murine Rauscher leukemia virus; AMV, avian myeloblastosis virus.

[b]The results of molecular hybridization between [³H]DNA complementary to the various viral RNAs and pRNA preparations from the indicated neoplastic tissues. The plus sign indicates that hybridizations were positive and the minus sign indicates that none could be detected (Hehlmann, Kufe, and Spiegelman, 1972a, b).

unique RNA found in the human neoplasias is in complete agreement with what has been described for the corresponding virus-induced malignancies in the mouse.

SIMULTANEOUS DETECTION TEST FOR REVERSE TRANSCRIPTASE AND HIGH MOLECULAR WEIGHT RNA

Needless to say, the existence of the remarkable concordance exhibited in Table 2 does not establish a viral etiology for these diseases in man. The next step required the performance of experiments designed to answer the second and third questions raised in the introduction, i.e., those relating to the size of the RNA being detected and whether or not it is associated with a reverse transcriptase in a particle possessing other features of complete or incomplete virus particles. We now turn our attention to the description of these techniques and their application to the analysis of human malignant tissue.

What we sought was a method of detecting the presence of particles similar to the RNA tumor viruses in human material that would be simple, sensitive, and sufficiently discriminating, so that a positive outcome could be taken as an acceptable signal for the presence of a virus-like agent. To achieve this goal, we devised a test that depended on the simultaneous detection of two diagnostic features of the animal RNA tumor viruses.

The oncornaviruses exhibit two identifying characteristics. They contain a large $(1 \times 10^7$ daltons) single-stranded RNA molecule having a sedimentation coefficient of 60 S to 70 S, often referred to as high molecular weight RNA. They also have reverse transcriptase (Baltimore, 1970; Temin and Mizutani, 1970), an enzyme that can use the viral RNA as a template to make a complementary DNA copy (Spiegelman et al., 1970).

The possibility of a concomitant test for both the enzyme and its template was suggested by studies of the early reaction intermediates (Spiegelman et al., 1970; Rokutanda et al., 1970). The initial DNA product was found complexed to the large 70 S RNA template. These structures can be detected by the unusual position of the newly synthesized small tritiated DNA products in Cs_2SO_4 density gradients, glycerol velocity gradients, and acrylamide gel electrophoresis (Bishop et al., 1971). The most informative assay is to subject the isotopically labeled product to sedimentation analysis prior to the removal of the RNA. If the labeled DNA product behaves as if it is a 70 S molecule, and if it can be shown that it does so because it is complexed to a 70 S RNA molecule, then evidence is provided for the presence of a reverse transcriptase using a 70 S RNA template. One may then tentatively conclude that the material examined contains particles similar to the RNA tumor viruses.

It was on this basis that Schlom and Spiegelman (1971) developed the simultaneous detection test that was used to demonstrate the presence in human milk of particles containing 70 S RNA and a reverse transcriptase (Schlom, Spiegelman, and Moore, 1972). The test was modified (Gulati, Axel, and Spiegelman, 1972) to be applicable to cancerous tissue using the MMTV as the experimental model.

Figure 3 diagrams the procedure used. Briefly, tumor cells are disrupted and fractionated by differential centrifugation. A high speed cytoplasmic pellet is isolated since, if virus is present, it is most likely to be found in this fraction. An endogenous reverse transcriptase reaction is then performed with this pellet. The product of the reaction with its RNA template is freed of protein and then analyzed in a glycerol velocity gradient to determine the sedimentation coefficient of the $[^3H]DNA$ as well as in a Cs_2SO_4 equilibrium gradient to determine its density.

The presence of particles encapsulating 70 S RNA and reverse transcriptase will be indicated by the appearance of a peak of newly

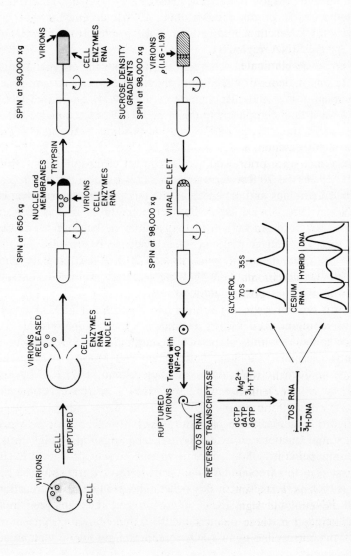

Figure 3. Simultaneous detection test for 70 S RNA and reverse transcriptase in neoplastic tissue (see text for further details).

synthesized DNA traveling at a speed corresponding to a 70 S RNA molecule. That its apparent large size is due to its being complexed to a 70 S RNA molecule can be readily verified by subjecting the purified nucleic acid to ribonuclease prior to velocity examination, and this should result in the disappearance of the "70 S" [³H]DNA. Similarly, if the reaction is positive, newly synthesized DNA should appear in the RNA region of a Cs_2SO_4 density gradient, and this again should be eliminated by prior treatment with ribonuclease.

The simultaneous detection test was first applied to human breast cancer. Figure 4 exemplifies a positive reaction with material obtained from a malignant adenocarcinoma of the breast and treated as outlined in Figure 3. Here we see the 70 S DNA complex observed with the P-100 fraction, and it is evident that this complex is an RNA-dependent one since prior treatment with ribonuclease eliminates the [³H]DNA from the 70 S region of the velocity gradient. In this series, 38 adenocarcinomas and 10 nonmalignant controls were examined in this manner. It was found that 79% of the malignant breast samples were positive for the simultaneous detection reaction, and all of the control samples from normal and benign tissues were negative.

It was further demonstrated (Axel, Gulati, and Spiegelman, 1972) that the breast carcinoma particles encapsulating the 70 S RNA and reverse transcriptase possess a density between 1.16 and 1.19 g/ml, the density characteristic of the oncogenic viruses. Identical experiments were undertaken (Baxt, Hehlmann, and Spiegelman, 1972; Kufe et al., 1973) with human leukemias, lymphomas, and sarcomas (Table 3).

It is noteworthy that positive outcomes were observed in more than 95% of the leukemic patients whether they were acute or chronic, lymphoblastic or myelogenous. Thus, despite their disparate clinical pictures and differing cellular pathologies, these various types of leukemias have similar, though probably not identical, virus-related information.

The experiments we have just summarized on human breast cancer, the leukemias, and the lymphomas were designed to probe further the etiologic significance of our exploratory investigations which identified in these neoplasias RNA that was homologous to those of the corresponding murine oncornaviruses. The data obtained with the simultaneous detection test established that at least a portion of the tumor-specific virus-related RNA that was detected was a 70 S RNA template physically associated with a reverse transcriptase

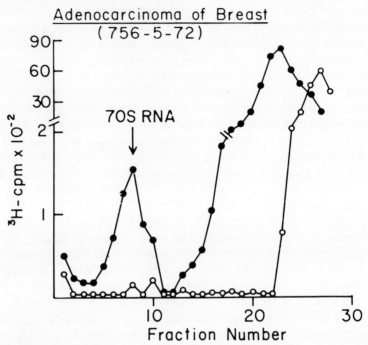

Figure 4. Effect of ribonuclease on the detection of the high molecular weight RNA-[³H]DNA complex. Breast tumor tissue (adenocarcinoma 756-5-72) was processed as described in Figure 2. The viral pellet (P-100) was suspended in 0.01 M Tris-HCl (pH 8.3) and divided into two equal parts. A standard RNA-instructed DNA polymerase reaction was performed on one part of the P-100 fraction; after incubation for 15 min at 37°C, the nucleic acid complex was extracted with phenol-cresol and was sized on a 10 to 30% linear glycerol gradient (●——●). After disruption with detergent, the other half of the P-100 fraction was incubated in the presence of RNase A (50 μg/ml) and RNase T₁ (50 μg/ml) for 15 min at 25°C. A standard RNA-instructed DNA polymerase reaction was then performed (0——0) (Axel, Gulati, and Spiegelman, 1972).

in a particle possessing a density between 1.16 and 1.19 g/ml, three of the diagnostic features of the animal RNA tumor viruses. Furthermore, the DNA synthesized in the particles found in each type of neoplasia hybridized uniquely to the RNA of the corresponding animal oncornavirus. Note that this last result is complementary to and completes the logic of our experimental approach. We started out by using animal tumor viruses to generate [³H]DNA probes that were used to find related RNA in human neoplastic tissue. We concluded

Table 3. Simultaneous detection tests with human tumors and controls[a]

Tissue	No. of positive reactions	Average "70 S" (cpm)	No. of negative reactions	Average "70 S" (cpm)	Positive reaction (%)
Carcinoma of the breast	28	668	10	20	74
Control (nonmalignant breast tissue)	0	0	10	8	0
Leukemia	22	481	1	0	95
Hodgkin's disease	22	379	6	14	79
Burkitt's lymphoma	9	369	2	14	82
Other lymphomas	7	347	1	24	88
Control (spleens)	0	0	14	14	0

[a]Results of simultaneous detection assays with human tumors and controls. The average of the cpm in the 70 S position monitored by external size markers is summarized. The reactions were designated as positive if the cpm exceeded 30 above background (Kufe et al., 1973).

by using analogous human particles to generate [³H]DNA probes that were then used to determine sequence relatedness to the RNA of the relevant oncornaviruses. None of the human probes hybridized to the avian viral RNA. The probe generated by the particles from human breast cancer was homologous only to the RNA of MMTV, whereas the human leukemic and lymphoma probes were related in sequence only to RLV RNA, the murine leukemic agent. The biologic logical consistency of these results adds further weight to their relevance to human disease.

GERM-LINE TRANSMISSION OF VIRAL INFORMATION

We now come to grips with the popular virogene (Todaro and Huebner, 1972) concept that derives from animal experiments and argues that all animals prone to cancer contain in their germ line at least one complete copy of the information necessary and sufficient to convert a cell from normal to malignant and produce the corresponding tumor virus. This hypothesis presumes that the malignant segment usually remains silent and that its activation by intrinsic or extrinsic factors leads to the appearance of virus and the onset of cancer.

There are various ways of testing the validity of the virogene hypothesis, but the pathways differ in the technical complexities entailed. One approach commonly used attempts to answer the question: "Does every normal cell contain at least one complete copy of the required virus-related malignant information?" The methodologies employed included the techniques of genetics, chemical-viral induction, and molecular hybridizations. However, for a variety of reasons, none of these gave, or could give, conclusive answers. Genetic experiments do not readily distinguish between susceptible genes and actual viral information. Furthermore, even if genetic data succeeded in identifying *some* structural viral genes, it would still be necessary to establish that *all* of the viral genes are represented in the genome. Attempts to settle the question by demonstrating that *every* cell of an animal can be chemically induced to produce viruses have thus far (for obvious reasons) not been tried. The best that has been achieved along these lines was to show that *cloned* cells do respond positively. However, the proportion of clonable cells is small and *clonability may well be a signal for prior infection with a tumor virus.*

Finally, the quantitative limitations of molecular hybridization make it almost impossible to provide definitive proof that each cell

contains one complete viral copy in its DNA. Although it is not difficult to show that 90% of the information is present, it is the last 10%
that constitutes the insurmountable barrier and 10% of 10^7 daltons
amounts to a far from trivial 10^6 daltons, the equivalent of about
three genes.

The experimental approach we adopted in an attempt to resolve
the question of the presence of complete and competent viral genomes
in normal cells again involves molecular hybridization (Figure 5).
Virtually all normal cells contain within their DNA at least a portion
of the murine leukemia virus genome. If a DNA copy of RLV RNA

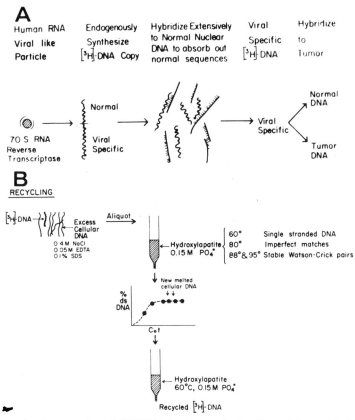

Figure 5. *A*, generation of [³H]DNA by human leukemic particles and hybridization of sequences shared with normal DNA; *B*, separation of leukemia-
specific sequences by hydroxyapatite chromatography. See text for further
details. *SDS*, sodium dodecyl sulfate.

is annealed exhaustively to a vast excess of cellular DNA (cDNA) from normal cells, about 30% of the cDNA fails to react. If this DNA is isolated, it reacts both with pure 70 S viral RNA and with DNA from cells transformed with RLV. These experiments show that some RLV sequences are missing from normal BALB/c DNA. These unique virus-specific sequences are present only in leukemic DNA (Sweet et al., 1974).

Identical experiments were simultaneously performed (Baxt and Spiegelman, 1972) in the case of human leukemias, with viral particles isolated from human leukemic buffy coats. These particles were used to generate [^{3}H]DNA probes from which normal sequences were moved by hybridization to normal leukocyte DNA in vast excess. The resulting residue of unpaired [^{3}H]DNA was then annealed alternatively to the white blood cell DNA from leukemic patients and to normal DNA (Figure 6).

A typical outcome of hybridizing such recycled tritiated DNA to normal and leukemic DNA is shown in Figure 6. It is evident that no complexes stable at temperatures above 88°C are formed with normal DNA. On the other hand, 57% of the recycled [^{3}H]DNA probe forms well paired duplexes with leukemic DNA. A series of such experiments was performed with particle-generated [^{3}H]DNA obtained from eight untreated patients with either acute or chronic myelogenous leukemia. In every case, the [^{3}H]DNA, after being subjected to exhaustive annealing to normal DNA, yielded a residue that forms stable duplexes only with leukemic DNA.

EVIDENCE AGAINST CHROMOSOMAL INHERITANCE OF VIRAL INFORMATION FROM STUDIES OF IDENTICAL TWINS

We now come to a biologically more precise and informative experiment on the question of the chromosomal inheritance of the necessary viral information. The comparison of leukemia and lymphoma patients with normals (Baxt and Spiegelman, 1972; Kufe, Peters, and Spiegelman, 1973) suggests that healthy individuals do not contain the neoplastic-specific sequences. However, the data do not rule out the possibility that those who develop the disease do so because they in fact inherit the required information in their germ line. One way to resolve this issue is to study the situation in identical twins. This was done in the case of leukemia. Since identical twins are monozygous, i.e., derive their genomes from the same fertilized egg, any chromo-

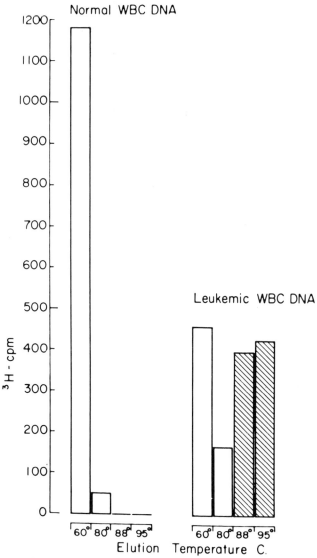

Figure 6. Hydroxyapatite elution profile of a hybridization reaction of recycled leukemic [³H]DNA to nuclear DNA from normal leukocytes and from leukemic leukocytes of the patient from which the [³H]DNA was derived.

somally transmitted information must be present in both. If the leukemic member of the pair contains the particle-related DNA sequences, and does so because he inherited them through his germ line, then these same sequences must be found in the leukocyte DNA of his healthy sibling. To perform the experiment, it was necessary to locate identical twins with completely convincing evidence for monozygosity and where only one twin was leukemic. Also, the twins had to be of adult age since at least 1 unit of whole blood is required to provide enough leukocyte DNA to carry out the required hybridization.

Two sets of identical twins satisfying all of these requirements were found and an experiment similar to the one outlined above was performed with each pair (Baxt et al., 1973). In each instance, particles containing the reverse transcriptase and 70 S RNA were again isolated from the leukocytes of the leukemic members and were used to generate the [³H]DNA endogenously. The [³H] DNA was purified, and sequences shared with normal DNA were removed by exhaustive hybridization in the presence of a vast excess of normal DNA from random, healthy blood donors. This was then followed by hydroxyapatite chromatography to separate paired from unpaired [³H]DNA. It is important to emphasize that in the recycling step the normal DNA used came from the leukocytes of healthy, random blood donors and not from the normal twin. To have used the latter would have obviously confused the issue. The residue of the tritiated DNA that did not pair with the normal DNA was then used to test for the presence of a sequence in the leukocyte DNA of the patient and that of his healthy sibling.

The results obtained with the two sets of twins are described in Figure 7 and it is evident that the same situation occurs between the members of the twin pairs that was observed in the comparison of unrelated leukemic patients and random normals. The leukemic twin contains particle-related sequences that cannot be detected in the leukocytes of his healthy sibling.

The fact that we could establish a sequence difference between identical twins implies that the additional information found in the DNA of the leukemic members was inserted after zygote formation. This finding argues against the applicability of the virogene hypothesis to this disease since it would demand that the leukemia-specific sequences found in the DNA of the individual with the disease must surely also exist in the genome of his identical twin. These results are

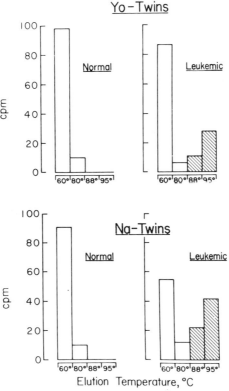

Figure 7. Hydroxyapatite elution profile of a hybridization reaction of the recycled leukemic twin [³H]DNA probe to nuclear DNA from normal leukocytes, normal twin leukocytes, and leukocytes from the same leukemic twin. The annealing reaction mixtures contained 20 A_{260} units of cellular DNA, 0.004 pmol of [³H]DNA, and 15 μmol of NaH PO⁴ (pH 7.2) in a final volume of 0.1 ml. The reaction was brought to 98°C for 60 sec and 0.04 mmol of NaCl was added. The reaction mixture was then incubated at 60°C for 50 hr. The reaction was stopped by the addition of 1 ml of 0.05 M NaH PO₄ (pH 6.8). The sample was then passed over a column of hydroxyapatite of 20-ml bed volume at 60°C. The column was washed with 40 ml of 0.15 M NaH PO₄ (pH 6.8) at 60, 80, 88, and 95°C. Fractions of 4 ml were collected, the A_{260} of each fraction was read, and the DNA was precipitated with 2 μg/ml of carrier yeast RNA and 10% trichloroacetic acid. The precipitate was collected on Millipore filters, which were dried and counted. In all cases, greater than 80% of the nuclear DNA reannealed. A background count of 8 cpm was subtracted in all instances (Baxt et al., 1973).

also inconsistent with the possibility that individuals who have leukemia have it because they inherit the complete viral genome.

CONCLUDING COMMENTS

The investigations summarized here were designed to see whether
molecular evidence could be found for a viral etiology of human
cancer. The experiments started out by using DNA probes synthesized with the aid of a variety of known RNA animal tumor viruses.
We found that human breast cancer contains RNA homologous only
to that of the murine mammary tumor virus. On the other hand,
human leukemias, sarcomas, and lymphomas all contain RNA homologous uniquely to that of the murine leukemia virus. The specificity
pattern of the RNA found in the human neoplasias examined is in
complete accord with that observed in the corresponding virus-
induced malignancies in the mouse.

The use of the simultaneous detection test permitted further
elucidation of the etiology significant in these findings. Thus, we have
shown that at least a portion of the virus-related RNA we were
detecting by hybridization is in the form of a 70 S RNA template
physically associated with a reverse transcriptase, two of the diagnostic features of the RNA tumor viruses. Furthermore, the DNA
synthesized by the human tumor cell reverse transcriptase on its own
endogenous template is related in sequence to the analogous murine
viral genome. Note that this last result is complementary to and
completes the logic of our earlier experiments in which the DNA
synthesized in murine particles was used as a probe to find the virus-
related information in human neoplasias.

It is important to emphasize that finding unique sequences in the
leukemias and lymphomas does not disprove the virogene hypothesis
in an absolute sense. Indeed, in a global biologic context, no collection of individual experiments can eliminate hypotheses that invoke
the germ-line transmission of a complete copy of some *unspecified*
viral information required for malignancy and the production of an
RNA tumor virus. The experiments we have described relevant to
this issue make this hypothesis unlikely only for those particular
neoplasias and associated particulate elements that were in fact subjected to experimental examination. Although not yet achieved, it
would not be terribly shocking if some day the virogene concept is
established with some neoplasia in man or in a laboratory animal
strain inbred for this or some other purpose.

What is evident is that our findings with the human leukemias
and lymphomas suggest more optimistic pathways for the control of

these diseases. The data suggest that in at least some instances we may not be forced to master the control of our own genes in order to cope with these neoplasias. The data also suggest that the malignant transformation involves the entry and the chromosomal insertion of new virus-related information. Either or both of these steps could provide additional and possibly more accessible targets for chemotherapy. Finally, the existence of the leukemia- and lymphoma-specific sequences and their protein products offers the clinician hitherto unsuspected parameters that could potentially be useful adjuncts in diagnosing and monitoring therapy.

REFERENCES

Axel, R., S. C. Gulati, and S. Spiegelman. 1972. Particles containing RNA-instructed DNA polymerase and virus-related RNA in human breast cancers. Proc. Natl. Acad. Sci. USA 69:3133–3137.

Axel, R., J. Schlom, and S. Spiegelman. 1972a. Presence in human breast cancer of RNA homologous to mouse mammary tumour virus RNA. Nature 235:32–36.

Axel, R., J. Schlom, and S. Spiegelman. 1972b. Evidence for translation of viral-specific RNA in cells of a mouse mammary carcinoma. Proc. Natl. Acad. Sci. USA 69:535–538.

Baltimore, D. 1970. RNA-dependent DNA polymerase in virions of RNA tumour viruses. Nature 226:1209–1211.

Baxt, W., R. Hehlmann, and S. Spiegelman. 1972. Human leukaemic cells contain reverse transcriptase associated with a high molecular weight virus-related RNA. Nature (New Biol.) 240:72–75.

Baxt., W. G., and S. Spiegelman. 1972. Nuclear DNA sequences present in human leukemic cells and absent in normal leukocytes. Proc. Natl. Acad. Sci. USA 69:3737–3741.

Baxt, W., J. W. Yates, H. J. Wallace, Jr., J. F. Holland, and S. Spiegelman. 1973. Leukemia-specific DNA sequences in leukocytes of the leukemic member of identical twins. Proc. Natl. Acad. Sci. USA 70:2629–2632.

Bishop, D. H. L., R. Ruprecht, R. W. Simpson, and S. Spiegelman. 1971. Deoxyribonucleic acid polymerase of Rous sarcoma virus: reaction conditions and analysis of the reaction product nucleic acids. J. Virol. 8:730–741.

Evans, R. M., M. A. Baluda, and M. Shoyab. 1974. Differences between the integration of avian myeloblastosis virus DNA in leukemic cells and of endogenous viral DNA in normal chicken cells. Proc. Natl. Acad. Sci. USA 71:3152–3156.

Gallo, R. C., N. R. Miller, W. C. Saxinger, and D. Gillespie. 1973. Primate RNA tumor virus-like DNA synthesized endogenously by RNA-dependent DNA polymerase in virus-like particles from fresh human acute leukemic blood cells. Proc. Natl. Acad. Sci. USA 70:3219–3224.

Gulati, S. C., R. Axel, and S. Spiegelman. 1972. Detection of RNA-instructed DNA polymerase and high molecular weight RNA in malignant tissue. Proc. Natl. Acad. Sci. USA 69:2020–2024.

Hehlmann, R., D. Kufe, and S. Spiegelman. 1972a. RNA in human leukemic cells related to the RNA of a mouse leukemia virus. Proc. Natl. Acad. Sci. USA 69:435–439.

Hehlmann, R., D. Kufe, and S. Spiegelman. 1972b. Viral-related RNA in Hodgkin's disease and other human lymphomas. Proc. Natl. Acad. Sci. USA 69:1727–1731.

Kufe, D., R. Hehlmann, and S. Spiegelman. 1972. Human sarcomas contain RNA related to the RNA of a mouse leukemia virus. Science 175:182–185.

Kufe, D., I. T. Magrath, J. L. Ziegler, and S. Spiegelman. 1973. Burkitt's tumors contain particles encapsulating RNA-instructed DNA polymerase and high molecular weight virus-related RNA. Proc. Natl. Acad. Sci. USA 70:737–741.

Kufe, D. W., W. P. Peters, and S. Spiegelman. 1973. Unique nuclear DNA sequences in the involved tissues of Hodgkin's and Burkitt's lymphomas. Proc. Natl. Acad. Sci. USA 70:3810–3814.

Rokutanda, M., H. Rokutanda, M. Green, K. Fujinaga, R. K. Ray, and C. Gurgo. 1970. Formation of viral RNA-DNA hybrid molecules by the DNA polymerase of carcoma-leukemia viruses. Nature 227:1026–1029.

Schlom, J., and S. Spiegelman. 1971. Simultaneous detection of reverse transcriptase and high molecular weight RNA unique to oncogenic RNA viruses. Science 174:840–843.

Schlom, J., S. Spiegelman, and D. H. Moore. 1972. Detection of high molecular weight RNA in particles from human milk. Science 175:542–544.

Spiegelman, S., A. Burny, M. R. Das, J. Keydar, J. Schlom, M. Travnicek, and K. Watson. 1970. Characterization of the products of RNA-directed DNA polymerases in oncogenic RNA viruses. Nature 227:563–567.

Sweet, R. W., N. C. Goodman, J. -R. Cho, R. M. Ruprecht, R. R. Redfield, and S. Spiegelman. 1974. The presence of DNA sequences following viral induction of leukemia in mice. Proc. Natl. Acad. Sci. USA 71:1705–1709.

Temin, H. M. 1964. Nature of the provirus of Rous sarcoma. Natl. Cancer Inst. Monogr. 17:557–570.

Temin, H. M., and S. Mizutani. 1970. RNA-dependent DNA polymerase in virions of Rous sarcoma virus. Nature 226:1211–1213.

Todaro, G. J., and R. J. Huebner. 1972. The viral oncogene hypothesis: new evidence. Proc. Natl. Acad. Sci. USA 69:1009–1015.

Varmus, Harold E., Peter K. Vogt, and J. Michael Bishop. 1973. Integration of deoxyribonucleic acid specific for Rous sarcoma virus after infection of permissive and nonpermissive hosts. Proc. Natl. Acad. Sci. USA 70:3067–3071.

Immunosurveillance of Cancer

Richmond T. Prehn, M.D.

The role of the immune system in oncogenesis and in the defense against neoplastic cell growth is one of continued controversy. It is now nearly 20 years since the demonstration that tumors are antigenic in their original hosts (Prehn and Main, 1957; Klein et al., 1960). However, the biologic function of these antigens and the role of immunity in tumor biology remain obscure.

There seems to be little controversy over the fact that the immune reaction can function to limit the spread and activity of oncogenic viruses; rather the controversy is over the role of the immune mechanism vis-à-vis the already transformed cell, the tumor cell per se. This role may be to limit tumor cell proliferation and to actually eliminate nascent tumors (immunologic surveillance); on the other hand, the immune reaction has the property, under some conditions, of stimulating target cell growth (immunologic stimulation) and it is possible that this activity may be of biologic importance. A third possibility is that the immune response, under natural conditions, may be essentially neutral with respect to tumor cell survival. Each of these possibilities is probably correct under certain

This investigation was supported by Public Health Service Research Grants CA-08856, CA-06927, CA-05255, CA-13456, and RR-05539 from the National Institutes of Health, and by an appropriation from the Commonwealth of Pennsylvania.

23

circumstances. The god of tumor immunology is Janus, the two-faced.

The evidence in favor of the surveillance function is largely derived from animal experiments which show that oncogenesis in response to potent chemical oncogens or laboratory viruses is sometimes, but not always, enhanced by measures designed to reduce the animal's immunologic reactivity (Burnet, 1970). These measures include thymectomy of the newborn, x-irradiation, and treatment with anti-lymphocyte serum, with cytotoxin, or with other immunodepressants. It is also to be noted in this context that the newborn, immunologically immature animal is usually more susceptible to oncogenesis than is the adult.

Further support of the surveillance hypothesis derives from the fact that there is a rather general relationship between the latency of tumor induction (i.e., the time between application of a strong oncogen and the gross appearance of tumor) and the immunogenicity of the tumor. On the average, late arising tumors have little capacity to immunize an animal against growth of a tumor implant in immunization-challenge type in vivo tests (Prehn, 1969). There is evidence suggesting that this relationship is probably due, at least in part, to immunoselection. If tumors are induced in an immunologically deficient environment, such as the interior of an intraperitoneal diffusion chamber, there is apparently no relationship between the latency and the average immunogenicity (Bartlett, 1972). It would seem that whenever tumors arise slowly in an immunocompetent animal, there are time and opportunity for immunoselection of less immunogenic tumor cell variants. The implication is therefore strong that some degree of immunologic surveillance actually occurs.

All of the evidence that has been cited here in favor of the surveillance hypothesis is derived from work with tumors induced by high concentrations of chemicals or laboratory viruses under conditions in which the tumor incidence is high. Tumors that result from such conditions tend to be highly immunogenic and would appear to be logical candidates for some degree of immunologic surveillance. Spontaneous tumors, i.e., tumors that arise sporadically in low incidence and without known cause or as a result of very low concentrations of oncogen, are quite different; they usually possess relatively minor capacities to immunize and in fact their levels of immunogenicity are often at or below the level of detectability (Prehn, 1975). Interference with the immunologic capacities of animals has apparently little or no effect on the incidence of such spontaneous tumors with one exception; both animals and humans that are grossly immunologically deficient may develop a high incidence of lymphoreticular tumors (Outzen et al., 1975). However, since this is the only type of tumor that definitely occurs in excess, this increased incidence is unlikely to be due to a lack of immunologic surveillance. A lack of the postulated surveillance function would be expected to produce an excess of all types of tumors. Rather, the lymphoreticular tumor excess is probably due more directly to the injury to the lymphoreticular system.

It might be argued that, just as in the case of carcinogen-induced tumors of longer latency, the lack of immunogenicity of spontaneous tumors might itself be a result of immunoselection and thus be evidence of surveillance. This is probably not the case. It was shown that tumors that arose in immune-free environments (such as a tissue culture dish) lacked immunogenicity unless transformation had been produced by a chemical or oncogenic virus. Spontaneous transformation in culture, either in vitro or in diffusion chambers in vivo, regularly resulted in nonimmunogenic tumors (Prehn, 1970; Parmiana, Carbone, and Prehn, 1971; Bartlett, 1972). Lack of immunogenicity among spontaneous tumors is thus a function of the lack of carcinogen, not immunologic surveillance. Apparently, some degree of immunoselection and immunosurveillance may occur when the tumors have been endowed by the oncogen with a high level of immunogenicity, but there is no likelihood nor evidence for surveillance among tumors of low immunogenicity, i.e., among spontaneous tumors or tumors induced in low frequency by low levels of oncogen (Nehlsen, 1971; Sanford et al., 1973; Outzen et al., 1975; Stutman, 1975).

The knowledge that an immune response can be cytotoxic to tumor cells derives from direct observation during in vitro tests, and this information has long been available. It was therefore natural to interpret the potentiating effects of immunosuppressive agents on chemical or viral oncogenesis as evidence of the effectiveness of immunosurveillance, at least in relation to tumors induced by high concentrations of oncogen. However, it is now known from similar in vitro observations that, under certain still poorly defined conditions, the immune reaction may have an exactly contrary effect, i.e., stimulation of the growth of the target tumor cells (Medina and Heppner, 1973; Fidler, 1973; Jeejeebhoy, 1974; Kall and Hellström, 1975; Bray and Keast, 1975; Bartholomaeus et al., 1974; Ilfeld et al.,

1973). The stimulation has both an immunologically specific and a nonspecific component. Antibody has been shown to possess the stimulatory property, but it is probable that other effector mechanisms can also operate to stimulate growth of target tumor cells. Whether inhibition or stimulation occurs is, at least to some extent, a function of dosage relationships, i.e., a low level of antibody tends to be stimulatory while a higher level is inhibitory (Shearer, Philpott, and Parker, 1973). Thus, the effect of the immune mechanism tends to be biphasic, being stimulatory when the immune response is "weak" and inhibitory when it is "strong" (Prehn and Lappé, 1971; Prehn, 1971, 1972). The "strength" of the response is probably governed by many factors including the nature and number of antibody receptors on the cell surface, the manner of immunization, the time after immunization at which the effects are measured, and the immunologic capacities of the animal and the nature of its immune reaction.

Since the immune reaction can be either stimulatory or inhibitory to target tumor cells, how should experiments showing an increased susceptibility to chemical tumor induction in immunodepressed animals be interpreted? The original interpretation of such data as evidence of immunologic surveillance may not be correct. It would be equally logical to assume that the immunodepressants lowered the immune reactivity from an essentially neutral level into the stimulatory range.

Be that as it may, both surveillance and stimulation depend upon the target tumors being immunogenic. I have already pointed out that so-called spontaneous tumors and those induced by very low levels of oncogen usually lack this property. It would seem therefore unlikely that either surveillance or stimulation plays a role in the biology of such tumors; however, if some naturally occurring tumors are actually due to environmental exposure to oncogens in sufficient concentrations to produce minimal degrees of tumor immunogenicity, stimulation of tumor growth may be the predominant effect of the weak immune reaction.

The hypothesis that neither surveillance nor stimulation is influential in spontaneous tumor systems seems to be supported by the data thus far obtained by study of the "nude" mouse. The nude mouse is a mutant that exhibits a congenital aplasia of the thymus. It seems to be completely devoid of functionally effective T-cell-dependent immune reactivity. For example, the nude mouse will accept any allo- or xenogeneic normal tissue graft yet attempted, even from donors as disparate as the amphibia. If kept under pathogen-free or bacteria-free conditions, the animals are long lived despite their immunologic handicap. Such animals would appear to have little or no capacity for either stimulation or surveillance. The evidence to date suggests that there is little or no difference in the spontaneous tumor incidence in these animals as compared with that in their immunologically normal heterozygous littermates (Outzen et al., 1975; Stutman, 1975). Similar results have been observed with normal animals that have been immunologically depressed throughout their lives by anti-lymphocyte serum (Nehlsen, 1971; Sanford et al., 1973). It therefore seems probable that the immune reaction plays little if any role in the biology of spontaneous tumors.

If the immune reaction has as little to do with the biology of spontaneous tumors as the above results suggest, how is it that evidence of immunologic reactions against human tumors is so widespread? I think the meaning of this evidence is very uncertain indeed. The types of tests usually employed, i.e., some modification of the original colony inhibition assay or the Takasugi and Klein cytotoxicity assay, give results that seem to have very little correlation with the behavior of the tumors in the patients. In animal systems these tests do not correlate with simultaneous in vivo assays (i.e., the growth of challenge tumor implants in immunized and control animals (Baldwin, 1973; Wahl et al., 1974)) very much more than could be accounted for by chance and sometimes there is no correlation at all. There does, however, seem to be an excellent correlation between the presence or absence of cytotoxic sera and the dissemination of malignant melanoma (Lewis et al., 1969; Bodurtha et al., 1975). Thus, the interpretation of the vast amount of data being accumulated about the immunology of human tumors must remain, for the present, very ambiguous.

Perhaps the most important immediately useful information that I wish to convey in this paper is the biphasic nature of the effects of the immune reaction on a tumor. If the tumor is of a type that can be influenced at all, it is not presently possible to predict in what direction that influence may act. Attempts to increase immune reactivity against a tumor could, under some circumstances, stimulate rather than retard tumor growth. It seems obvious that immunotherapy must therefore be approached with great caution.

REFERENCES

Baldwin, R. T. 1973. Immunological aspects of chemical carcinogenesis. Adv. Cancer Res. 18:1–76.

Bartholomaeus, W. N., A. E. Bray, J. M. Papadimitriou, and D. Keast. 1974. Immune response to a transplantable malignant melanoma in mice. J. Natl. Cancer Inst. 53:1065–1072.

Bartlett, G. L. 1972. Effect of host immunity on the antigenic strength of primary tumors. J. Natl. Cancer Inst. 49:493–504.

Bodurtha, A. J., D. O. Chee, J. F. Laucius, M. J. Mastrangelo, and R. T. Prehn. 1975. Clinical and immunological significance of human melanoma cytotoxic antibody. Cancer Res. 35:189–193.

Bray, A. E., and D. Keast. 1975. Changes in host immunity following excision of a murine melanoma. Brit. J. Cancer 31:170–175.

Burnet, F. M. 1970. Immunological Surveillance. Pergamon Press, Oxford.

Fidler, I. J. 1973. *In vitro* studies of cellular-mediated immuno-stimulation of tumor growth. J. Natl. Cancer Inst. 50:1307–1312.

Ilfeld, D., C. Carnaud, I. R. Cohen, and N. Trainin. 1973. *In vitro* cytotoxicity and *in vivo* tumor enhancement induced by mouse spleen cells autosensitized *in vitro*. Int. J. Cancer 12:213–222.

Jeejeebhoy, H. 1974. Stimulation of tumor growth by the immune response. Int. J. Cancer 13:665–678.

Kall, M. A., and I. Hellström. 1975. Specific stimulatory and cytotoxic effects of lymphocytes sensitized *in vitro* to either alloantigens or tumor antigens. J. Immunol. 114:1083–1088.

Klein, G., H. O. Sjögren, E. Klein, and K. E. Hellström. 1960. Demonstration of resistance against methylcholanthrene-induced sarcomas in the primary autochthonous host. Cancer Res. 20:1561–1572.

Lewis, M. G., R. L. Ikonopisov, R. C. Nairn, T. M. Phillips, G. Hamilton-Fairley, D. C. Bodenham, and P. Alexander. 1969. Tumor specific antibodies in human malignant melanoma and their relationship to extent of disease. Brit. Med. J. 3:547–552.

Medina, D., G. Heppner. 1973. Cell-mediated "immunostimulation" induced by mammary tumor virus-free Balb/c mammary tumors. Nature 242:329–330.

Nehlsen, S. L. 1971. Prolonged administration of antithymocyte serum in mice. Clin. Exp. Immunol. 9:63–77.

Outzen, H. C., R. P. Custer, G. J. Eaton, and R. T. Prehn. 1975. Spontaneous and induced tumor incidence in germfree "nude" mice. J. Reticuloendothel. Soc. 17:1–9.

Parmiana, G., G. Carbone, and R. T. Prehn. 1971. *In vitro* "spontaneous" neoplastic transformation of mouse fibroblasts in diffusion chambers. J. Natl. Cancer Inst. 46:261–268.

Prehn, R. T. 1969. The relationship of immunology to carcinogenesis. Ann. N. Y. Acad. Sci. 164:449–457.

Prehn, R. T. 1970. Discussion. *In* R. T. Smith and M. Landy (eds.), Immune Surveillance, pp. 451–462. Academic Press, New York.

Prehn, R. T. 1971. Perspectives on oncogenesis: Does immunity stimulate or inhibit neoplasia? J. Reticuloendothel. Soc. 10:1–16.

Prehn, R. T. 1972. The immune reaction as a stimulator of tumor growth. Science 176:170.

Prehn, R. T. 1975. Relationship of tumor immunogenicity to concentration of the oncogen. J. Natl. Cancer Inst. 55:189–190.

Prehn, R. T., and M. A. Lappé. 1971. An immunostimulation theory of tumor development. Transplantation Rev. 7:26–54.

Prehn, R. T., and J. M. Main. 1957. Immunity to methylcholanthrene-induced sarcomas. J. Natl. Cancer Inst. 18:769–778.

Sanford, B. H., H. I. Kohn, J. J. Daily, and S. F. Soo. 1973. Long-term spontaneous tumor incidence in neonatally thymectomized mice. J. Immunol. 110:1437–1439.

Shearer, W. T., G. W. Philpott, and C. W. Parker. 1973. Humoral immunostimulation of tumor cell growth. Clin. Res. 21:839.

Stutman, O. 1975. Delayed tumour appearance and absence of regression in nude mice infected with murine sarcoma virus. Nature 253:142–144.

Wahl, D. V., W. H. Chapman, I. Hellström, and K. E. Hellström. 1974. Transplantation immunity to individually unique antigens of chemically induced bladder tumors in mice. Int. J. Cancer 14:114–121.

Immunodiagnosis of Human Neoplasia

J. Bruce Smith, M.D., F.A.C.P.

The use of immunologic methods to demonstrate the presence of malignant cells is a young discipline in science, and much of what looks promising one day is often discarded the next. However, the possibilities of either developing rapid means of diagnosis and staging of cancer or, perhaps, devising a form of immunotherapy for selected patients are real ones and at least partially justify the zeal with which tumor immunology is currently pursued. Although the occurrence of tumor-associated antigens (TAA) had been postulated long before the mid-1950's, the notion was not generally accepted until after the work of Foley (1953), who demonstrated that syngeneic mice could be immunized to chemically induced tumors; and that of Prehn and Main (1957) whose studies of methyl cholanthrene–induced sarcomata in mice clearly established the existence of TAAs. Since these initial investigations, immunologists have amassed a vast armamentarium of sophisticated weaponry with which to take aim at and attack the TAA.

It should be noted at the outset that except in the case of chemically induced tumors (Prehn, 1965) TAAs are not necessarily

This work was supported by United States Public Health Service Grants CA-06551, CA-06927, and RR-05539 from the National Institutes of Health and by an appropriation from the Commonwealth of Pennsylvania.

31

tumor specific. The same virus-induced antigens can occur not only in several disease entities but also can cross species lines (Old and Boyse, 1965). Many TAAs, including some virus-coded antigens (Pearson and Freeman, 1968; Hellman and Fowler, 1971), have been found to cross-react with macromolecules normally present in embryonic tissue or serum (Alexander, 1972). This re-expression of onco-fetal antigens (OFA) in cancer may be a phenomenon associated with the de-repression of a structural gene during malignant transformation.

The development of immunologic tests for malignancy is based on the notion that TAAs are either produced (or shed) in sufficient quantity to be measurable in the serum or other body fluids or are sufficiently different from normal cell constituents that the host mounts a measurable immune response to them (Table 1).

This paper discusses some immunologic tests currently in use in the diagnosis and follow-up of cancer and some tests which may, in the future, prove to be clinically useful.

TESTS BASED ON OCCURRENCE OF CIRCULATING OR FIXED TUMOR CELL PRODUCTS

α-1 Fetoprotein (AFP)

This normal α-1 globulin of fetal serum gradually falls in concentration until it is undetectable, by conventional methods, in the immediate postnatal period. Similar embryonic α-globulins have been found in all species tested (Gitlin and Boesman, 1967). Although the exact function of AFP is not known, it binds estrogen and may serve as a carrier for that hormone (Uriel, de Nechaud, and Dupiers, 1972).

AFP was first found in adult mammalian serum by Abelev et al. (1963) who noted high levels of AFP in the serum of mice with transplanted hepatomas. Tatarinov (1966) later confirmed that patients with primary hepatocellular carcinoma also had AFP detectable in their serum. Using simple and relatively insensitive techniques of detection, i.e., precipitation of AFP in gel by antiserum after either double diffusion or cross-electrophoresis tests, several studies showed that AFP could be found in 50 to 90% of serum samples from adult patients with hepatoma (Alpert, Uriel, and de Nechaud, 1968; Smith and Todd, 1968; Purves, Bersohn, and Geddes, 1970), and the usefulness of AFP detection in areas such as Africa and the Orient, where hepatoma is common, seemed clearly established. Subsequent

Table 1. Major categories of diagnosis associated with positive immunologic tests

Tests	Disease
Tests based on detection of tumor-associated antigens	
α-1 fetoprotein	Hepatoma
	Germinal cell tumors
Carcinoembryonic antigen	Gastro-intestinal cancer
	Alcoholic liver disease
Fetal sulphoglycoprotein antigen	Gastric cancer
Hodgkin's S and F antigens	Hodgkin's disease
Virus-associated antigens	Leukemia
Tests based on occurrence of anti-tumor antibody in the serum	
Anti-EB virus	Infectious mononucleosis
	Burkitt's lymphoma
	Nasopharyngeal carcinoma
Anti-cell surface antibody	Sarcoma
	Melanoma
Tests based on cell-mediated immunologic methods	
Delayed hypersensitivity	Melanoma
	Burkitt's lymphoma
	Colon cancer
	Lung cancer
	Breast cancer
Makari skin test	Many cancers
	Inflammatory disorders
Macrophage electrophoretic mobility test	All cancers tested
	Inflammatory disorders
	Neurologic diseases

studies showed that AFP also occurred in high frequency in serum from patients with certain germinal cell tumors (Smith and O'Neill, 1971; Elgort et al., 1973). However, with the development of radioimmunoassay and other sensitive techniques AFP was found in normal adult serum (Ruoslahti and Seppala, 1971) and raised levels were found in serum of pregnant women (Smith, 1971a), in serum from patients with cirrhosis (Hulbert et al., 1973), viral hepatitis (Smith 1971a, 1971b, 1971c), and ataxia telangiectasia (Waldmann and McIntire, 1972), and after partial hepatectomy (Smith, 1971c).

The diagnostic usefulness of AFP determination is dependent on the assay used (Table 2). For mass screening programs and for testing individual serum samples where hepatoma is suspected, the use of double diffusion or counter-electrophoresis techniques is reasonably specific, as these tests do not usually detect AFP in the low concentrations occurring in non-neoplastic conditions. The differential diagnosis between hepatoma and most germinal cell tumors is generally not a problem and one must be aware of only the unusual case of another type of cancer being associated with high concentrations of AFP in the serum (Alpert, Pinn and Isselbacher, 1971; Kozower et al., 1971; Mehlman, Bulkley, and Wiernik, 1971). Once the diagnosis of hepatoma or germinal cell tumor is established, then serial AFP determinations can be useful in evaluating response to therapy.

A recent report (Mizejewski and Allen, 1974) indicated that administration of anti-AFP antiserum to mice with transplanted hepatomas resulted in retardation of growth of the tumors. Thus, it is possible that AFP will eventually be useful in therapy as well as diagnosis and follow-up.

Table 2. Occurrence of α-1 fetoprotein (AFP) according to method of detection used[a]

I. Double diffusion (2 μg/ml)
Hepatocellular carcinoma
Embryonal carcinoma—testis
Choriocarcinoma—ovary
Yolk sac carcinoma[a]
Occasional other nonhepatic tumors
Hepatitis
Partial biliary atresia[b]
II. Immunoradioautography, Sandwich counter-electrophoresis, aggregate hemagglutination (100 ng/ml)
Acute viral hepatitis
Partial hepatectomy
Pregnancy
III. Radioimmunoassay (> 10 ng/ml)
Ataxia telangiectasia
Hepatic cirrhosis
Normal

[a]Numbers in parentheses indicate lower limits of detectable concentrations.
[b]J. B. Smith, previously unpublished.

Carcinoembryonic Antigen (CEA)

This carcinofetal glycoprotein was first described by Gold and Freedman (1965a, 1965b) and was found using an antiserum raised in rabbits to a perchloric acid extract of a colon cancer. Using this antiserum, CEA was found in extracts of all gastrointestinal tumors tested and, while not detected in adult tissue extracts, was found in fetal gut. Radioimmunoassay measured CEA in the serum of patients with colon and other G.I. cancers (Thompson et al., 1969); however, various studies employing radioimmunoassay subsequently showed that CEA could also be found in serum from patients with a variety of neoplastic and non-neoplastic conditions. These include carcinoma of the lung and breast (LoGerfo, Krupey, and Hansen, 1971; Lawrence et al., 1972), genito-urinary system (Reynoso et al., 1972), sarcoma, neuroblastoma, and various other tumors (Reynoso et al., 1972), alcoholic liver disease (Moore et al., 1971), and macroglobulinemia (Reynoso et al., 1972). Martin and Martin (1970) have also demonstrated small amounts of CEA in normal tissues.

Because of the several techniques used for purifying CEA and various modifications of the radioimmunoassay for CEA, it is probable that some of the apparent nonspecificity of the test is due to laboratory artifact and that the manipulations may cause the occurrence of subspecificities of CEA which have a wider range of occurrence than the original material isolated by Gold and Freedman. Until questions of diagnostic and antigenic specificity are resolved, however, CEA measurements will not be a useful diagnostic tool and the current clinical usefulness of the CEA test is limited to follow-up evaluation.

Fetal Sulfoglycoprotein Antigen (FSA)

Hakkinen (1966) reported that rabbit antiserum to a pool of mucoproteins isolated from gastric juice from cancer patients detected an antigen in gastric secretions from all patients with stomach cancer but not in gastric secretions from normal control individuals. FSA was subsequently shown to be present in fetal gut tissue (Hakkinen, Jarvi, and Gronroos, 1968) and not to be related to blood group antigens. FSA was shown to have some antigenic relationship to CEA (Hakkinen, 1972); unabsorbed antiserum detected both CEA and FSA. Absorption of antiserum with colon tissue removed CEA cross-reactivity but left anti-FSA.

Hakkinen (1974) has completed a large scale screening study for the presence of FSA in gastric secretions of volunteer individuals in Finland. A total of 13,612 volunteers (7,567 male and 6,045 female) between the ages of 40 and 69 were studied, and 461 FSA secretors underwent gastroscopy. Five surgery-requiring lesions were found: polyposis, ulcer, cancer in situ, obvious cancer, and malignant ulcer. Unfortunately, gastroscopy was not done on a control population of nonsecretors of FSA and thus the results are difficult to interpret. Since the average annual incidence rate of gastric cancer in Finland is 51 cases per 100,000 population (Hakkinen, 1974), it is possible that asymptomatic FSA secretors form a group of individuals at high risk for developing gastric cancer and thus earlier diagnosis of this lesion may be possible.

Hodgkin's S and F Antigens

Order and co-workers (Order, Porter, and Hellman, 1971; Order, Chism, and Hellman, 1972; Katz et al., 1973), in a series of papers, have described two TAAs in Hodgkin's disease (HD). These antigens, termed "F" and "S" for their fast and slow electrophoretic mobility, were initially found by an immunofluorescence test using rabbit antiserum to extracts of HD nodules from two patients (Order et al., 1971). Cells of the HD nodule showed fluorescence with the antiserum while normal autologous tissue did not. F antigen was found mainly in HD involved spleen while S antigen was more predominant in involved lymph nodes. A subsequent study (Order et al., 1972) showed that the S and F antigens occurred in 18 of 19 spleens from Hodgkin's disease patients but that F, and occasionally S, antigen could be found in spleens involved with disease processes other than HD. F antigen was also found in cultured Burkitt's lymphoma cells (Order, Colgan, and Hellman, 1974). Purification of these TAAs by Katz et al. (1973) and the study of their tissue distribution indicated that the F antigen was present in small amounts in normal spleen and that it was also readily demonstrated in fetal spleen and liver and neonatal thymus. Most recently, F antigen has been found to be normal tissue ferritin (Eshhar, Order, and Katz, 1974) and the suggestion was made that ferritin levels in tissue might be helpful as a diagnostic index of activity in HD. Further studies will be necessary to clarify the usefulness of these TAAs in Hodgkin's disease and other malignancies.

Virus-associated Antigens in Human Tumors

Tumors induced by both DNA and RNA viruses may be highly antigenic in mice (Old and Boyse, 1965) and a number of antigens associated with these oncogenic viruses have been found in cultured or fresh human malignant cells (see references below). Whether the detection of these virus-associated antigens indicates that the same or similar agents are responsible for both animal and human tumors is a question yet to be resolved. Several lines of evidence strengthen the notion that RNA C-type viruses are associated with human tumors. Cross-reactive antigens between the murine-leukemia virus of the Rauscher strain (MuLV-Rauscher) and human acute leukemia cells (two myelogenous and three lymphocytic) have been found (Mann, Haltermann, and Leventhal, 1973) and MuLV-Rauscher RNA has been demonstrated to occur in 68% of human sarcomas (Kufe, Hehlmann, and Spiegelman, 1972). Also, a high percentage (67%) of human breast cancers contain RNA with sequences in common with the RNA of mouse mammary tumor virus (MMTV) (Axel, Schlom, and Spiegelman, 1972). Recent studies on the occurrence of RNA tumor virus antigens in human leukemia have shown that the major structural protein (p-30) of both the woolly monkey (SSAV) and gibbon ape (GALV) leukemia viruses occurs in human acute leukemia cells. Sherr and Todaro (1975) reported that leukemia cells from 5 patients with acute leukemia (2 myelocytic, 1 myelomonocytic, 1 histocytic, and 1 unknown) contained the p-30 antigen of some RNA tumor virus known to produce leukemia in lower mammals. These workers also reported that extracts of spleen from patients with lymphocytic leukemia and ovarian carcinoma also contained the p-30 antigen of SSAV C-type virus (Sherr and Todaro, 1974). Gallagher and Gallo (1975) have recently reported the isolation of C-type RNA virus from cultures of human acute myelogenous leukemia cells.

Although the major contribution of these studies is in the areas of etiology and pathogenesis of leukemia, the use of tests to determine the presence of virus or viral antigens might in the future prove useful in identifying populations or individuals at high risk for the development of leukemia.

TESTS BASED ON MEASUREMENT OF
ANTI-TUMOR OR OTHER ANTIBODIES IN SERUM

Anti-tumor Antibodies

Antibodies to several antigenic determinants associated with EB virus infection have been found in serum from patients with infectious mononucleosis, Burkitt's lymphoma, and nasopharyngeal carcinoma (Henle, Henle, and Diehl, 1968; Henle et al., 1970). These antibodies are directed at EB virus capsid antigen, "early" antigen, or a soluble EB antigen. In patients with infectious mononucleosis antibody to "early" antigen is often in highest titer during and just after active infection. Titers of antibody to "early" antigen in patients with Burkitt's lymphoma often fall when patients are in remission and may thus be of predictive value in this disease.

Wood and Morton (1971) also have reported cytotoxic antibody in the serum of 70% of patients with sarcoma. This antibody was detected by complement-dependent lysis of autologous and allogeneic sarcoma cells in tissue culture and indicates a common antigen in sarcoma. Moore and Hughes (1973), using an immunofluorescence test, showed anti-sarcoma antibodies in the serum of sarcoma patients and found that antibodies were more likely to occur if the malignancy was localized.

Several studies have now confirmed that antibodies to melanoma TAAs occur with higher frequency in the serum of patients with melanoma than in control individuals (Morton et al., 1968; Muna, Marcus, and Smart, 1969). Lewis et al. (1969) found that anti-melanoma antibodies were directed toward two separate antigens, one a melanoma cell surface TAA for which a complement-dependent cytotoxic assay was used and the other a cytoplasmic antigen detected by immunofluorescence. They found that antibody of either type was more prevalent in patients with localized disease. These findings were confirmed by Bodurtha et al. (1975) who demonstrated cytotoxic antibody in 9 of 10 melanoma patients with localized disease and only in 1 of 11 patients with disseminated melanoma. This study also showed that little cross-reactivity occurred since allogeneic cells were often not affected by antibody. Lewis and Phillips (1972) have made similar observations.

It seems possible that detection of these various types of antibodies may yield valuable information on the clinical staging of certain cancer patients and may have diagnostic potential as well.

Autoantibodies in Cancer

The two main types of autoantibodies detectable in serum of cancer patients are anti-nuclear factor (ANF) and anti-smooth muscle antibody (SMA). Whitehouse (1973) found SMA in 68% of cancer patients and 20% of control sera and ANF in 27% and 2% of cancer and control sera, respectively. Patients with neuroblastoma were notable for the complete absence of ANF. Moore and Hughes (1973) also found that SMA was more prevalent in serum from sarcoma patients (45%) than from carcinoma patients (36%) or control individuals (35%) while ANF occurred in 8, 22, and 23% of sarcoma, carcinoma, and control sera, respectively. The significance of these findings is not known at present.

TESTS BASED ON OCCURRENCE
OF CELL-MEDIATED IMMUNITY TO TAAs

Delayed Hypersensitivity

The delayed hypersensitivity (DH) reaction to an antigen is often representative of a strong and usually specific cell-mediated immune response and such a test for TAAs would be useful for both diagnosis and follow-up evaluation. Skin tests in several human cancers have been studied. Fass et al. (1970) found that Ugandan melanoma patients had positive DH to autologous melanoma cell extracts if the disease was localized but negative tests when the disease was widespread. Hollinshead, Stewart, and Herberman (1974) found DH reactions to melanoma cell membrane extracts in patients with melanoma when either autologous or allogeneic tumor cell extracts were used, and they also found that positive reactions were more frequent in patients with localized disease than in those with metastases (17 of 22 and 7 of 19 patients, respectively).

Similar findings have been reported in patients with Burkitt's lymphoma. Fass, Herberman, and Ziegler (1970) noted that a patient with localized Burkitt's tumor had DH to extracts of autologous tumor but not to an extract of autologous normal lymphocytes. After treatment, 7 of 12 patients manifested DH to autologous Burkitt's tumor extracts and remained in remission for an average 31 weeks compared to the 5 negative DH patients who all relapsed within 14 to 20 weeks.

Skin tests in patients with colon carcinoma (Hollinshead et al., 1970) also showed DH to membrane extracts of autologous tumor cells and to extracts of normal embryonic gut. Seventeen of 19 patients studied in the postoperative period had DH to an antigen extract containing CEA.

Skin test reactivity of a DH nature was also found in breast cancer patients by Hughes and Lytton (1964) and confirmed by Stewart (1969), who reported that 9 of 49 patients with breast cancer had DH to breast cancer cell extracts. As opposed to the findings in other tumors, Stewart and Orizaga (1971) found that breast cancer patients with DH fared worse than those without positive skin tests. Fractionation of soluble antigens of breast carcinoma by Hollinshead et al. (1974) indicated that two antigens were able to elicit DH. One antigen caused DH in patients with both localized and metastatic cancer and the other, present in cancer tissue and benign breast lesions, caused DH only in cancer patients with localized disease.

Antigens from lung cancer cells but not from normal lung tissue have also been shown to elicit DH responses (Hollinshead, Stewart, and Herberman, 1974).

While these tests sound promising, much work on the specificity along with serial studies in individual patients will be necessary prior to their general use for cancer detection or staging.

Makari Skin Test

This rather special test is not a delayed hypersensitivity reaction but an immediate one after the interdermal injection of tumor polysaccharides plus autologous serum. The test is based on observations by Makari and Huck (1955), who used the Schultz-Dale technique to demonstrate antigens in the serum of cancer patients. Makari (1960) later developed a skin test for use in patients with cancer, and Tee (1973) recently completed a double-blind prospective study using the Makari skin test. He found that patients with malignancy and with noncancerous inflammatory disorders both had a high rate of positivity. This nonspecificity makes the Makari test unsuitable for use as an immunodiagnostic test for cancer.

Macrophage Electrophoretic Mobility (MEM) Test

Field and Caspary (1970) found that a basic protein extracted from human brain could induce lymphocytes from patients with various types of malignancy to produce a substance which slowed the migration of normal macrophages in an electrophoresis test (MEM test). Work on the nature of the antigens (encephalitogenic factor, EF; cancer-basic protein, CaBP) in this system has shown them to be proteolipids common to all malignant tumors and normal brain (Dickinson and Caspary, 1973). Presumably lymphocytes from cancer patients become sensitized to cancer-basic protein and produce the macrophage slowing factor when exposed to CaBP in vitro. Field and Caspary (1970) reported that the MEM test was positive (i.e., showed macrophage slowing) in all cancer patients tested, and their observations were confirmed by other studies (Pritchard et al., 1972; Goldstone, Kerr, and Irvine, 1973). Recently, Field, Caspary, and Smith (1973) reported that, using the MEM test, they were able to diagnosis correctly the presence of cancer in 463 of 464 serum samples from patients with various malignancies but cautioned that patients with neurologic disease, sarcoidosis, Crohn's disease, ulcerative colitis, asthma, myasthenia gravis, and influenza may be sensitive to cancer-basic protein. Further studies should clarify the usefulness of the MEM test as a diagnostic tool in cancer.

Cytotoxicity Assays

The ability of lymphoid cells to lyse or prevent the growth of tumor cells in vitro has been demonstrated by several groups of investigators (Hellstrom et al., 1968; Bubenik et al., 1971; O'Toole et al., 1973; Cohen, Ketcham, and Morton, 1973) and the colony inhibition technique and other assays for target cell destruction by lymphocytes have been useful in the study of the nature and mechanism of target cell destruction and serum factors that modify the reaction. It appears that tumor antigen in excess and complexes of antibody and TAA are both able to block effectively cell-mediated cytotoxicity (Baldwin, Price, and Robins, 1973). While assays for cell-mediated lysis of target cells have been used to demonstrate immunity in several human tumor systems, other studies have shown that lymphoid cells from normal individuals are better able to kill tumor target cells than are lymphoid cells from patients with cancer (Takasugi, Mickey, and Terasaki, 1973). It appears at this time that the usefulness of these tests is not in the area of tumor diagnosis but rather in the study of the host response to cancer and possibly in follow-up evaluation of patients on therapy.

CONCLUSIONS

The results of any immunodiagnostic test for cancer must be interpreted with circumspection. One must be aware not only of the
fallibility of these tests but also of the specificity of the test relative
to the disease state in question and to the sensitivity of the method
used.

REFERENCES

Abelev, G. I., S. D. Perova, N. I. Khramkova, Z. A. Postnikova, and I. S.
    Irlin. 1963. Production of embryonal α-globulin by transplantable mouse
    hepatomas. Transplantation 1:174–180.
Alexander, P. 1972. Foetal "antigens" in cancer. Nature 235:137–140.
Alpert, E., V. W. Pinn, and K. Isselbacher. 1971. Alpha-fetoprotein in a
    patient with gastric carinoma metastatic to the liver. New Eng. J.
    Med. 285:1058–1059.
Alpert, M. E., J. Uriel, and B. de Nechaud. 1968. Alpha-1 fetoglobulin
    in the diagnosis of human hepatoma. New Eng. J. Med. 278:984–986.
Axel, R., J. Schlom, and S. Spiegelman. 1972. Presence in human breast
    cancer of RNA homologous to mouse mammary tumor virus RNA.
    Nature 235:32–36.
Baldwin, R. W., M. R. Price, and R. A. Robins. 1973. Significance of
    serum factors modifying cellular immune responses to growing tu-
    mours. Brit. J. Cancer 28(Suppl. I):37–47.
Bodurtha, A. J., D. O. Chee, J. F. Laucius, M. J. Mastrangelo, and R. T.
    Prehn. 1975. Clinical and immunological significance of human mela-
    noma cytotoxic antibody. Cancer Res. 35:189–193.
Booth, S. N., G. C. Jamieson, J. P. G. King, J. Leonard, G. D. Oates,
    and P. W. Dykes. 1974. Carcinoembryonic antigen in management of
    colorectal carcinoma. Brit. Med. J. 4:183–187.
Bubenik, J., J. Jakoubkova, P. Krakora, M. Baresova, P. Helbich, V.
    Viklicky, and V. Malaskova. 1971. Cellular Immunity to Renal Car-
    cinomas in man. Int. J. Cancer 8:503–513.
Cohen, A. M., A. S. Ketcham, and D. L. Morton. 1973. Specific inhibition
    of sarcoma-specific cellular immunity by sera from patients with grow-
    ing sarcomas. Int. J. Cancer 11:273–279.
Dickinson, J. P., and E. A. Caspary. 1973. The chemical nature of cancer
    basic protein. Brit. J. Cancer 28(Suppl. I):224–228.
Elgort, D. A., G. I. Abelev, D. M. Levina, E. V. Marienbach, G. A. Mar-
    tochkina, A. V. Laskina, and E. A. Solovjeva. 1973. Immunoradio-
    autography test for alpha fetoprotein in the differential diagnoses of
    germinogenic tumors of the testis and in the evaluation of effectiveness
    of their treatment. Int. J. Cancer 11:586–594.
Eshhar, Z., S. E. Order, and D. H. Katz. 1974. Ferritin, a Hodgkin's
    disease associated antigen. Proc. Natl. Acad. Sci. USA 1:3956–3960.

Fass, L., R. B. Herberman, and J. Ziegler. 1970. Delayed certaneous hypersensitivity reactions to autologous extracts of Burkitt-lymphoma cells. New Eng. J. Med. 282:776–780.

Fass, L., J. L. Ziegler, R. B. Herberman, and J. W. M. Kiryabwire. 1970. Cutaneous hypersensitivity reactions to autologous extracts of malignant melanoma cells. Lancet i:116–118.

Field, E. J., and E. A. Caspary. 1970. Lymphocyte sensitization: an in vitro test for cancer? Lancet ii:1337–1341.

Field, E. J., E. A. Caspary, and K. S. Smith. 1973. Macrophage electrophoretic mobility (MEM) test in cancer: a critical evaluation. Brit. J. Cancer 28:(Suppl. I):208–214.

Foley, E. J. 1953. Antigenic properties of methylcholanthrene-induced tumors in mice of the strain of origin. Cancer Res. 13:835–837.

Gallagher, R. E., and R. C. Gallo. 1975. Type C RNA tumor virus isolated from cultured human acute myelogenous leukemia cells. Science 187:350–353.

Gitlin, D., and M. Boesman. 1967. Fetus specific serum proteins in several mammals and their relation to human α-fetoprotein. Comp. Biochem. Physiol. 21:327–336.

Gold, P., and S. O. Freedman. 1965a. Demonstration of tumor-specific antigens in human colonic carcinomata by immunological tolerance and absorption techniques. J. Exp. Med. 121:439–462.

Gold, P., and S. O. Freedman. 1965b. Specific carcinoembryonic antigens of the human digestive system. J. Exp. Med. 122:467–481.

Goldstone, A. H., L. Kerr, and W. J. Irvine. 1973. The macrophage electrophoretic mobility test in cancer. Clin. Exp. Immunol. 14:469–472.

Hakkinen, I. P. T. 1966. An immunochemical method for detecting carcinomatous secretions from human gastric juice. Scand. J. Gastroenterol. 1:28–32.

Hakkinen, I. P. T., O. Jarvi, and J. Gronroos. 1968. Sulphoglycoprotein antigens in the human alimentary canal and gastric cancer. An immunohistological study. Int. J. Cancer 3:572–581.

Hakkinen, I. P. T. 1972. Immunological relationship of the carcinoembryonic antigen and the fetal sulfoglycoprotein antigen. Immunochemistry 9:1115–1119.

Hakkinen, I. P. T. 1974. A population screening for fetal sulfoglycoprotein antigen in gastric juice. Cancer Res. 34:3069–3072.

Hellman, A., and A. K. Fowler. 1971. Hormone-activated expression of C-type RNA tumour virus genome. Nature (New Biol.) 233:142–144.

Hellstrom, I., K. E. Hellstrom, G. E. Pierce, and J. P. S. Yang. 1968. Cellular and humoral immunity to different types of human neoplasms. Nature 220:1352–1354.

Henle, G., W. Henle, and V. Diehl. 1968. Relation of Burkitt's tumor-associated Herpes-type virus to infectious mononucleosis. Proc. Natl. Acad. Sci. USA 59:94–101.

Henle, W., G. Henle, B. A. Zajac, G. Pearson, R. Waubke, and M. Scriba. 1970. Differential reactivity of human serums with early antigens induced by Epstein-Barr virus. Science 169:188–190.

Hollinshead, A., D. Glew, B. Bunnag, P. Gold, and R. Herberman. 1970. Skin-reactive soluble antigen from intestinal cancer-cell membranes and relationship to carcinoembryonic antigens. Lancet i:1191–1195.

Hollinshead, A., W. T. Jaffurs, L. K. Alpert, J. E. Harris, and R. B. Herberman. 1974. Isolation and identification of soluble skin reactive membrane antigens of malignant and normal human breast cells. Cancer Res. 34:2961–2968.

Hollinshead, A. C., T. H. M. Stewart, and R. B. Herberman. 1974. Delayed hypersensitivity reactions to soluble membrane antigens of human malignant lung cells. J. Natl. Cancer Inst. 52:327–338.

Hughes, L. E. and B. Lytton. 1964. Antigenic properties of human tumors: delayed cutaneous hypersensitity reactions. Brit. Med. J. 1:209–212.

Hulbert, K., B. Silver, P. Gold, S. Feder, S. O. Freedman, and J. Shuster. 1973. Radioimmunoassay for Human alpha-1 fetoprotein. Proc. Natl. Acad. Sci. USA 70:526–530.

Katz, D. H., E. Order, M. Graves, and B. Benacerraf. 1973. Purification of Hodgkin's disease tumor-associated antigens (spleen/lymphnodes/fetal liver/F and S antigens). Proc. Natl. Acad. Sci. USA 70:396–400.

Kozower, M., K. A. Fawaz, H. M. Miller, and M. M. Kaplan. 1971. Positive alpha-fetoglobulin in a case of gastric carcinoma. New Eng. J. Med. 285:1059–1060.

Kufe, D., R. Hehlmann, and S. Spiegelman. 1972. Human sarcomas contain RNA related to the RNA of a mouse leukemia virus. Science 175:182–185.

Lawrence, D. J. R., U. Stevens, R. Bettelheim, D. Darcy, C. Leese, C. Turberville, P. Alexander, E. W. Johns, and A. M. Neville. 1972. Role of plasma carcinoembryonic antigen in diagnosis of gastrointestinal, mammary and bronchial carcinoma. Brit. Med. J. 3:605–609.

Lewis, M. G., R. L. Ikonopisov, R. C. Nairn, T. M. Phillips, G. Hamilton-Fairley, D. C. Bodenham, and P. Alexander. 1969. Tumor-specific antibodies in human malignant melanoma and their relationship to the extent of the disease. Brit. Med. J. 3:547–552.

Lewis, M. G., and T. M. Phillips. 1972. The specificity of surface membrane immunofluorescence in human melanoma. Int. J. Cancer 10:105–111.

LoGerfo, P., J. Krupey, and H. J. Hansen. 1971. Demonstration of an antigen common to several varieties of neoplasia; assay using zirconyl phosphate gel. New Eng. J. Med. 285:138–141.

Mackay, A. M., S. Patel, S. Carter, U. Stevens, D. J. R. Laurence, E. H. Cooper, and A. M. Neville. 1974. Role of serial plasma C.E.A. assays in detection of recurrent and metastatic colorectal carcinomas. Brit. Med. J. 4:382–385.

Makari, J. G. 1960. Recent studies in the immunology of cancer. Detection of tumors in man by the skin testing of polypaccheride-antibody complexes. J. Amer. Geriatr. Soc. 8:675–688.

Makari, J. G., and M. G. Huck. 1955. Use of Schultz-Dale test for detection of specific antigen in sera of patients with carcinoma. Brit. Med. J. ii:1291–1295.

Mann, D., R. Haltermann, and B. G. Leventhal. 1973. Crossreactive antigens or human cells infected with Rauscher Leukemia virus and on human acute leukemia cells. Proc. Natl. Acad. Sci. USA 70:495–497.

Martin, F., and M. S. Martin. 1970. Demonstration of antigens related to colonic cancer in the human digestive system. Int. J. Cancer 6:352–360.

Mehlman, D. J., B. H. Bulkley, and P. H. Wiernik. 1971. Serum alpha-1 fetoglobulin with gastric and prostatic carcinomas. New Eng. J. Med. 285:1060–1061.

Mizejewski, G. J., and R. P. Allen. 1974. Immunotherapeutic suppression in transplantable solid tumors. Nature 250:50–51.

Moore, M., and L. A. Hughes. 1973. Circulating antibodies in human connective tissue malignancy. Brit. J. Cancer 28(Suppl. I):175–184.

Moore, T. L., H. Z. Kupchik, N. Marcon, and N. Zamcheck. 1971. Carcinoembryonic antigen assay in cancer of the colon and pancreas and other digestive disorders. Amer. J. Digest. Dis. 16.1–7.

Morton, D. L., R. A. Malmgren, E. C. Holmes, and A. S. Ketcham. 1968. Demonstration of antibodies against human malignant melanoma by immunofluorescence. Surgery 64:233–240.

Muna, N. M., S. Marcus, and C. Smart. 1969. Detection by immunofluorescence of antibodies specific for human malignant melanoma cells. Cancer 23:88–93.

Oettgen, H. F., T. Aoki, L. J. Old, E. A. Boyse, E. deHarven, and G. Mills. 1968. Suspension culture of a pigment producing cell line derived from a human malignant melanoma. J. Natl. Cancer Inst. 41:827–843.

Old, L. J., and E. A. Boyse. 1965. Antigens of tumors and leukemias induced by viruses. Fed. Proc. 24:1009–1017.

Order, S. E., S. E. Chism, and S. Hellman. 1972. Studies of antigens associated with Hodgkin's disease. Blood 40:621–633.

Order, S. E., J. Colgan, and S. Hellman. 1974. Distribution of fast- and slow-migrating Hodgkin's tumor-associated antigens. Cancer Res. 34:1182–1186.

Order, S. E., M. Porter, and S. Hellman. 1971. Hodgkin's disease: Evidence for a tumor associated antigen. New Eng. J. Med. 285:471–474.

O'Toole, C., P. Perlmann, H. Wigzell, B. Unsgaard, and C. G. Zetterlund. 1973. Lymphocyte cytotoxicity in bladder cancer. No requirement for thymus derived effector cells? Lancet i:1085–1088.

Pearson, G., and G. Freeman. 1968. Evidence suggesting a relationship between polyemia virus-induced transplantation antigen and normal embryonic antigen. Cancer Res. 28:1665–1673.

Prehn, R. T., and J. M. Main. 1957. Immunity to methylcholanthrene-induced sarcomas. J. Natl. Cancer Inst. 18:769–778.

Prehn, R. T. 1965. Cancer antigens in tumors induced by chemicals. Fed. Proc. 24:1018–1022.

Pritchard, J. A. V., J. L. Moore, W. H. Sutherland, and C. A. F. Joslin. 1972. Macrophage-electrophoretic-mobility (MEM) test for malignant disease, an independent confirmation. Lancet ii:627–629.

Purves, L. R., I. Bersohn, and E. W. Geddes. 1970. Serum alpha-fetoprotein and primary cancer of the liver in man. Cancer 25:1261–1270.

Ravry, M., C. G. Moertel, A. J. Schutt, and V. L. W. Go. 1974. Usefulness of serial serum carcinoembryonic antigen (CEA) determinations
during anti-cancer therapy or long-term follow-up of gastrointestinal
carcinoma. Cancer 34:1230–1234.

Reynoso, G., T. M. Chu, D. Holyoke, E. Cohen, T. Nemoto, J. J. Wang,
J. Chuang, P. Guinan, and G. P. Murphy. 1972. Carcinoembryonic
antigen in patients with different cancers. JAMA 220:361–365.

Ruoslahti, E., and M. Seppala. 1971. Studies of carcino-fetal proteins. III.
Development of a radioimmunoassay for α-fetoprotein. Demonstration of
fetoprotein in serum of healthy human adults. Int. J. Cancer 8:374–
383.

Sherr, C. J., and G. J. Todaro. 1974. Type C viral antigens in man. I.
Antigens related to endogenous primate virus in human tumors. Proc.
Natl. Acad. Sci. USA 71:4703–4707.

Sherr, C. J., and G. J. Todaro. 1975. Primate type C virus p30 antigen in
cells from humans with acute leukemia. Science 187:855–856.

Smith, J. B., and D. Todd. 1968. Foetoglobin and primary liver cancer.
Lancet 2:833.

Smith, J. B. 1971a. Alpha-fetoprotein in neoplastic and non-neoplastic
conditions. In N. G. Anderson and J. H. Coggin (eds.), Proceedings of
the First Conference and Workshop on Embryonic Antigens in Cancer,
pp. 305–312.

Smith, J. B. 1971b. Occurrence of alpha-fetoprotein in acute viral hepatitis. Int. J. Cancer 8:421–424.

Smith, J. B. 1971c. Dynamics of alpha-fetoprotein (AFP) synthesis in
non-neoplastic hepatic disorders. Clin. Res. 19:739.

Smith, J. B., and R. T. O'Neill. 1971. Alpha-fetoprotein: Occurrence in
germinal cell and liver malignancies. Amer. J. Med. 51:767–771.

Stewart, T. H. M. 1969. The presence of delayed hypersensitivity reactions
in patients toward cellular extracts of their malignant tumors. I. The
role of tissue antigen, nonspecific reactions of nuclear material, and
bacterial antigen as a cause of this phenomenon. Cancer 23:1368–1379.

Stewart, T. H. M., and M. Orizaga. 1971. The presence of delayed hypersensitivity reactions in patients toward cellular extracts of their malignant tumors. 3. The frequency, duration and cross reactivity of this
phenomenon in patients with breast cancer, and its correlation with
survival. Cancer 28:1472–1478.

Takasugi, M., M. R. Mickey, and P. I. Terasaki. 1973. Reactivity of
lymphocytes from normal persons on cultured tumor cells. Cancer Res.
33:2898–2902.

Tatarinov, Y. S. 1966. Content of embryo-specific α-globulin in fetal and
neonatal sera and sera from adult humans with primary carcinoma of
the liver. Fed. Proc. (Trans. Suppl. Pt. 2)25:T344–T346.

Tee, D. E. H. 1973. Clinical evaluation of the Makari tumour skin test.
Brit. J. Cancer 28(Suppl. I):187–197.

Thompson, D. M. P., J. Krupey, S. O. Freedman, and P. Gold. 1969. The radioimmunoassay of circulating carcinoembryonic antigen of the human digestive system. Proc. Natl. Acad. Sci. USA 64:161–167.

Uriel, J., B. de Nechaud, and M. Dupiers. 1972. Estrogen-binding properties of rat, mouse and man fetospecific serum proteins. Demonstration by immunoautoradiographic methods. Biochem. Biophys. Res. Commun. 46:1175–1180.

Waldmann, T. A., and R. K. McIntire. 1972. Serum-alpha-fetoprotein levels in patients with ataxia-telangiectasia. Lancet ii:1112–1115.

Whitehouse, J. M. A. 1973. Circulating antibodies in human malignant disease. Brit. J. Cancer 28(Suppl I):170–174.

Wood, W. C., and D. L. Morton. 1971. Host immune response to a common cell-surface antigen in human sarcomas. New Eng. J. Med. 284:569–572.

E pidemiology of Cancer and Host Susceptibility Factors: Breast Cancer

W. Thomas London, M.D., F.A.C.P.

Epidemiology is a set of methods for the study of the distributions and determinants of diseases in human populations. Historically it developed as an approach to the study of infectious diseases, particularly epidemic infectious disease; hence, the name epidemiology. In recent years, as the cause and methods of prevention and/or cure of most infectious diseases became known, epidemiology as a discipline went into decline. Many medical schools in the 1950's and early 1960's had three or four lectures on epidemiology in the entire 4-year curriculum. In part as a response to this situation, attempts were made to apply epidemiologic methods to the study of the major chronic diseases of man: heart disease, cancer, and stroke.

Although epidemiology has contributed to an understanding of cancer (and other chronic diseases) in man, it has faced a number of

This work was supported by USPHS grants CA-06551, RR-05539, and CA-06927 from the National Institutes of Health and by an appropriation from the commonwealth of Pennsylvania.

49

difficulties not encountered in the study of infectious diseases. These can be enumerated as follows:

1. The etiologic agent or agents or even the class of agents is not known with certainty. In the study of communicable diseases, either the agent was already identified or epidemiologic methods permitted the identification of the source of the infectious agent, e.g., water supply, contaminated salad, infected mosquitoes, etc.

2. It is likely that cancer is the result of an interaction of several factors, each of which must be present to produce the disease. In the case of communicable diseases even if other factors come into play, the infectious agent is the overriding causative factor. The study of several factors concurrently is very difficult and the methodology to solve this problem has not been fully developed.

3. The incubation period for most infectious diseases is days to weeks, or in some instances (hepatitis B) months, or in very rare instances (Kuru) years. As the period between exposure to an agent and onset of disease gets longer, the demonstration of an etiologic association becomes more difficult. The latent (or incubation) periods for cancers in man are very long (2 to 20 years or more).

4. The clinical manifestations of pathologically defined cancers are often vague or absent. Precancerous lesions or carcinomas in situ are usually asymptomatic. Hence, finding epidemiologic relationships between early cancer and causative agents requires development of new techniques.

5. If an association is demonstrated between a particular agent and a neoplastic disease, determining whether the association is a cause or an effect of the disease can be extremely difficult.

6. In the study of communicable diseases, epidemiology generally centers on careful comparisons of exposed and unexposed groups with respect to the incidence or prevalence of a particular disease. In the study of cancer in man it is not clear what constitutes an adequate control. Because of the long latent period and the problems of early diagnosis, some or many members of the control group may already have or will develop the disease under study.

If there are such major problems in the study of the epidemiology of cancer, why bother with epidemiology at all? The answer is simply that the significance of basic biologic research on agents which may cause cancer in man cannot be evaluated until the effects of such agents on human populations are assessed. Since we cannot deliberately expose humans to potential carcinogens, it is necessary to study the experiments of nature on existing human populations. Epidemiology is the tool for these studies.

It must be emphasized that epidemiology cannot stand alone. It must relate directly to research in the laboratory and to clinical observations at the bedside. Progress is made when the flow rate of information and ideas between these different approaches to cancer research is high.

There are basically two types of epidemiologic studies: retrospective and prospective. Retrospective studies are usually performed first. They involve identification of cases, patients with the disease under study, and controls (see item 6 above). An investigation is then made to see whether there was a difference in exposure to the factor under study between the cases and controls. The retrospective approach is used by a physician whenever he takes a history. In fact, the best leads to agents which may cause cancer in man have been collected by alert clinicians taking careful histories. To mention only three recent examples: the associations of carcinoma of the vagina in women with exposure to diethylstilbesterol in utero, lung cancer in men with exposure to chlormethyl methyl ether, and angiosarcomas of the liver with exposure to vinyl chloride were discovered by clinicians who were not epidemiologists or professional cancer researchers.

The second method is a prospective study. Two groups (commonly called cohorts by epidemiologists) are identified, neither of which at present has the disease under study, but one group has been exposed to the suspect agent and the other has not. The two groups are then followed and the number of persons in each group developing the disease are compared. If associations are found in prospective studies, the cause and effect relationship is much more likely. Because of the long latent period and relatively low incidence of most cancers, true prospective studies of cancer are rarely done (Mausner and Bahn, 1974).

There is a third approach which utilizes elements of both retrospective and prospective studies. This is called an historical prospective study. It requires the identification of exposed and unexposed groups from reliable past records. For example, if the telephone company from their medical records identified operators who were or were not treated with estrogens for menopausal symptoms between 1950 and 1960, it would then be possible to ascertain the current prevalence of breast cancer in each group and to estimate the yearly incidence of breast cancer in each group. The weakness of this approach is that if an association of estrogen therapy with breast cancer were found, it would still not be certain whether the estrogens were responsible or the factors which originally caused only certain women to be treated with estrogens.

With this background an attempt has been made to summarize the available epidemiologic data for the major cancers of man (Table 1). This kind of data needs to be combined with available laboratory and clinical data in order to formulate testable hypotheses. In the remainder of this paper I have tried to do this for one human cancer, breast cancer.

Table 1. Risk factors for common malignant neoplasms

Lung (Smoking and Health, 1964; Wynder and Hoffman, 1968)
- Age—direct association
- Male 6 × Female
- Cigarette smoking 10–50 ×
- Uranium miners 10 ×
- Asbestos workers 90 ×
- Nickel refiners 5–10 ×
- Smelter workers 3 ×
- Urban 2–3 × rural
- Bullous disease 2–6 ×
- Pulmonary Tbc 5–9 ×

Cervix (Lundin, Erickson, and Sprunt, 1964; Rotkin, 1967)
- Blacks 4–5 × whites
- Jewish 0.25 ×
- Ever married 3 ×
- Number of sexual partners—direct
- Age at first intercourse—inverse
- Venereal diseases
- Herpes virus type 2 infection 2–3 ×

Colon (Burkitt, 1971; Haenzel and Corren, 1971)
- Geography—U.S., U.K., Canada 6 × Asia, Africa
- Ulcerative colitis 8–30 ×
- Familial polyposis syndromes 6 ×
- Close relatives 3 ×
- Asbestos workers
- Shoe workers   degrees of risk
- Machinists   not estimated
- Diet-? fat, beef, low fiber

Uterus (Stewart et al., 1966)
- Whites 1.4 × blacks
- Never married 1.3–2.4 ×
- Parity—inverse
- Age of menopause—direct
- Japan, Austria, Chile 3 × Norway, New Zealand, Australia
- Close relatives 5 ×
- Hypertension 1.5 ×
- Diabetes 1.5 ×
- Obesity 1.5–3 ×

Breast cancer is the most common neoplastic disease of women in the United States and Europe and is a major cause of mortality among women age 40 and older. Six of every 100 women in the U.S. will develop breast cancer in their lifetime. The annual incidence in the U.S. of new cases approaches 90,000 which ultimately produces about 35,000 deaths per year (Third National Cancer Survey, 1974).

Risk factors which have been identified and the degrees of increased risk incurred are shown in Table 2. This is an impressive array of factors associated with increased risk. The risks resulting from interactions of these factors have not been studied. Nevertheless, some grouping of factors can be suggested. Ages at first pregnancy, menarche, and menopause, marital status, and androgen and estrogen excretion form one possible group. Geographic distribution and obesity may reflect a common nutritional factor. Familial aggregation, pre-existing benign breast disease, and prior occurrence of cancers of other sites may all reflect some common intrinsic factors.

In the past, these various risk factors have been explained by the action of viruses, genes, or hormones or various combinations of these agents (MacMahon, Cole, and Brown, 1973); the available data favoring each of these agents can be examined in the light of the known risk factors.

Since 1936, when Bittner described a filterable agent, that caused breast cancer, in the milk of certain mouse strains, a search has continued for such an agent in man. The mouse mammary tumor virus (MMTV) is a type B RNA virus which is vertically transmitted not only through the milk but also genetically; the genome of the virus is carried in the genome of the host (Bentvelzen et al., 1970). Moore and his colleagues (1969) have demonstrated that particles similar in several respects to MMTV can be found in human milk. The particles contain 70 S RNA and RNA-dependent DNA polymerase (reverse transcriptase, RT); both are characteristics of RNA tumor viruses (Schlom, Spiegelman, and Moore, 1971).

If an MMTV-like virus is associated with human breast cancer, it might be expected that evidence of such a virus would be found in families with several cases of breast cancer. Electron microscopic studies of milk samples obtained from women from high risk and low risk families did not show differences in particle counts. About 5% of each group showed particles of the MMTV type (Sarkar and Moore, 1972). Recently, assays for RT have been carried out and 74% of all human milk samples were found to have RT activity

Table 2. Breast cancer risk factors[a]

Risk factors	Degree of risk
1. Age at first pregnancy	> 35 yr, 1.3–1.5 × nulliparous < 18 yr, 0.5 × nulliparous
2. Age at menarche	< 16 yr, 1.8 × > 16 yr
3. Marital status	Single 1.5 × married
4. Age at menopause Natural Artificial Oophorectomy	 > 55 yr, 2 × < 45 yr menopause 0.4 × natural > 35 yr, 0.3 × all women
5. Geography	U.S., Northern Europe 5 × Asia, Africa
6. Body mass—height and weight	20% overweight 2–3 × general population (g.p.) > 170 cm 3 × < 160 cm dietary fat? risk
7. Androgen excretion	Etiocholanolone < 1.2 mg/24 hr, 2–5 × > 1.5 mg/24 hr, also androsterone
8. Estrogen metabolite	Low estriol (E_3)/estrone (E_1) + estradiol (E_2) risk unknown
9. Family aggregation	Sisters or daughters of proband 2–4 × g.p. Sisters of sister and mother with bilateral premenopausal b.c. 47 × g.p.
10. Benign breast disease	Cystic mastitis 4 × g.p.
11. Cancers of other sites	Ca of the endometrium 1.3–2.0 × g.p. Ca of the salivary gland 4 × g.p. Ca of the colon 2 × g.p.

[a]See Stewart et al., 1966; Anderson, 1972; MacMahon, Cole, and Brown, 1973; de Waard, 1974; Sherman and Korenman, 1974.

(Moore, 1975). Henderson et al. (1974), in a careful case-control study, examined the question of whether patients with breast cancer had been breast fed, i.e., exposed to a virus in maternal milk as infants. The prevalence of breast feeding among the patients did not differ from controls. Moore (1975) also found that 25% of sera from women regardless of their breast cancer status neutralize MMTV in infectivity tests in mice. Thus, these studies do not support a milk-transmitted viral etiology of breast cancer.

They do not, however, rule out other forms of vertical trans-mission. Moore (1975) found evidence of RNA sequences, homolo-gous to the MMTV genome, in 5 of 15 human mammary cancers. These RNA sequences hybridized 18 to 77% of MMTV DNA probes. Such RNA sequences were not found in normal breast tissue. Whether DNA homologous to MMTV RNA is present in human breast tissue is unclear at present.

A second virus, which may be related to human breast cancer, is the Mason-Pfizer monkey virus (MPMV). This virus was isolated from a spontaneous tumor originating in the breast of a rhesus mon-key. MPMV is also an RNA virus that contains RT and 70 S RNA. DNA probes from the RNA of this virus hybridize to about two-thirds of human breast cancers (Colcher, Spiegelman, and Schlom, 1975). Thus far, hybridization to the RNA of benign breast tissue has not been reported. It will be important to find out whether DNA homolo-gous to MPMV RNA is present in human tissues. If the genome of the virus were integrated into the genome of the host then viral DNA should be present in both benign and malignant tissues. Should testing for integrated viral DNA become available it would then be possible to test high risk and low risk families for its presence. As it stands, the virus hypothesis alone does not explain the known risk factors. Therefore, other factors must be considered.

Family aggregation of cases of breast cancer is compatible with either a genetic or environmental mechanism. Although many fami-lies have now been described showing multiple cases of breast cancer in several generations, I am not aware of any reports of formal segre-gation analysis on these families.

Anderson (1972) has made a major contribution by identifying a subset of very high risk breast cancer families. In these families breast cancer is bilateral, occurs in premenopausal women (frequently in their 20's and 30's), and affects a large proportion of the women in each generation. Anderson has estimated that the risk of a sister of a premenopausal woman with bilateral breast cancer developing breast cancer is 6–9 $\times$ the general population. If her mother and a sister had bilateral, premenopausal breast cancer then the risk is 47 $\times$ the general population.

Knudson (1971) has suggested a genetic model for cancer based primarily on observations of familial and nonfamilial retinoblastoma. The model states that there is a cancer gene which can be inherited or acquired by mutation. When the cancer genes are present at the same loci in homologous chromosomes (alleles), that cell will be transformed into a cancer cell. Knudson suggests that familial forms of cancer are explained by inheritance of one of the pair of necessary genes from one of the parents. Some cells as a result of random mutation are likely to have a mutant gene at the "cancer" locus on the homologous normal chromosome. Since mutational events happen randomly it is likely, according to this acquired-inherited model, that cancer will arise in multiple sites in the same organ or in the case of mammary cancer in both breasts. If this gene is relatively rare in the germ-line of the general population, then we can assume that bilateral breast cancer will behave like a dominant trait. Therefore, female offspring of women with bilateral breast cancer would have a 50% chance of developing breast cancer and the disease in these women would tend to occur bilaterally. As far as I am aware, the Knudson hypothesis has not been formally tested in families with multiple cases of breast cancer.

Hormones have been considered in the etiology of breast cancer because of observations relating menstrual history, reproductive experience, and estrogen and androgen excretion to risk of breast cancer. Sherman and Korenman (1974) have proposed an hypothesis which could explain and connect these seemingly unrelated observations.

Estrogens act on the breast primarily by causing development and elongation of ducts, whereas progesterone produces alveolar proliferation and development. During pregnancy large amounts of both estrogen and progesterone are produced, causing marked proliferation of glandular tissue.

During the normal menstrual cycle, estrone (E1) and estradiol (E2) are produced in increasing quantities until ovulation. There is a sudden drop in estrogen production postovulation followed by a secondary rise in estrogen production in the luteal phase followed by a decline prior to menses. Progesterone is produced by the corpus luteum only in the post ovulatory (luteal) phase of the cycle. In anovulatory cycles the corpus luteum does not develop and hence very little progesterone is produced. Also during the normal luteal phase the androgen metabolites androsterone and etiocholanolone are excreted in the urine in increased amounts and the estriol $(E_3)/(E_1 + E_2)$ ratio is increased. (Estriol is a metabolite of estrone.) Presumably in anovulatory cycles the excretion of androgen is reduced and the $E_3/E_1 + E_2$ ratio is low.

Thus, the Sherman-Korenman hypothesis states that estrogen secretion, in the absence of progesterone, either because of failure to develop corpora lutea and/or failure to become pregnant, results in unopposed estrogenic stimulation and ultimately in malignant transformation of the breast ductal epithelium.

It may well be that these three hypotheses (viral, genetic, endocrine) are all, at least in part, correct. Anderson's (1972) and other data support the notion that premenopausal and postmenopausal breast cancer are different diseases. Medullary and lobular breast cancers, morphologically distinct entities, appear to be associated with familial and bilateral cases. They may differ in other ways from the usual ductal forms.

I would like to suggest that familial medullary or lobular carcinoma of the breast conforms to the Knudson hypothesis. It may well be that the required mutational event is produced by a virus, thus combining the viral-genetic etiologies. This hypothesis can be tested by comparing the epidemiology of medullary and lobular carcinomas with that of ductal cancer. Differences should be found with respect to family incidence, age of onset, and bilaterality. In families with more than one case of medullary or lobular cancer, segregation analysis should be compatible with dominant inheritance.

The endocrine hypothesis may be associated primarily with postmenopausal breast cancer but also premenopausal cases associated with infertility, irregular menstrual cycles, and anovulatory cycles. The endocrine abnormality may be aggravated by obesity and increased fat in the diet. deWaard's data suggest that nutritional factors apply primarily to postmenopausal cases (deWaard, 1974). I am not aware of any data showing that estrogens alone are capable of transforming cells in vitro. My guess is that at least one other factor, a virus or a chemical carcinogen, is needed. If a virus is involved it probably is very common in the environment and the endocrine factors interact with the virus to produce malignant transformation. Testing of this hypothesis is more difficult, but Sherman and Korenman (personal communication) are doing a retrospective-prospective study on women whose menstrual cycles were carefully recorded when they were college students in the 1930's. These women are now 55 to 70 years old. The prediction is that women with irregular cycles and/or amenorrhea when they were young will have higher rates of breast cancer in their postmenopausal years.

The ultimate test of whether an agent (or factor) is causally related to a disease is what happens when the suspect agent is removed or a possible predisposing condition is corrected. For example, the most powerful evidence in favor of cigarettes causing lung cancer is the marked decrease in incidence of this disease in persons who were smokers but have stopped smoking. In the case of breast cancer the several hypotheses suggested above offer a few possibilities for intervention. If overnutrition or consumption of fat is causally related to one form of breast cancer, it would be possible to test the effect of weight reduction in premenopausal women on their development of breast cancer during the postmenopausal years. The virus-genetic hypothesis offers the possibility of a vaccine or immunologic manipulation. Recently, Moore (1975) has shown that immunization is effective in preventing MMTV-induced breast cancer in mice. The estrogen hypothesis suggests that hormonal therapy for certain women during their reproductive years might reduce their risk.

Thus, there is reason to hope that epidemiology coupled with observations at the bedside and basic laboratory research will lead to an understanding of breast cancer in humans and ultimately to the prevention of this disfiguring and often lethal disease.

REFERENCES

Anderson, D. E. 1972. A genetic study of human breast cancer. J. Natl. Cancer Inst. 48:1029–1034.
Bentvelzen, P., J. H. Daams, P. Hageman, and J. Calatal. 1970. Genetic transmission of viruses that incite mammary tumour in mice. Proc. Natl. Acad. Sci. USA 67:379–384.
Biometry Branch, N.C.I. 1974. Third National Cancer Survey. Advanced Three Year Report, 1969-1971, Incidence. DHEW Publication No. (NIH) 74-637.
Bittner, J. J. 1936. Some possible effects of nursing on the mammary gland tumor incidence in mice. Science 84:162–163.
Burkitt, P. P. 1971. Epidemiology of cancer of the colon and rectum. Cancer 28:3–13.
Colcher, D., S. Spiegelman, and J. Schlom. 1975. Relationship of Mason-Pfizer virus to human breast cancer. Program of the Breast Cancer Task Force, Division of Cancer Biology and Diagnosis, National Cancer Institute, p. 49.

deWaard, F. 1974. Diet and nutrition as environmental factors in the pathogenesis of breast cancer. Report to the Profession—Breast Cancer September 30, 1974. Division of Cancer Biology and Diagnosis. Natl. Cancer Inst., NIH, US, DHEW.

Haenzel, W., and P. Corren. 1971. Cancer of colon and rectum and adinomatous polyps. A review of the epidemiologic findings. Cancer 28: 14–24.

Henderson, B. E., D. Powell, I. Rosario, C. Keys, R. Hanisch, M. Young, J. Casogrande, V. Gerkinn, and M. C. Pike. 1974. An epidemiologic study of breast cancer. J. Natl. Cancer Inst. 53:609–614.

Knudson, A. G. 1971. Mutation and cancer: statistical study of retinoblastoma. Proc. Natl. Acad. Sci. USA 68:820–823.

Lundin, F. F., C. C. Erickson, and P. H. Sprunt. 1964. Socioeconomic distribution of cervical cancer in relation to early marriage and pregnancy. Public Health Monograph 73 (PHSP No. 1209).

MacMahon, B., P. Cole, and J. Brown. 1973. Etiology of Human Breast Cancer: A review. J. Natl. Cancer Inst. 50.

Mausner, J. S., and A. K. Bahn. 1974. Epidemiology—An introductory test, pp. 312–326. W. B. Saunders, Philadelphia.

Moore, D. H. 1975. Studies of human milk and mammary tumors. Programs of the breast cancer task force. Division of cancer biology and diagnosis. National Cancer Institute, p. 198.

Moore, D. H., N. H. Sarkar, C. E. Kelly, N. Pillsbury and J. Charney. 1969. Type B particles in human milk. Tex. Rep. Biol. Med. 27:1027–1039.

Report of the advisory committee to the Surgeon General of the Public Health Service. 1964. Smoking and Health (PHSP No. 1103).

Rotkin, I. D. 1967. Adolescent coitus and cervical cancer: Associations of related events with increased risk. Cancer Res. 27:603–617.

Sarkar, N. H., and D. H. Moore. 1972. On the possibility of a human breast cancer virus. Nature 236:103–106.

Schlom, J., S. Spiegelman, and D. H. Moore. 1971. RNA- dependent DNA polymerase activity in virus-like particles isloated from human milk. Nature 231:97–100.

Sherman, B. M., and S. G. Korenman. 1974. Inadequate corpus luteum function: A pathophysiological interpretation of human breast cancer epidemiology. Cancer 33:1306–1312.

Stewart, H., L. Dunham, J. Casper, H. Dorn, L. Thomas, J. Edgcomb, and A. Symeonidis. 1966. Epidemiology of cancers of uterine cervix, corpus, breast and ovary in Israel and New York City. J. Natl. Cancer Inst. 37:1–95.

Wynder, E. L., and D. Hoffman. 1968. Current studies on etiology and prevention. In W. L. Watson (ed.), Lung Cancer. C. V. Mosby, St. Louis.

Neuroblastoma and Host Defense Mechanisms

James M. Gerson, M.D.,
and Audrey E. Evans, M.D.

Neuroblastoma and possible host defenses have long been a subject of clinical interest and speculation, and have been offered as one explanation for the many unique characteristics observed in patients with this tumor. The overall accumulation of facts pertaining to host defense mechanisms has been biased toward tumor-specific type reactions, and only recently has interest developed in immune profiling of the patient with neuroblastoma. This presentation reviews the unique characteristics demonstrated in patients with neuroblastoma and the information accumulated regarding host defense.

Neuroblastoma is a malignant tumor of sympathetic nervous tissue. It is the fourth most common pediatric malignancy and has an annual incidence rate of 9.6 per million children (Young and Miller, 1975). The peak age at diagnosis is 2 years, and males are affected slightly more than females (Miller, Fraumeni, and Hill, 1968). Over 60% of the patients have disseminated disease at diagnosis. The overall 2-year survival rate for this tumor has remained unchanged in the past 20 years despite the use of multimodal therapy and new drug regimens. The accumulation of facts pertaining to the immune-related pathogenesis of this tumor may be helpful in devising new therapeutic approaches for patients with neuroblastoma.

Many of the unique characteristics observed in patients with neuroblastomas may partly be explained by assuming an immune response by the patient to his tumor. Studies of such patients have provided much of the data which are accumulating regarding human tumor host interactions. The following characteristics of neuroblastoma are those which may be associated with host defense mechanisms: 1) spontaneous regression; 2) neuroblastoma in situ; 3) the prognosis related to the pattern of metastatic spread; 4) survival related to age; 5) the relationship of lymphocytes to prognosis; and 6) normal delayed hypersensitivity skin reactions associated with a better survival experience.

SPONTANEOUS REGRESSION

Neuroblastoma has long been cited as the prime example of a tumor which can undergo spontaneous regression. Everson and Coles' monograph (1966) included 29 cases of neuroblastoma patients considered to have true spontaneous regression; this group comprised 17% of the total 176 cases reported. More recently, Evans, Gerson, and Schnaufer (in press) surveyed the 22 member institutions of the Children's Cancer Study Group. Twenty-four additional case reports were obtained. It is difficult to arrive at a rate of spontaneous regression since the patient base from which these data were derived was unknown. However, utilizing the Children's Hospital of Philadelphia data, this phenomenon occurred in 13 of 174 patients reviewed, giving a rate of 8%. The patients exhibiting spontaneous regression did so in two ways—either by complete disappearance of their disease or to a lesser extent by maturation of the tumor to benign ganglioneuroma. The regression occurred in three ways—following no treatment of any kind, following treatment (usually radiation therapy) to only one area of disease leaving other areas untreated, or as a result of unusual or inadequate treatment such as a short course of corticosteroids or antimetabolites. The latter group cannot truly be identified as spontaneous regression. From the above reviews one can surmise that the patient most likely to have spontaneous regression of his tumor will 1) probably be under 6 months of age and nearly always under 2 years at diagnosis and 2) will in all likelihood have stage II or stage IV-S disease according to Evans' staging criteria (1971).

NEUROBLASTOMA IN SITU

Beckwith and Perrin (1963), Guinn, Gilbert, and Jones (1969), and Shanklin and Sotela-Avila (1969) have reported on the presence of adrenal neuroblastoma in situ found at autopsy in infants, less than 3 months of age, who had died from causes unrelated to neoplasia. They have been estimated to occur at an incidence ranging from 1:23 to 1:1000 infant autopsies—much higher than the incidence figures for clinically overt neuroblastoma. The question has been raised whether the appearance is that of true neuroblastoma or simply persistance of immature fetal neuroblasts (Turkel and Itabashi, 1974). The evidence suggests that neuroblastoma in situ does indeed occur more often than it is clinically diagnosed and that it disappears spontaneously.

PROGNOSIS RELATED TO PATTERN OF METASTATIC SPREAD

Patients with metastases to only skin and/or liver (stage IV-S) have a higher cure rate than those with regional disease (stage III) or those who have bone metastases (stage IV) (D'Angio, Evans, and Koop, 1971). To what extent skin involvement augments delayed hypersensitivity responses against tumor remains to be answered. The extent of disease, or antigenic load, and how the antigenic load is distributed also seem to be important. Usually the greater the antigenic load, stage, or tumor burden, the worse the survival experience (Breslow and McCann, 1971). This does not hold true, however, for the patients with stage IV-S disease; some infants can have a large volume of tumor in the liver which will disappear with little or no therapy, whereas a similar amount of residual tumor elsewhere in the abdomen has a very poor prognosis. The distribution of neuroblastoma cells in the stage IV-S patient may implicate a greater role for the regional lymph node or perhaps other augmenting nonspecific immune factors. This conjectural appraisal needs a data base, for the patients with stage IV-S disease may hold a key to understanding the interrelationship between host immune response and neoplasia.

SURVIVAL RELATED TO AGE

Age is inversely related to survival; the younger the patient, the better the survival (Breslow and McCann, 1971). Age appears to influence both the stage of disease at diagnosis and the prognosis for each stage. For children under 1 year 17%, 23%, and 29% are in stages I, II, and IV-S, respectively, as compared to 12% and 72% in stages III and IV in children 2 years and more. The overall survival rate by age, and irrespective of stage, is 73%, 26%, and 12% for patients 0 to 11 months, 12 to 23 months, and 24 months or more. Four factors stand out in appraising the younger patient: 1) a normally present relative lymphocytosis, 2) the possible presence of circulating maternal antibody, 3) different nutritional habits, and 4) a shorter latent period between the initiation of oncogenesis and its clinical expression. To what extent, if any, these factors play a part and how they interact remain to be seen.

LYMPHOCYTE COUNTS

Patients with increased peripheral blood lymphocytes (Bill and Morgan, 1970), increased lymphocytic infiltration of the tumor (Martin and Beckwith, 1968), and increased bone marrow "lymphoblasts" at diagnosis have a better survival experience (Evans and Hummeler, 1973). To what extent these lymphocytes are thymus derived (T-cells), bone marrow derived (B-cells), or null cells is not known. One reported abstract studied 4 patients at diagnosis and found increased B cells and decreased T-cells present (Falletta, Mukhopadhyay, and Fernbach, 1974). Accumulation of this type of information on more patients, correlation with stage, and in vitro cytotoxicity or blocking tests are needed.

NORMAL DELAYED HYPERSENSITIVITY SKIN REACTIONS

Helson et al. (1971) has shown that patients who are able to recognize and develop a delayed hypersensitivity skin reaction to topical dinitrochlorobenzene have a more favorable prognosis. There is no reported series evaluating the ability of neuroblastoma patients to respond to standard intradermal antigens such as mumps and monilia.

ACUTE PHASE REACTANTS

Studies of patients at the Children's Hospital of Philadelphia have shown that patients who have marked elevations of serum acute phase reactants at diagnosis and whose levels stay elevated despite therapy have a worse prognosis (Gerson, Evans, and Rosen, 1975). What nonspecific feedback effects are exerted on cellular and humoral reactions is unknown. However, one acute phase reactant located in the α-2 globulins and designated immunoregulatory alpha (IRA) has been reported, and is postulated as having a role in normal suppressive immune feedback mechanisms (Milton, 1971). Its role in neuroblastoma is undefined.

Studies of patients with the above characteristics have provided and will continue to provide significant data regarding the roles and interactions of specific and nonspecific host defense mechanisms engaged in tumor rejection or enhancement. These studies in human tumor immunology primarily depend upon the results from in vitro assay systems. Most of the accumulated immunologic data pertaining to human neuroblastoma centers on tumor-specific phenomena—specifically the balance between cell-mediated cytotoxicity and blocking factor(s). Information concerning the direct presence of tumor-specific antigens (TSA), the role of humoral complement-dependent cytotoxicity, the role of antibody-dependent lymphocytotoxicity, and the possible roles of lymphokines is scarce.

TUMOR-SPECIFIC IMMUNE REACTIONS

Presence of Human Tumor-specific Antigens

The immune surveillance theory for neoplastic cells as proposed by Thomas (1959) and Burnet (1961) embraces two fundamental concepts: 1) the neoplastic cell develops new antigenic determinants which can be recognized by the immune system as foreign; and 2) the host can mount an effective immunologic response to these new tumor antigens and thus eliminate the neoplastic cell. This theory has been supported by subsequent demonstrations that patients with immune deficiency disease (Gatti and Good, 1971) or patients who are immunosuppressed (Penn and Starzl, 1972; Schneck and Penn, 1971) have an increased risk of developing malignancy. In addition, tumor-specific transplantation antigens (TSTA) have been demonstrated for most animal systems studied (Klein, 1968), and human tumor-specific antigens (TSA) have been shown to be present for several tumors (Klein et al., 1967; Morton et al., 1968; Eilber and Morton, 1970; Hellstrom et al., 1968). It can be generally stated that chemical carcinogen-induced tumors have TSTA unique for each tumor (Klein, 1968) and only occasionally induce tumors with less reactive common antigens on their surface (Reiner and Southam, 1969). On the other hand, virus-induced tumors have been shown to possess TSTA shared by all tumors induced by the same virus regardless of the morphology of the tumor (Sjogren and Bansal, 1971).

The immunosurveillance theory of neoplasia seems to be well established. However, Prehn's (1972) recent work has demonstrated that a degree of immunity may be stimulatory for tumor growth. His interpretation of the findings and how they relate to the immuno-surveillance theory is presented earlier in this monograph.

Immune Response to Human Neuroblastoma

It has been inferred from cytotoxicity experiments (Hellstrom, Hell-strom, and Pierce, 1968; Hellstrom et al., 1970) that neuroblastomas possess shared antigens, and according to Jose and Seshadri (1974) these TSA are located in the membrane turnover fraction. A recent report by Wang, Sinks, and Chu (1974) describes the presence of carcinoembryonic antigen in the plasma of neuroblastoma patients. Most in vitro studies for this tumor have been done by the Hellstroms (1968, 1970) using their colony inhibition (CI) assay. Since then their findings have been confirmed by Jagarlamoody et al. (1971) and Jose and Seshadri (1974) using radioisotope release assays and also by Kumar et al. (1972) utilizing reduction in target cell number as a parameter of effector cell cytotoxicity. All assays utilized incubation times for targets and effectors of 3 to 5 days at 37°C, 5% CO_2, and the effector to target cell ratio varied from 1000:1 to 50,000:1. Freshly cultured neuroblastoma cells were used in each instance.

Time does not permit a discussion of each particular assay, and it is difficult to make direct extrapolations from one assay system to another, so only the results are summarized.

Cellular Immunity

Nearly all of the patients' lymphocytes which were tested against neuroblastoma target cells were found to be either inhibitory or cyto-toxic. Allogeneic and autochthonous reactions were of equal intensity, and this effect was not related to extent of disease. Matched target fibroblasts were not affected. Interestingly, Hellstrom, Hell-strom, and Pierce (1968) found that lymphocytes from 7 of 12 mothers, 1 of 4 fathers, and 5 of 10 siblings of neuroblastoma patients significantly inhibited neuroblastoma colony formation in vitro. Maternal controls matched for age and parity were nonreactive.

Lymphocytes from other tumor patients and normal donors were only occasionally inhibitory.

Humoral Immunity

There is insufficient evidence to make a strong comment regarding the role of complement-dependent cytotoxic antibody. The only reported results were by Hellstrom, Hellstrom, and Pierce (1968) using their CI test. They tested plasma from 6 patients and 5 mothers, using human unabsorbed complement, and found 3 out of 6 patients and 4 out of 5 mothers to have positive inhibition assays.

Most studies with sera have been concerned with demonstrating the presence or absence of blocking factors. These blocking factors were described in animal systems (Hellstrom et al., 1969; Kaliss, 1964) and subsequently identified as being either antibody (Ran and Witz, 1972; Jose and Skvaril, 1974) or antigen-antibody complexes (Jose and Seshadri, 1974; Sjogren, 1971). Furthermore, their presence correlated with extent of disease (Hellstrom et al., 1970, 1973). Hellstrom et al. (1970), seeking to understand why all patients tested had inhibitory lymphocytes, and yet had overt clinical disease, were the first to search for blocking factors in neuroblastoma patients. They found that 6 of 6 sera from patients with progressive disease had blocking factor—a factor which could abrogate the inhibitory effect of lymphocytes in vitro, whereas 0 of 4 patients who were symptom free had blocking sera. Jose and Skvaril (1974) have identified this factor to reside in the IgG1, and IgG3 fractions of patients' sera, and it has since been demonstrated that blocking occurs most efficiently at antigen-antibody equilibrium, less so at antigen excess, and minimally at antibody excess (Jose and Seshadri, 1974).

COMMENT

If, as has been shown above, neuroblastoma has tumor-specific antigen and all patients regardless of stage have inhibitory or cytotoxic lymphocytes against neuroblastoma cells in vitro, how does the tumor manage to resist rejection in vivo? In light of Wang's data perhaps the antigen expressed is a common blast or embryonic antigen, which initiates the formation of blocking antibody which prevents an autoimmune reaction. Or perhaps the present data must be more cautiously interpreted considering the recent report by Takasugi, Mickey, and Terasaki (1973) that showed a high percentage of nonspecific cytotoxicity of control lymphocytes against established tumor cell lines. A third possibility is that in vitro correlates of host immunity can't be extrapolated to the in vivo circumstance, although better clinical correlative studies may rule against this.

Atlhough much of the evidence for spontaneous initiation of tumor growth and regression in humans must be inferred, much can be learned by correlating the results of serial in vitro immune testing with the patient's response to therapy or recurrence of disease and using these results as a guide for therapy. It is conceivable that immunodiagnosis will also become a very useful tool once neuroblastoma TSA is directly identified and characterized.

REFERENCES

Beckwith, J. B., and E. V. Perrin. 1963. In situ neuroblastomas: A contribution to the natural history of neural crest tumors. Amer. J. Pathol. 43:1089–1100.

Bill, A. H., and A. Morgan. 1970. Evidence for immune reactions to neuroblastoma and future possibilities for investigation. J. Pediatr. Surg. 5:111–116.

Breslow, N., and B. McCann. 1971. Statistical estimation of prognosis for children with neuroblastoma. Cancer Res. 31:2098–2103.

Burnet, F. M. 1961. Immunological recognition of self. Science 133: 307–311.

D'Angio, G. J., A. E. Evans, and C. E. Koop. 1971. Special pattern of widespread neuroblastomas with a favorable prognosis. Lancet 1046. Vol. 1.

Eilber, F. R., and D. L. Morton. 1970. Sarcoma specific antigens: detection by complement fixation with serum from sarcoma patients. J. Natl. Cancer Inst. 44:651–656.

Evans, A. E., G. J. D'Angio, and J. Randolph. 1971. A proposed staging for children with neuroblastoma. Cancer 27:324.

Evans, A. E., J. M. Gerson, and L. Schnaufer. Spontaneous regression of neuroblastoma. J. Natl. Cancer Inst. Monogr. In press.

Evans, A. E., and K. Hummeler. 1973. The significance of primitive cells in marrow aspirates of children with neuroblastoma. Cancer 32:906.

Everson, T. C., and W. H. Cole. 1966. Spontaneous Regression of Cancer, pp. 11–87. W. B. Saunders, Philadelphia.

Falletta, J., N. Mukhopadhyay, and D. H. Fernbach. 1974. Clin. Res. 22: abstract 84-a.

Gatti, R. A., and R. W. Good. 1971. Occurrence of malignancy in immunodeficiency disease. A literature review. Cancer Res. 28:89–98.

Gerson, J. M., A. E. Evans, and F. Rosen. 1975. Acute phase reactants as indicators of prognosis in patients with neuroblastoma. Proc. Amer. Assoc. Cancer Res. 16:abstract 76.

Guinn, G., E. Gilbert, and B. Jones. 1969. Incidental neuroblastoma in infants. Amer. J. Clin. Pathol. 51:126–136.

Hellstrom, I., K. E. Hellstrom, A. H. Bill, G. E. Pierce, and J. P. S. Yang. 1970. Studies on cellular immunity to human neuroblastoma cells. Int. J. Cancer. 6:172.

Hellstrom, I., K. E. Hellstrom, A. C. Evans, G. H. Heppner, G. E. Pierce, and J. P. S. Yang. 1969. Serum mediated protection of neoplastic cells from inhibition by lymphocytes immune to their tumor-specific antigens. Proc. Natl. Acad. Sci. USA 62:362–368.

Hellstrom, I., K. E. Hellstrom, G. E. Pierce, and A. H. Bill. 1968. Demonstration of cell bound and humoral immunity against neuroblastoma cells. Proc. Natl. Acad. Sci. USA 60:1231–1238.

Hellstrom, I., K. E. Hellstrom, G. E. Pierce, and J. P. S. Yang. 1968. Cellular and humoral immunity to different types of human neoplasms. Nature 220:1352–1354.

Hellstrom, I., G. A. Warner, K. E. Hellstrom, and H. O. Sjögren et al. 1973. Sequential studies on cell mediated tumor immunity and blocking serum activity in ten patients with malignant melanoma. Int. J. Cancer 11:280–292.

Helson, L., C. Ramos, H. Oettgen, et al. 1971. DNCB reactivity in children with neuroblastoma. Proc. Amer. Assoc. Cancer Res. 12:86.

Jagarlamoody, S. M., R. August, R. H. Tew, and C. F. McKhann. 1971. In Vitro Detection of Cytotoxic Cellular Immunity against Tumor Specific Antigens by a Radioisotope Technique. Proc. Natl. Acad. Sci. USA 68:1345–1350.

Jose, D. G., and R. Seshadri. 1974. Circulating immune complexes in human neuroblastoma: direct assay and role in blocking specific cellular immunity. Int. J. Cancer 13:824–38.

Jose, D. G., and F. Skvaril. 1974. Serum inhibitors of cellular immunity in human neuroblastoma. IgG subclass of blocking activity. Int. J. Cancer 13:113–118.

Kaliss, N. 1964. The elements of immunological enhancement: A consideration of mechanisms. Ann. N.Y. Acad. Sci. 101:64–79.

Klein, G. 1968. Tumor specific transplantation antigens. GHA Clowes Memorial Lecture. Cancer Res. 28:625–635.

Klein, G., P. Clifford, E. Klein, et al. 1967. Membrane immunofluorescence reactions of Burkitt's lymphoma cells from biopsy specimens and tissue cultures. J. Natl. Cancer. Inst. 39:1027–1044.

Kumar, S., G. Taylor, S. K. Steward, M. A. Waghe, and D. Pearson. 1972. Cellular immunity in Wilms' tumor and neuroblastoma. Int. J. Cancer 10:36–43.

Martin, R. F., and J. B. Beckwith. 1968. Lymphoid infiltrates in neuroblastomas, their occurrence and prognostic significance. J. Pediatr. Surg. 3:161.

Miller, R. W., J. F. Fraumeni, Jr., and J. A. Hill. 1968. Neuroblastoma: Epidemiologic approach to its origin. Amer. J. Dis. Child 115:253–261.

Milton, J. D. 1971. Effect of an immunosuppressive serum α-2 glyco-protein with ribonuclease activity on the proliferation of human lympho-cytes in culture. Immunology 20:205.

Morton, D. L., R. A. Malmgren, E. C. Holmes, and A. S. Ketcham. 1968. Demonstration of antibodies against human malignant melanoma by immunofluorescence. Surgery 64:233–240.

Penn, I., and T. E. Starzl. 1972. A summary of the status of de-novo can-cer in transplant recipients. Trans. Proc. 4:723.

Prehn, R. T. 1972. The immune reaction as a stimulator of tumor growth. Science 176:170–171.

Ran, M., and I. P. Witz. 1972. Tumor associated immunoglobulins. En-hancement of syngenic tumors by IgG2-containing tumor eluates. Int. J. Cancer 9:242–247.

Reiner, J., and C. M. Southam. 1969. Further evidence of common anti-genic properties in chemically induced sarcomas of mice. Cancer Res. 29:1814–1820.

Schneck, S. A., and I. Penn. 1971. De-novo brain tumors in renal trans-plant recipients. Lancet 1:983–986.

Shanklin, D. R., and C. Sotela-Avila. 1969. In situ tumors in fetuses, newborns and young infants. Biol. Neonate 14:286–316.

Sjogren, H. O., and S. C. Bansal. 1971. Antigens in virally induced tumors. In B. Amos (ed.), Immunology. pp. 921–938. Academic Press, Inc., New York.

Sjogren, H. O., I. Hellstrom, S. C. Bansal, and K. E. Hellstrom. 1971. Sug-gestive evidence that "blocking antibodies" of tumor bearing individuals may be antigen-antibody complexes. Proc. Natl. Acad. Sci. USA 68: 1372–1375.

Takasugi, M., M. R. Mickey, and P. I. Terasaki. 1973. Reactivity of lymphocytes from normal persons in cultured tumor cells. Cancer Res. 33:2898–2902.

Thomas, L. 1959. Discussion in Cellular and Humoral Aspects of Hyper-sensitivity States, pp. 529–532. H. S. Lawrence (ed.). H. Hoeber, New York.

Turkel, S. B., and H. Itabashi. 1974. The natural history of neuroblastic cells in the fetal adrenal gland. Amer. J. Pathol. 76:225–244.

Wang, J. J., L. F. Sinks, and T. M. Chu. 1974. Carcinoembryonic antigen in patients with neuroblastoma. J. Surg. Oncol. 6:211–217.

Young, J. L., Jr., and R. W. Miller. 1975. Incidence of malignant tumors in U.S. children. J. Pediatr. 86:254–258.

Immunotherapy of Malignant Melanoma: a Review

Michael J. Mastrangelo, M.D., F.A.C.P.,
Robert E. Bellet, M.D.,
J. Frederick Laucius, M.D.,
and Jane Berkelhammer, Ph.D.

For over a decade human cutaneous malignant melanoma has served as a signal tumor type for the testing of a wide variety of immuno-therapeutic modalities. Malignant melanoma has captured the interest of immunotherapists for several reasons. There are well documented cases of spontaneous regression of primary melanomas as well as metastatic disease indicating that tumor growth may be under host control (Everson and Cole, 1966; Lewis, 1972). A recently reported case of spontaneous regression of dermal melanoma metastases provided ancillary evidence to indicate that, in some cases, the host control mechanisms may be immunologic (Bodurtha et al., in press). Second, a tumor-associated antigen has been described for human malignant melanoma and it has been demonstrated by a variety of

This research was supported by United States Public Health Service Grants CA-13456, CA-05255, CA-06927, and RR-05539 from the National Institutes of Health and by an appropriation from the Commonwealth of Pennsylvania.

immunologic techniques (Gutterman et al., 1975). It soon became apparent that the host could mount both cellular (Hellström et al., 1971) and humoral (Muna, Marcus, and Smart, 1969; Bodurtha et al., 1975) immune responses against the melanoma-associated antigens. Clinically useful augmentation of this host immune response is the chief objective of immunotherapy.

In this review we discuss our own experiences with immunotherapy in patients with malignant melanoma as well as selected reports of other investigators so as to provide a representative overview of research activity in this area. Although a variety of immunotherapeutic modalities is discussed, emphasis is placed on bacillus Calmette-Guerin (BCG), the immunologic adjuvant which has been most widely tested in human malignant melanoma.

LOCAL IMMUNOTHERAPY

The animal studies of Zbar, Bernstein, and Rapp (1971) stimulated interest in the use of intralesional bacillus Calmette-Guerin (BCG) in the treatment of cancer. Working with an inbred strain of guinea pigs and a transplantable hepatocarcinoma, these investigators demonstrated that intralesional BCG can induce regression of established dermal tumor transplants as well as stimulate tumor-specific cell-mediated immunity. They found that tumor regression requires an intact immune system and direct contact between BCG and tumor cells. Subsequent studies in this system indicated that intralesional BCG treatment of dermal tumor transplants can control nodal and visceral metastases in selected situations (Hanna and Peters, in press).

Following the pioneering work of Morton (1971), a number of investigators studied the therapeutic efficacy of intralesional BCG in patients with metastatic melanoma. The results of these studies were recently reviewed (Nathanson, 1974) and indicate that approximately 58% of injected dermal and subcutaneous lesions regress as do 13% of uninjected lesions. We have also used intralesional BCG in the treatment of patients with metastatic melanoma. The objectives of our studies were to define the melanoma patient population that could benefit from this therapeutic modality and to define toxicity. In the initial study (Mastrangelo et al., in press b), patients with surgically incurable melanoma which was accessible for injection were entered. Treatment consisted of injecting a single lesion with one immunizing dose of BCG (Research Foundation, Chicago, Ill.).

Therapy was repeated at 2-week intervals with a minimum adequate trial consisting of three to five treatments. Of 19 patients entered, 15 received sufficient therapy to be evaluable for response. Two patients achieved complete remissions (CR) of 12 and 37+ months duration. An additional three patients achieved partial remissions (PR) ($\geq$ 50% reduction in tumor burden) of 2, 4, and 6 months duration. The remaining 10 patients failed to respond favorably.

The tumor profiles of these two groups (responders and non-responders) are summarized in Table 1. Responders appeared to have a substantially smaller mean tumor burden than did non-responders. This difference, however, was not statistically significant. Of the 15 patients evaluable for response, five patients had dermal melanoma metastases. All five patients experienced regression of injected dermal lesions. Uninjected dermal lesions regressed completely in two patients and partially in three. Injected and uninjected dermal lesions which underwent complete regression did not recur. Two patients with dermal lesions also had subcutaneous nodules at the initiation of immunotherapy. Only when the resultant abscess completely enveloped the injected lesion was significant regression noted and these lesions frequently recurred. In one of these two patients uninjected subcutaneous lesions underwent modest partial regression of short duration. An additional nine patients had sub-

Table 1. Pretreatment tumor profile of melanoma patients undergoing intralesional BCG therapy

	Responders	Nonresponders
Total patients	5	10
Tumor burden(G)		
Mean	7.9	124.4
Range	0.3–18.2	0.8–725
Distribution		
Regional	4/5	7/10
Disseminated	1/5	3/10
Tissue involvement		
Dermis	5/5	0/10
Subcutaneous	2/5	9/10
Nodes	1/5	4/10
Viscera	0/5	2/10

cutaneous lesions which failed to respond to intralesional BCG therapy. The nonresponding subcutaneous lesions were substantially larger (> 1 cm diameter) than the responding lesions. One responder had dermal, subcutaneous, and histologically documented contralateral inguinal lymph node metastases from a melanoma of the dorsum of the left foot. Following cessation of intralesional BCG injection of the dermal and subcutaneous metastases, the lymph nodes were excised. The presence of melanin-laden macrophages in the subcapsular areas of these nodes provided circumstantial evidence of tumor regression in uninjected lymph nodes. This case has been reported in detail (Mastrangelo et al., 1974).

Prior to therapy the functional status of each patient's cellular and humoral immune systems was evaluated as follows: quantitation of immunoglobulins, response to typhoid vaccination (Eli Lilly and Co.), DNCB (dinitrochlorobenzene) sensitization, and skin testing with microbial antigens. The results of these studies are summarized in Table 2. Three of five responders were PPD negative prior to therapy and all three converted to purified protein derivative (PPD) positive after treatment. Seven of 10 nonresponders were PPD negative prior to therapy and only two converted following therapy.

Table 2. Pretreatment status immune system of melanoma patients undergoing intralesional BCG therapy[a]

	Responders	Nonresponders
Total patients	5	10
DNCB: number positive	5/5	9/10
Skin tests		
Mean positive of 6	1.4	1.5
PPD +	2/5	3/10
PPD conversion	3/3	2/7
Typhoid immunization: number reacting	5/5	9/9
Immunoglobulins		
G	4 (N), 1 (↑)	9 (N), 1 (↓)
A	4 (N), 1 (↓)	6 (N), 2 (↑), 2 (↓)
M	2 (N), 3 (↑)	6 (N), 2 (↑), 2 (↓)

[a]DNCB, dinitrochlorbenzene; PPD, purified protein derivative; N, normal; ↑, increased; ↓, decreased.

Whether this represents a relative state of energy or is simply the result of the ineffectiveness of the nondermal route of BCG injection in producing PPD conversion remains to be determined.

It was apparent from these initial observations that dermal metastases responded favorably (5 of 5) to intralesional BCG therapy whereas subcutaneous lesions were considerably more resistant (2 of 11), and recurred frequently. Injection of lymph node metastases also appeared ineffective (0 of 4). As a result, intralesional BCG therapy was continued only for patients with dermal melanoma metastases in an effort to define further the responsiveness of these patients. We also wished to test in melanoma patients the observations of Hanna and Peters (in press) in animals that intralesional BCG treatment of dermal metastases could control visceral disease in selected cases.

Data from an additional nine treated patients have been pooled with the data from the five previously treated patients with dermal melanoma metastases. Six of 14 (43%) patients achieved CR and 5 of 14 (36%) achieved PR. Three of 14 (21%) patients failed to respond. The tumor profile of these patients is detailed in Table 3. All three nonresponders had disseminated disease as opposed to only 2 of 11 responders. The tumor burden of the nonresponders was sub-

Table 3. Pretreatment tumor profile of melanoma patients undergoing intralesional BCG therapy[a]

	CR	PR	NR
Total patients	6	5	3
Stage			
Regional	5/6	4/5	0/3
Disseminated	1/6	1/5	3/3
Tumor burden(G)			
Mean	4.4	10.7	350
Range	0.3–11.8	0.3–30	50–500
Distribution:			
Skin	6	5	3
Subcutaneous	1	1	2
Lymph node	1	0	2
Lung	0	1	1
Liver	0	0	1

[a]CR, complete remission; PR, partial remission; NR, no response.

stantially greater than responders. Indeed, the sole nonresponder with a modest tumor burden developed extensive pulmonary metastases shortly after initiation of therapy, suggesting that she harbored substantial occult disease at initial evaluation.

The clinical responses are detailed in Table 4. Complete responses were of longer duration than partial responses. Though responders lived substantially longer than nonresponders, there is as yet no real difference in survival between complete and partial responders. This may simply reflect the limited tumor burden of these patients. However, all six CRs remain alive as opposed to 2 of 5 PRs. Three of six CRs relapsed. Two of three patients developed new dermal metastases and were reinduced. One patient developed visceral metastases, necessitating initiation of chemotherapy, which resulted in a CR.

Response by site of metastasis is detailed in Table 5. Regression of injected dermal metastases was noted in 12 of 14 patients. Two patients with advanced disseminated melanoma failed to exhibit regression of injected dermal metastases. Thirteen of 14 patients were evaluable for regression of uninjected dermal metastases with one patient having only a single metastasis. Three patients with disseminated disease and larger tumor burdens showed no evidence of regression of uninjected dermal metastases. All of the remaining 10

Table 4. Response profile of melanoma patients undergoing intralesional BCG therapy[a]

	CR	PR	NR
Total patients	6	5	3
Duration			
Mean (mos.)	12.6+	4.2+	
range	2+–41+	2–6	
Survival			
Mean (mos.)	23.3+	19.2+	4.6+
Range	7+–48+	4+–39+	3–8+
Alive (3/75)	6/6	2/5	1/3
Relapsed	3/6	4/5	
Reinduced	2/3		
Total in remission (3/75)	5/6	1/5	

[a]CR, complete remission; PR, partial remission; NR, no response.

Table 5. Lesion response profile of melanoma patients undergoing intralesional BCG therapy[a]

	CR	PR	NR
Total patients	6	5	3
Skin			
Injected	6/6	5(2P)/5	1/3
Uninjected	5/5	5(3P)/5	0/3
Subcutaneous (UI)	0/1	1(P)/1	0/2
Lymph node (UI)	1/1		0/2
Lung		1/1	0/1
Liver			0/1

[a]CR, complete remission; PR, partial remission, NR, no response; P, partial; UI, uninjected.

patients with more modest tumor burdens (≤ 30 G) exhibited regression of uninjected lesions. In three patients this was only partial. In these three patients the dermal metastases were large (> 1 cm) with substantial involvement of the subcutaneous tissues. This objective response rate of uninjected dermal lesions of 10 of 13 (76%) is considerably higher than the 13% reported in the literature. This may be the result of several factors. First, our treatment regimen extends over a minimum of 6 to 8 weeks, thus allowing greater opportunity for uninjected lesions to regress when compared to single treatment regimens. Second, considerable effort was made to include patients with intracutaneous dermal metastases and to exclude those patients with dermal metastases which extended into the subcutaneous tissue. Only 1 of 4 patients with subcutaneous metastases experienced partial regression of these uninjected lesions and this was of brief duration (2 months). Of three patients with lymph node metastases only one patient (previously described) showed evidence of tumor regression. The two nonresponders differed from the responder in having massive nodal and total body tumor burdens. Of two patients with pulmonary metastases, one patient exhibited regression of a solitary pulmonary nodule. This is the first documented instance of a visceral metastasis regressing with the intralesional injection of dermal melanoma metastases and was reported in detail (Mastrangelo et al., in press).

Systemic toxicity consisted of a flu-like syndrome characterized by fever (up to 104°F), chills, anorexia, and occasional vomiting. Generally symptoms began within 4 to 6 hours of therapy and subsided within 36 to 48 hours. Aspirin or Tylenol provided prompt relief. These side effects generally increased in intensity with continued therapy but were not treatment limiting.

Twelve of 21 patients (20 melanoma; 1 breast cancer) treated with BCG developed hepatic abnormalities (hepatomegaly, abnormal scan, abnormal liver chemistries) and as a result underwent percutaneous liver biopsy. Hepatic granulomas were noted in six. The indications for biopsy in these six were hepatomegaly (1) or an abnormal scan (5). None of these six patients showed significant clinical or biochemical evidence of deteriorating liver function and no antituberculous therapy was needed. These data were reported in detail (Bodurtha et al., 1974). More serious hepatic toxicity has been noted by other investigators (Pinsky et al., in press). Two fatalities have been reported which were associated with intralesional BCG therapy for malignant melanoma (McKhann et al., 1975). In both cases hypersensitivity to BCG was suspected because of the clinical picture of fever, major clotting abnormalities, hypotension, and anuria. Pinsky et al. (in press) also noted severe hypersensitivity reactions in three patients but in only one was this life threatening. The absence of clinically significant systemic toxicity in our own studies might be due to the modest doses of BCG used.

The histology of BCG-associated tumor regression has been described by several investigators (Mastrangelo et al., in press; Lieberman, Wybran, and Epstein, 1975). As expected, the initial response is one of acute inflammation which evolves over several weeks to a chronic granulomatous response with melanin-laden macrophages. Pinsky et al. (in press) suggested that the histology of a regressing lesion following intratumoral BCG differs from that of a nonregressing lesion. In the latter group, in addition to residual tumor, caseation and plasma cell infiltration are prominent.

In summary, several investigators documented the efficacy of intralesional BCG in controlling dermal melanoma metastases. The relative effectiveness compared to chemotherapy remains to be determined. Intralesional BCG is of questionable value in the direct therapy of subcutaneous melanoma metastases and probably of no value in the direct therapy of lymph node metastases. This latter finding is in agreement with the observations of Smith et al. (1975) who were unable to induce regression by direct injection of BCG into tumor-bearing nodes in guinea pigs. In almost all cases, patients with visceral metastases responded poorly to intralesional BCG therapy of dermal lesions. We documented one case in which a pulmonary metastasis regressed in excess of 50% following intralesional BCG therapy of dermal metastases. This observation as well as those of Hanna and Peters (1975) in an animal model suggests that this modality of therapy may be effective in controlling visceral metastases in selected patients with a limited tumor burden and an intact immune system. We are pursuing the study of patients with dermal and visceral metastases to define further the patient population that can benefit from this type of treatment.

Other agents have been evaluated, although considerably less extensively, as local immunotherapy in patients with malignant melanoma. Klein and Holterman (1972) sensitized melanoma patients to DNCB and subsequently applied DNCB to cutaneous melanoma metastases. They noted tumor regression in 4 of 6 immunocompetent patients. Stjernsward and Levin (1971) have also had success with this modality of therapy.

Hunter-Craig et al. (1970) employed live vaccinia virus in the local immunotherapy of malignant melanoma and noted regression in 9 of 10 treated lesions. Roenigk et al. (1974) treated 20 patients with either regional or disseminated metastatic melanoma with intratumoral injections of vaccinia virus. They found positive cellular cytotoxicity in all patients responding to immunotherapy and could detect no blocking factors. Patients with systemic disease did not respond. There were five complete responses in patients with disease confined to the skin.

Cheema and Hersh (1972) injected metastatic melanoma nodules with autologous lymphocytes which had been activated in vitro with phytohemagglutinin. Tumor regression was noted and may well have been the result of lymphocyte mediators released locally. In the future, investigators will most probably study the therapeutic efficacy of a variety of lymphocyte factors injected intratumorally. In addition, intralesional injection of lectins could be employed to activate lymphocytes present in tumors. Lin, Bruce, and Walcroft (1975) demonstrated that the use of concanavalin A might be limited by an unusual toxicity, a generalized vasculitis.

SYSTEMIC IMMUNOTHERAPY

Active

Micrometastatic Disease   The term micrometastatic disease is used to identify that clinical circumstance in which the patient has had all clinically evident disease removed, most often surgically, but remains at high risk of recurrence. Examples of such clinical situations are the following: 1) patients with stage I (local) melanoma who have had a deeply invasive (level IV or V as defined by Clark et al., 1969) primary lesion surgically excised; 2) patients with stage II (regional) melanoma who have had definitive surgical therapy; and 3) patients with stage III (disseminated) melanoma who have had all known disease removed. Patients in all three categories remain at high risk for recurrence despite potentially curative surgery. The objectives of immunotherapy in this setting are to increase the surgical cure rate or to prolong the disease-free interval by killing or retarding the growth of clinically occult residual tumor cells.

BCG is the immunologic adjuvant which has been most thoroughly evaluated in this clinical circumstance. Bluming et al. (1972) studied a group of 12 African patients who underwent definitive surgical therapy for stage I and II melanoma of the extremity. They evaluated the relative efficacy of two methods of BCG administration (Pasteur Institute BCG by scarification versus Glaxo BCG intradermally) in stimulating delayed type hypersensitivity and prolonging the disease-free interval. Although 6 of 6 patients who received the intradermal Glaxo BCG recurred by 30 weeks, only 1 of 6 who received the Pasteur Institute BCG relapsed by 52 weeks. The prolonged disease-free interval of the Pasteur Institute BCG-treated group was attributed to the increased quantity of viable BCG units administered. Unfortunately, an untreated control was not included, thus making interpretation of the results difficult.

Gutterman et al. (1975) studied the therapeutic efficacy of two BCG preparations (fresh liquid Pasteur BCG and Tice BCG) and several dose schedules in patients with lymph node recurrence (stage II) of melanoma who underwent definitive surgery. At a dose of 6 × 10^8 viable units given weekly for 3 months, then every other week for 3 months and subsequently monthly until relapse (low dose), the Tice BCG was more effective in prolonging the disease-free interval than was the fresh liquid Pasteur BCG. Furthermore, patients receiving high dose BCG therapy (6 × 10^8 viable units weekly for 3 months, then every other week until relapse) had a significant improvement in prognosis when compared to patients on low dose BCG therapy and to historical controls. Although this study employed historical controls, both the current treatment groups and the historical controls were rigorously analyzed and appear comparable.

Morton (1974) has also initiated a study of BCG immunotherapy in patients with stage II and III melanoma who have had definitive surgical therapy. Immunotherapy consists of either Tice strain BCG alone (Tine technique adjacent to each axilla and given weekly for 1 year, biweekly for 6 months, then monthly, until recurrence) or in combination with irradiated autologous or allogeneic tissue culture melanoma cells (1×10^8 cells) at the same intervals as BCG. For stage II and III melanoma patients receiving immunotherapy both disease-free interval and survival have been improved as compared to historical controls. Unfortunately, a majority of these patients have been followed for less than 2 years and thus a definite statement regarding the efficacy of these modalities of immunotherapy cannot as yet be made. In addition, a simultaneous control group is currently being established which might allow for a clearer interpretation.

Several studies have been initiated in the United States and in Europe which will compare BCG to an untreated control group in stage II melanoma patients. Two studies include a chemotherapy adjuvant treatment group as well. Within 5 years a definite statement regarding the efficacy of postoperative BCG immunotherapy for stage II melanoma patients may be made.

Corynebacterium parvum is a gram-positive anaerobe with a potent stimulating effect on the reticuloendothelial system (Adlam and Scott, 1973) when administered as a killed vaccine. The demonstration of anti-tumor effects in animal tumor systems (Likhite and Halpern, 1973) led to a number of clinical trials in cancer patients. The Southeastern Cancer Study Group is currently evaluating *C. parvum* as a postsurgical adjuvant in stage II and III melanoma patients. The use of *C. parvum* in tumor immunotherapy has been recently reviewed (Scott, 1974).

Levamisole is a sulfur-containing antihelminthic which is widely used in veterinary and human medicine. This agent was shown to have immuno-stimulating activity in humans (Brugman et al., 1973). A study by Rojas et al. (1976) in breast cancer patients (T_{3-4}, N_2 M_0) utilized Levamisole as a postirradiation adjuvant. The median disease-free interval was 9 months for 23 control patients and 25 months for the Levamisole-treated cases. A postsurgical adjuvant trial in melanoma patients is currently being conducted.

Macrometastatic Disease

Tumor-specific Immunotherapy Though immunization with tumor cells or cell fractions is effective in animal systems in inducing resistance to subsequent tumor transplants (Prehn and Main, 1957), such procedures are inffective in suppressing the growth of established tumors. This lack of therapeutic benefit in the animal models was confirmed in clinical trials. Ikonopisov et al. (1970), Krementz et al. (1971), and Currie, Lejeune, and Hamilton-Fairley (1971) attempted to immunize melanoma patients with irradiated autologous tumor cells. Of 39 patients treated only one objective response was noted.

The failure to achieve successful therapy by active specific immunization with tumor cells may be related in part to the low degree of antigenicity of the immunizing material. Attempts to enhance the antigenicity of tumor cells have included: coupling a highly antigenic protein to the tumor cells and chemical modification with iodoacetate and neuraminidase. Rios and Simmons (1972) demonstrated regression of established tumors after active immunization of mice with neuraminidase-treated sarcoma cells. Levy, Siegler, and Shingleton (1974) employed subcutaneous inoculation of irradiated neuraminidase-treated autochthonous tumor cells and BCG as part of a four-stage immunotherapy regimen for melanoma patients with surgically incurable disease. Other stages included vaccination with BCG, intratumor injection of dermal and subcutaneous metastases with BCG, and subcutaneous or intratumor injection of specifically sensitized autologous lymphocytes. Of 111 patients followed for at least 1 year, 32% remained alive and free of detectable disease. However, no patients with visceral metastases had complete regression. This treatment regimen is of prolonged duration and consequently significant numbers of patients are lost prior to completion of therapy. The complexity of the regimen makes definition of the therapeutically effective stages difficult.

Our experience with intralesional BCG therapy of patients with dermal melanoma metastases described in preceding paragraphs raised the question of the possible efficacy of this therapeutic modality in patients with dermal as well as lymph node and visceral metastases. However, there are insufficient numbers of patients with dermal as well as lymph node and/or visceral metastases to test adequately this hypothesis. We have attempted to circumvent this problem by treating patients with lymph node and visceral metastases with the intradermal injection of a vaccine containing irradiated (15,000 rads) autochthonous tumor cells ($1-2 \times 10^8$) + 0.5 ml of BCG (Glaxo). Tumor tissue is obtained from each patient prior to the initiation of therapy. Tumor cells are mechanically dispersed (40 mesh wire screen), frozen in liquid nitrogen, and irradiated immediately prior to use. Therapy is continued at 2-week intervals for a minimum of five treatments in nonresponders or until the vaccine is exhausted in responders.

There are presently 17 evaluable patients; four patients responded favorably, two with complete disappearance of tumor and two with a greater than 50% reduction in tumor burden. The clinical profiles of both responding and nonresponding patients are detailed in Table 6. Responders were more likely to be female and have smaller tumor burdens with disease limited to the lymph nodes and subcutaneous tissues. Responses were of short duration (4, 3, 3, and 2 months) and relapse occurred soon after exhaustion of the vaccine.

Table 6. Clinical profile of melanoma patients immunized with tumor cells plus BCG[a]

	Responders	Nonresponders
Total	4	13
Sex (M:F)	1/3	7/6
Age (yr)		
Mean	59	50
Range	38–86	23–72
Prior therapy	1/4 (C)	5/13 (C)
Tumor burden (G)		
0–50	3/4	1/13
51–100	1/4	4/13
> 100	0/4	8/13
Tissue		
Nodes	4/4	9/13
Subcutaneous	1/4	11/13
Lung	0/4	5/13
Miscellaneous	0/4	2/13 (O, D)

[a]C, chemotherapy; O, osseous; D, dermal.

Sequential in vitro studies were performed on lymphocytes from eight melanoma patients to assess the change in reactivity during immunotherapy. Melanoma patients were bled every 2 weeks prior to injection with tumor cells + BCG. Lymphocytes were prepared from heparinized blood by centrifugation on a Ficoll-Hypaque gradient and were stored in liquid nitrogen until use. Following the fifth vaccine treatment, lymphocyte samples from each donor were thawed and tested simultaneously against an allogeneic melanoma cell line by the microcytotoxicity assay (Takasugi and Klein, 1970). All eight patients tested exhibited increased lymphocyte reactivity after immunotherapy (Table 7). This lymphocyte reactivity was not specific for the immunizing melanoma antigen, because when lymphocytes from melanoma patients were tested simultaneously against melanoma cells and against bladder carcinoma cells, the pattern of reactivity

Table 7. In vitro reactivity against allogeneic melanoma cells of lymphocytes from melanoma patients receiving irradiated tumor cells + BCG[a]

Lymphocyte donor	Mean No. cells ± S.D. after incubation with		Percent reduction
	Medium	Donor Ly.	
*M119	65 ± 12	53 ± 10	18 (A)
		37 ± 5	43 (B)
M115	117 ± 28	94 ± 11	20 (A)
		59 ± 14	50 (B)
*M82	77 ± 8	54 ± 6	30 (A)
		43 ± 10	44 (B)
M118	104 ± 26	78 ± 18	25 (A)
		63 ± 10	40 (B)
*M136	95 ± 20	56 ± 11	41 (A)
		47 ± 11	50 (B)
M23	145 ± 21	35 ± 16	76 (A)
		18 ± 7	88 (B)
M225	68 ± 10	37 ± 6	46 (A)
		7 ± 6	90 (B)
M141	62 ± 8	52 ± 13	16 (A)
		46 ± 6	26 (B)

[a]Ly, lymphocyte; *, responder; (A), pretreatment value; (B), post-treatment value.

against bladder carcinoma closely paralleled that against the melanoma cell line.

Striking correlations between lymphocyte reactivity and clinical course of disease were not apparent after five vaccine treatments. Only in extreme cases, i.e., when disease was rapidly progressive (e.g., M141), did lymphocytes show relatively little reactivity throughout the period tested.

To date the quality of tumor response has been disappointing. Remissions were of short duration and occurred only in patients with small tumor burdens confined to lymph nodes and subcutaneous tissue. The enhancement of lymphocyte cytotoxicity demonstrated by all treated patients who were studied and the timing of relapse with the cessation of immunotherapy suggested that therapeutic efficacy might be improved by prolonging treatment. This possibility is currently being investigated. Nonetheless, the restrictions of a small, nonvisceral tumor burden, sufficient accessible tumor to allow preparation of a large amount of vaccine and sufficiently indolent disease to allow for protracted therapy, virtually preclude application of this therapy modality to a significant portion of the melanoma patient population.

A new and exciting area of tumor-specific active immunotherapy is the use of informational molecules such as transfer factor and "immune" RNA to stimulate specifically the host's immune system. Transfer factor is a low molecular weight, nonimmunogenic molecule capable of transferring delayed type hypersensitivity from an immune donor to a nonimmune recipient (Neidhart and LoBuglio, 1974). Based on the successful use of transfer factor in the therapy of chronic infectious diseases (Bullock, Fields, and Brandiss, 1972; Whitcomb and Rocklin, 1973), clinical therapy trials have been initiated for a variety of tumor types. Lack of a good source of transfer factor is a deterrent to more widespread clinical trials. An excellent source would be patients who have undergone tumor resolution, the mechanism of which is thought to be immunologic, e.g., spontaneous tumor regression or tumor regression associated with immunotherapy. Unfortunately, such patients are few in number and investigators are reluctant to tamper with their immune systems for fear of inducing relapse. When a tumor-specific antigen preparation is available, this will allow donor immunization. In the trials conducted to date, transfer factor donors have generally been cohabitants of the patients who have a positive in vitro assay of immunity against the tumor. In some instances, a cross-immunization technique has been used to obtain transfer factor donors. Patient B is immunized with tumor from patient A and then serves as a donor of transfer factor for patient A. There are several limitations to this technique. The most problematic is the immunization not only against the tumor but HLA antigens as well. There is little published data on the therapeutic efficacy of transfer factor in melanoma patients. Spitler et al. (1973), Smith et al. (1973), Krementz et al. (1974), and Brandes, Galton, and Wiltshaw (1971) employed transfer factor in 21 patients with metastatic melanoma and noted improvement in eight. Individual series were small and the criteria for response varied. Although additional studies are in progress, definitive evaluation of this treatment modality will not be possible until a potent source of transfer factor becomes available.

"Immune" RNA (Pilch and deKernion, 1974) is a second informational molecule which differs from transfer factor in having the ability to transfer both humoral and cellular immunity from the sensitized donor to the nonsensitized recipient. A second important difference is the ability of "immune" RNA to effect interspecies transfer. The "immune" RNA obtained from a sensitized animal could possibly be used to treat patients. If therapists are to avoid transfer of immunity against transplantation antigens, a pure source of tumor-specific antigen will have to be available. Clinical trials with immune RNA are in preliminary stages and no data are presently available on it as a treatment of malignant melanoma.

In syngeneic animal systems, tumor immunotherapy is readily achieved by the passive transfer of lymphocytes from immunized donors to nonimmunized recipients. A significant immunotherapeutic effect is dependent on the persistence of the transferred lymphocytes in the recipient. In the clinical setting, HLA differences between donor and host virtually preclude the successful application of this modality. To circumvent this problem, several techniques were developed to enhance the therapeutic effect of autologous lymphocytes in vitro. Some investigators reasoned that the inability of autologous lymphocytes to control tumor growth may be related to an inadequate lymphocyte to tumor cell ratio. In an attempt to improve this ratio Moore and Gerner (1970) cultivated large numbers of autologous lymphocytes from melanoma patients and reinfused them. Tumor regression was noted in two of three patients who received more than 450 g of cultured lymphocytes. In one patient, cultured lymphocytes were labeled with radioactive chromium. Postinfusion studies indicated that these lymphocytes were sequestered largely in the lungs with only minimal localization around tumor nodules.

Other investigators attempted to enhance the therapeutic efficacy of autologous lymphocytes through in vitro activation by exposure to tumor-specific antigen. Golub and Morton (1974) have successfully sensitized lymphocytes in vitro against human melanoma-associated antigens. Clinical trials in melanoma patients with autologous lymphocytes are limited. Levy, Siegler, and Shingleton (1974) employed intratumor injection of specifically sensitized autologous lymphocytes as part of the four-stage immunotherapy regimen described in a preceding section. Because of the complexity of the therapy regimen, the contribution of the sensitized lymphocyte to the overall clinical results cannot be defined. In vitro "education" of lymphocytes against tumor-associated antigens, though appealing, is as yet only a potential modality of tumor immunotherapy.

Frenster and Rogoway (1968) devised a technique for reinfusion of autologous lymphocytes which have been nonspecifically activated in vitro by exposure to phytohemagglutinin (PHA). Clinical trials are currently underway in which the PHA-activated lymphocyte technique is employed in patients with sarcomas and melanomas who have had partial regression or stabilization of their disease on chemotherapy. Insufficient data are now available to evaluate the therapeutic merits of this modality of active immunotherapy.

Nonspecific Active Immunotherapy   Gutterman et al. (1974) evaluated the efficacy of dimethyltriazeno imidazole carboxamide (DTIC) plus fresh Pasteur BCG by scarification in 89 patients with disseminated melanoma. The results were compared with an historical control treated with DTIC alone. DTIC-BCG-treated patients with regional lymph node metastases had a remission rate of 55% compared to 18% in the historical controls. No difference in response rates was noted for patients with pulmonary and/or other visceral metastases. Survival, however, was prolonged for all patient categories treated with DTIC-BCG when compared to those treated with DTIC alone. Other investigators (Laucius et al., 1974), however, demonstrated response rates of 50% for melanoma patients with lymph node metastases treated with DTIC alone. This study made two points. First, BCG can be given safely in combination with therapeutic doses of DTIC. Second, the prolongation of survival for all categories of patients treated with DTIC-BCG when compared to DTIC alone in the absence of improved objective remission rates in some of these same patients indicates that trials which assess only objective response may well be overlooking a valuable therapeutic effect in prolonged survival.

Israel and Edelstein (1974) used *C. parvum* in combination with chemotherapy in melanoma patients with visceral metastases. Preliminary data revealed that at 12 months there were twice as many survivors in the chemoimmunotherapy group as in the chemotherapy alone group.

Adoptive Immunotherapy

This modality of immunotherapy involves the transfer of anti-tumor lymphocytes to a tumor-bearing recipient and the successful adoption by and function in the recipient of these lymphocytes. This technique is ideally suited to syngeneic animal models, but has been minimally effective in clinical studies. The most extensively investigated approach entails the cross-immunization of pairs of patients who are matched for both blood and tumor type. Both patients in each pair are actively immunized with subcutaneous transplants of their partner's tumor. White cells are then removed from the "immunized" tumor transplant recipient and transfused into the tumor donor. Nadler and Moore (1966, 1969), Krementz et al. (1974), and Curtis (1971) evaluated this modality of immunotherapy in 80 patients with metastatic melanoma and noted objective improvement in only 10. There are several obstacles to the effective utilization of this form of therapy: 1) immunization is attempted in patients who themselves have advanced cancer and are thus unlikely to mount a maximum immune response; 2) the recipients' lymphocytes are immunized against HLA antigens as well as tumor-associated antigens; 3) the transfused lymphocytes differ antigenically (HLA) from the donor and are probably rapidly eliminated from the donor; 4) the technique is complicated and time consuming.

Passive Immunotherapy

Passive immunotherapy is achieved by transferring specifically cytotoxic effector elements to a tumor-bearing recipient. Presently serotherapy with antibody is not being actively pursued for a variety of reasons. Mitchison (1955) demonstrated that cellular immunity plays a dominant role in tumor inhibition. Klein et al. (1960) further demonstrated that anti-tumor immunity can be transferred to a non-immunized animal by the transfer of lymphocytes, but not by transfer of serum. Second, in the absence of a pure tumor antigen preparation for immunization, anti-tumor antisera will also contain antibodies against normal transplantation antigens. Third, noncomplement-fixing tumor-specific antibodies may exhibit an enhancing or protective effect by blocking antigenic sites from recognition by cytotoxic antibodies or lymphocytes. Hellström et al. (1971) found that cytotoxic lymphocytes were present in patients with growing neoplasms and that in certain cases the serum of these patients contained blocking factors (i.e., tumor antigen or antigen-antibody complexes) which abrogated the cytotoxic effects of these lymphocytes. In turn, the effects of the blocking factors could be abrogated by "deblocking antibodies" present in the serum of patients rendered tumor-free. Further confirmation of these observations may cause a resurgence of interest in passive serotherapy.

Other potential adaptations of passive serotherapy involve the coupling of potent anti-tumor chemicals to tumor-specific antibody. Philpott et al. (1974) demonstrated selected cytotoxicity with coupled arsphenamine antibody and peroxidase in two in vitro tumors. Davies and O'Neill (1973) investigated chlorambucil coupled to anti-tumor antibody demonstrating "homing" in vitro but not in vivo. Clinical data are not yet available.

In summary, intralesional BCG is clearly effective in the treatment of dermal melanoma metastases. The relative merits of this modality compared to chemotherapy remain to be determined in a randomized prospective trial. The preliminary data on the use of BCG as a post surgical adjuvant in melanoma patients who are at high risk of recurrence and the combination of BCG and chemotherapy in patients with clinically evident metastases are encouraging but must await confirmation before these therapies can be routinely recommended. Appropriate studies are in progress. The other tumor immunotherapy techniques discussed must await considerable further study before final judgment of their merits.

REFERENCES

Adlam, C., and M. T. Scott. 1973. Lymphoreticular stimulatory properties of *Corynebacterium parvum* and related bacteria. J. Med. Microbiol. 6:261–274.

Bluming, A. Z., C. L. Vogel, J. L. Ziegler, N. Mody, and G. Kamya. 1972. Immunological effects of BCG in malignant melanoma. Two modes of administration compared. Ann. Intern. Med. 76:405–411.

Bodurtha, A. J., J. Berkelhammer, Y. K. Kim, J. F. Laucius, and M. J. Mastrangelo. A clinical, histological and immunological study of a case of metastatic malignant melanoma undergoing spontaneous remission. Cancer. In press.

Bodurtha, A. J., D. O. Chee, J. F. Laucius, M. J. Mastrangelo, and R. T. Prehn. 1975. Clinical and immunological significance of human melanoma cytotoxic antibody. Cancer Res. 35:189–193.

Bodurtha, A., Y. K. Kim, J. F. Laucius, R. A. Donato, and M. J. Mastrangelo. 1974. Hepatic granulomas and other hepatic lesions associated with BCG immunotherapy of cancer. Amer. J. Clin. Pathol. 61:747–752.

Brandes, L. J., D. A. G. Galton, and W. Wiltshaw. 1971. New approach to the immunotherapy of melanoma. Lancet 2:293–295.

Brugman, S. J., V. Schuermans, W. DeCock, D. Thienpont, P. Janssen, H. Verhaegen, L. Van Nimmen, A. C. Lovwagie, and E. Stevens. 1973. Restoration of host defense mechanisms in man by levamisole. Life Sci. 13:1499–1504.

Bullock, W. E., J. P. Fields, and M. W. Brandiss. 1972. An evaluation of transfer factor as immunotherapy for patients with lepromatous leprosy. New Eng. J. Med. 287:1053–1059.

Cheema, A. R., and E. M. Hersh. 1972. Local tumor immunotherapy with in vitro activated autochthonous lymphocytes. Cancer 29:982–986.

Clark, W. H., Jr., L. From, E. A. Bernardino, and M. C. Mihm. 1969. The histogenesis and biologic behavior of primary human malignant melanomas of the skin. Cancer Res. 29:705–727.

Currie, G. A., F. Lejeune, and G. Hamilton-Fairley. 1971. Immunization with irradiated tumor cells and specific lymphocyte cytotoxicity in malignant melanoma. Brit. Med. J. 2:305–310.

Curtis, J. E. 1971. Adoptive immunotherapy in the treatment of advanced malignant melanoma. Proc. Amer. Assoc. Cancer Res. 12:52.

Davies, D. A. L., and G. J. O'Neill. 1973. In vivo and in vitro effects of tumor specific antibodies with chlorambucil. Brit. J. Cancer 28(Suppl. 1):285–298.

Everson, T. C., and W. H. Cole. 1966. Spontaneous Regression in Cancer. W. B. Saunders, Philadelphia.

Frenster, J. H., and W. M. Rogoway. 1968. In vitro activation and reinfusion of autologous human lymphocytes. Lancet 2:978–980.

Golub, S. H., and D. L. Morton. 1974. Sensitization of lymphocytes in vitro against human melanoma associated antigens. Nature 251:161–163.

Gutterman, J. U., G. Mavligit, J. A. Gottlieb, M. A. Burgess, C. E. McBride, L. Einhorn, J. Freireich, and E. M. Hersh. 1974. Chemoimmunotherapy of disseminated malignant melanoma with dimethyl triazeno imidazole carboxamide and bacillus Calmette-Guerin. New Eng. J. Med. 291:592–597.

Gutterman, J. U., G. Mavligit, R. Reed, C. E. McBride, and E. M. Hersh. 1975. Immunology and immunotherapy of human malignant melanoma. Semin. Oncol. In press.

Hanna, M. G., Jr., and L. C. Peters. Efficacy of intralesional BCG therapy in guinea pigs with disseminated tumors. Cancer. In press.

Hellström, I., K. E. Hellström, H. O. Sjögren, and G. A. Warner. 1971. Demonstration of cell mediated immunity to human neoplasms of various histological types. Int. J. Cancer 7:1–16.

Hunter-Craig, I., K. A. Newton, G. Westbury, and B. W. Lacey. 1970. Use of Vaccinia Virus in the treatment of metastatic malignant melanoma. Brit. Med. J. 2:512–515.

Ikonopisov, R. L., M. G. Lewis, I. D. Hunter-Craig, D. C. Bodenham, T. M. Phillips, C. I. Cooling, J. Proctor, G. Hamilton-Fairley, and P. Alexander. 1970. Autoimmunization with irradiated tumor cells in human malignant melanoma. Brit. Med. J. 2:752–754.

Israel, L., and R. L. Edelstein. 1974. Nonspecific immunostimulation with Corynebacterium parvum in human cancer. In Immunological Aspects of Neoplasia, M. D. Anderson Hospital and Tumor Institute at Houston. Williams & Wilkins Co., Baltimore.

Klein, E., and O. A. Holterman. 1972. Immunotherapeutic approaches to the management of neoplasms. J. Natl. Cancer Inst. Monogr. 35:370–402.

Klein, G., H. O. Sjögren, E. Klein, and K. E. Hellström. 1960. Demonstration of resistance against methylcholanthrene induced sarcomas in the primary autochthonous host. Cancer Res. 20:1561–1572.

Krementz, E. T., P. W. A. Mansell, M. O. Hornung, M. S. Samuels, C. A. Sutherland, and E. V. Benes. 1974. Immunotherapy of malignant disease: The use of viable sensitized lymphocytes or transfer factor prepared from sensitized lymphocytes. Cancer 33:394–401.

Krementz, E. T., M. S. Samuels, J. H. Wallace, and E. N. Benes. 1971. Clinical experience in the immunotherapy of cancer. Surg. Gynec. Obstet. 133:209–217.

Laucius, J. F., A. J. Bodurtha, R. H. Creech, and M. J. Mastrangelo. 1974. Randomized prospective trial comparing BCNU plus vincristine versus imidazole carboxamide in patients with malignant melanoma. Proc. XI Int. Cancer Cong. 3:540.

Levy, N. L., H. F. Siegler, and W. W. Shingleton. 1974. A multiphase immunotherapy regimen for human melanoma: Clinical and laboratory results. Cancer 34:1548–1557.

Lewis, M. G. 1972. Immunology of human malignant melanoma. Ser. Haematol. 5:44–65.

Lieberman, R., J. Wybran, and W. Epstein. 1975. The immunologic and histopathologic changes of BCG-mediated tumor regression in patients with malignant melanoma. Cancer 35:756–777.

Likhite, V. V., and B. N. Halpern. 1973. The delayed rejection of tumors formed from the administration of tumor cells mixed with killed Corynebacterium parvum. Int. J. Cancer 12:699–704.

Lin, H., W. R. Bruce, and M. J. Walcroft. 1975. Concanavalin A (NSC-143504): Its action on experimental tumor cells and possible use in cancer chemotherapy. Cancer Chemother. Rep. 59:319–326.

Mastrangelo, M. J., R. E. Bellet, J. Berkelhammer, and W. H. Clark, Jr. 1975. Regression of pulmonary metastatic disease associated with intralesional BCG therapy of dermal melanoma metastases. Cancer. 36: 1305–1308.

Mastrangelo, M. J., Y. H. Kim, R. S. Bornstein, D. O. Chee, H. L. Sulit, J. W. Yarbo, and R. T. Prehn. 1974. Clinical and histologic correlation of melanoma regression after intralesional BCG therapy: A case report. J. Natl. Cancer Inst. 52:19–24.

Mastrangelo, M. J., H. L. Sulit, L. M. Prehn, R. S. Bornstein, J. W. Yarbro, and R. T. Prehn. Intralesional BCG in the treatment of metastatic melanoma. Cancer. In press.

McKhann, C. F., C. G. Hendrickson, L. E. Spitler, A. Gunnarsson, D. Banerjee, and W. R. Nelson. 1975. Immunotherapy of melanoma with BCG: Two fatalities following intralesional injection. Cancer 35:514–520.

Mitchison, N. A. 1955. Studies on the immunological response to foreign tumor transplants in the mouse. I. The role of lymph node cells in conferring immunity by adoptive transfer. J. Exp. Med. 102:157–177.

Moore, G. E., and R. E. Gerner. 1970. Cancer immunity-hypothesis and clinical trial of lymphocytotherapy for malignant diseases. Ann. Surg. 172:733–739.

Morton, D. L. 1971. Immunological studies with human neoplasms. J. Reticuloendothel. Soc. 10:137–160.

Morton, D. L. 1974. Cancer Immunotherapy: An Overview. Semin. Oncol. 1:297–310.

Muna, N. M., S. Marcus, and C. Smart. 1969. Detection by immunofluorescence of antibodies specific for human melanoma cells. Cancer 23:88–93.

Nadler, S. H., and G. E. Moore. 1966. Clinical immunologic study of malignant disease: Response to tumor transplants and transfer of leukocytes. Ann. Surg. 164:482–489.

Nadler, S., and G. E. Moore. 1969. Immunotherapy of malignant disease. Arch. Surg. 99:376–381.

Nathanson, L. 1974. Use of BCG in the treatment of human neoplasms: A review. Semin. Oncol. 1:337–350.

Neidhart, J. A., and A. F. LoBuglio. 1974. Transfer-factor therapy of malignancy. Semin. Oncol. 1:379–385.

Philpott, G. W., R. J. Bower, K. L. Parker, and W. T. Shearer. 1974. Affinity cytotoxicity of tumor cells with antibody-glucose oxidase conjugation, peroxidase and arsphenamine. Cancer Res. 34:2159–2164.

Pilch, Y. H., and J. B. deKernion. 1974. Immunotherapy of cancer with "immune" RNA: Current status. Semin. Oncol. 1:387–395.

Pinsky, C. M., Y. Hirshaut, J. M. Woodruff, R. Costello, and H. F. Oettgen. Intralesional injection of BCG in patients with malignant melanoma. Cancer. In press.

Prehn, R. T., and J. M. Main. 1957. Immunity to methylcholanthrene-induced sarcomas. J. Natl. Cancer Inst. 18:769–778.

Rios, A., and R. L. Simmons. 1972. Comparative effect of *mycobacterium bovis* and neuraminidase-treated tumor cells on the growth of established methylcholanthrene fibrosarcomas in syngeneic mice. Cancer Res. 32:16–21.

Roenigk, H. H., S. Deodhar, R. St. Jacques, and K. Burdick. 1974. Immunotherapy of malignant melanoma with vaccinia virus. Arch. Dermatol. 109:668–674.

Rojas, A. F., E. Mickiewicz, J. N. Feierstein, H. Glait, and A. J. Olivari. 1976. Levamisole in advanced human breast cancer. Lancet 1:211–215.

Scott, M. T. 1974. *Corynebacterium parvum* as an immunotherapeutic anticancer agent. Semin. Oncol. 1:367–378.

Smith, G. V., P. A. Morse, G. D. Deraps, S. Raju, and J. D. Hardy. 1973. Immunotherapy of patients with cancer. Surgery 74:59–68.

Smith, H. G., R. C. Bast, Jr., B. Zbar, and H. S. Rapp. 1975. Eradication of microscopic axillary lymph node metastasis after injection of living *mycobacterium bovis* into established intradermal tumors: Lack of efficacy of alternate routes of BCG administration. J. Natl. Cancer Inst. 55:1345–1352.

Spitler, L. E., J. Wybran, H. H. Fudenberg, A. S. Levin, and M. Lewis. 1973. Transfer factor therapy of malignant melanoma. Clin. Res. 21:221.

Stjernsward, J., and A. Levin. 1971. Delayed hypersensitivity-induced regression of human neoplasm. Cancer 28:628–640.

Suk, D., J. Pickren, and G. E. Moore. 1973. Unusual cellular reaction to malignant melanoma in patients infused with cultured autochthonous lymphocytes. N.Y. State J. Med. 73:2479–2483.

Takasugi, M., and E. Klein. 1970. A microassay for cell mediated immunity. Transplantation 9:219–227.

Whitcomb, M. E., and R. E. Rocklin. 1973. Transfer factor therapy in a patient with progressive pulmonary tuberculosis. Ann. Intern. Med. 79:161–166.

Zbar, B., I. D. Bernstein, and H. J. Rapp. 1971. Suppression of tumor growth at the site of injection with living Bacillus Calmette-Guerin. J. Natl. Cancer Inst. 46:831–839.

Topical Treatment of Cutaneous Neoplasms

Eugene J. Van Scott, M.D.

Neoplasms of the skin, because of their being readily accessible and detectable, have provided the opportunity of administering treatment early. This circumstance alone in large measure has accounted for the excellent control rates of epidermal cancers by means of conventional techniques, which have consisted of physical removal or destruction of clinically apparent lesions one by one. These techniques, however, have not been applicable to clinically imperceptible lesions, nor have they been of substantial usefulness in control of lymphomas of the skin.

Within recent years topical drug therapy has been found to be effective against both epidermal cancers and lymphomas and has been particularly useful in treating early lesions, even before such lesions have become clinically apparent, and in treating multiple lesions simultaneously. Such topical drug therapy has been of two types, namely chemotherapeutic and immunotherapeutic.

EPIDERMAL CANCERS

Virtually all basal cell carcinomas and squamous cell carcinomas of epidermal origin can be eradicated by means now available if these

This research was supported in part by National Institute of Health Grant PO1 CA 11536.

means are properly applied early. More important, however, is the fact that virtually all such cancers are preventable by treatment of precancerous lesions.

Precancerous lesions, by far the most common of which are actinic keratoses resulting from chronic overexposure to sunlight, are today routinely treated by topical chemotherapy with solutions or creams containing 5-fluorouracil (5-FU) in 1% or 5% concentration. The treatment technique, first introduced over a decade ago (Klein et al., 1962; Dillaha et al., 1963), today is recognized as one of the major advances in skin cancer control. Prior to its introduction lesions were obliterated by grossly destructive techniques, mainly thermal cautery, surgery, or x-irradiation. The use of topical 5-FU now permits a rather selective eradication, for the drug enters the skin only at sites of lesions where the epidermal barrier is impaired due to its faulty formation by the abnormal epidermal cells. The treatment has the distinct advantage of its being self-administered by the patient and its being relatively inexpensive. Adequate instructions for its application, and precautions to be followed, are given in the package inserts accompanying the products and from supplemental information which may be obtained from the product manufacturers.

Once actinically damaged skin manifests its first precancerous lesion, emergence of subsequent lesions may be expected over the course of time. Repeated topical treatments with 5-FU are therefore usually necessary and desirable at appropriate intervals, determined by close inspection of the skin and obtaining biopsy specimens if necessary to confirm diagnoses histopathologically.

Topical 5-FU chemotherapy is today judged to be adequate treatment of cancerous lesions as well as precancerous lesions, provided the lesions are sufficiently superficial and noninvasive as to be reached by the drug. Such lesions usually can be identified clinically by the experienced therapist, but doubts regarding lesion depth should be resolved by histopathologic monitoring via biopsy specimens.

As with cancer therapy generally, under-treatment should be avoided, and despite cosmetic considerations that concern both patient and physician it is best to continue daily topical application of drug until complete destruction of lesions is apparent, times varying from 2 to several weeks. Eroded sites caused by the drug's destruction of both normal and abnormal cells, although striking in appearance at peak of reaction, heal quite satisfactorily and provide results cosmetically more acceptable than those usually achieved by other treatment means.

The demonstrated efficacy of topical chemotherapy of epidermal neoplastic lesions with 5-FU has probably discouraged extensive explorations of therapeutic potential of topical immunotherapeutic procedures against these lesions. Nevertheless a substantial amount of work in this area has been reported by Klein and his associates (Williams and Klein, 1970) who have indeed been able to eradicate epithelial cancers by topical imposition of delayed hypersensitivity reactions to involved areas of skin. Candidate drugs for topical immunotherapeutic use must of course be sufficiently antigenic to provoke its immunologic recognition by the host when applied topically. One such agent has been dinitrochlorobenzene (DNCB), which has been used by the author in limited trials of immunotherapy of epidermal lesions in patients who can be sensitized to this chemical. Figures 1 and 2 illustrate how superficially located early epidermal cancerous lesions can be eradicated by topical imposition of delayed hypersensitivity reactions to DNCB.

The value of topical immunotherapy of epidermal cancers, however, remains largely untested because topical chemotherapy with

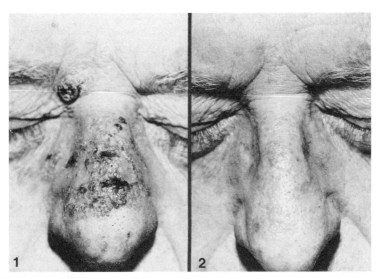

Figure 1. Actinic keratoses of nose and Bowenoid epidermal cancer of brow at peak of delayed hypersensitivity reaction 72 hours after application of DNCB. Figure 2. One month later lesions are not clinically detectable.

5-FU has been so effective and is now so widely used. Few patients present a need for a therapeutic alternative.

CUTANEOUS LYMPHOMA

Mycosis fungoides (MF) accounts for the vast majority of cases of lymphoma involving the skin. Initiated within the skin, often as a benign-appearing dermatitis and diagnosed as such at this early time, this disease progresses through successive cutaneous stages, whereupon, following the stage when tumors appear, the disease involves lymph nodes and thereafter may involve any internal organ (Block et al., 1963). Until recent years MF was uniformly fatal, even though temporary partial remissions were achievable with systemic chemotherapy, usually administered in the later stages of the disease (Epsten et al., 1972). Within the past few years advances against the disease have been achieved so that prognosis today, particularly of early stage disease, can be optimistically projected.

Intensive topical chemotherapy with nitrogen mustard (HN2) has proved to be one means of controlling this disease (Van Scott and Kalmanson, 1973). The drug has particular properties that permit it to have dual usefulness in topical therapy of MF. Its primary cytotoxic properties appear to account for resolution of lesions when the drug is applied as a chemotherapeutic agent, and its antigenicity permits it to be used for topical immunotherapy since delayed hypersensitivity reactions elicited on lesions of mycosis fungoides by HN2 can effect complete resolution of such lesions, much like the resolution of lesions due to delayed hypersensitivity reaction induced by DNCB (Ratner, Waldorf, and Van Scott, 1968).

Use of HN2 in topical therapy of MF has led to some additional findings of immunologic interest, ancillary to both its use as a chemotherapeutic drug and its use as an immunotherapeutic agent.

Topical Use of HN2 Primarily for Its Chemotherapeutic Effects

Sipos and Jasko (1956) and Haserick, Richardson, and Grant (1959) were first to observe that lesions of mycosis fungoides could be successfully eradicated by topical application of HN2. Repeatedly confirmed by others, it was not until later (Van Scott and Winters, 1970) that intensive whole body applications of the drug were shown to induce resolution of all cutaneous lesions in some patients. Such remissions were achievable in the absence of delayed hypersensitivity to the drug. Emergence of delayed hypersensitivity in the course of such topical therapy constituted an annoyance, and because of this ways were explored to desensitize patients after their becoming allergic, as well as ways to induce specific immunologic tolerance to HN2 prior to its topical use for its direct chemotherapeutic effect. Both objectives were achieved, i.e., it was found that allergic patients could be desensitized by daily intravenous infusions of HN2 over 2 or more weeks, and specific immunologic tolerance to HN2 could be induced by several weekly intravenous injections of similarly small amounts of the drug, given for at least 3 weeks prior to initiating topical HN2 chemotherapy (Van Scott and Kalmanson, 1973).

In the course of our studies on the antigenicity of HN2 it was found that nor-HN2, a structurally similar analogue of HN2, did not cross-react antigenically with HN2 in most patients (Van Scott and Yu, 1974) and could be used as a topical therapeutic substitute for HN2 in those patients allergic to HN2 and in whom desensitization procedures could not be carried out. Whereas HN2 is usually topically applied as a 0.02% solution, nor-HN2 has been used in a 0.5% concentration. Therapeutic results with topical nor-HN2 have been roughly equivalent to those obtained with HN2. Unfortunately nor-HN2, although usually not cross-reacting antigenically with HN2, is antigenic itself and several patients have become allergic to it.

These ancillary and alternate techniques have permitted treating large numbers of patients with topical HN2 for extended periods. At this time, after a median follow-up time of approximately 2 years approximately 50% of patients are in a disease-free status; and approximately 75% of patients first treated during the early stages of their disease (stages I and II) are disease free (Vonderheid, Grekin, and Van Scott, in preparation).

Topical Use of HN2 or DNCB for Immunotherapeutic Effects

These two materials, both highly antigenic, have been tested as topical immunotherapeutic agents in patients who are sensitized to them. In 14 such patients one or the other has been topically applied either to the entire body surface or to lesions only and the degree of improvement following the delayed hypersensitivity reactions has been evaluated. The amount topically administered has been determined by first titrating the degree of sensitivity elicited by applications of measured quantities of each material in solution to measured areas of unaffected skin. Such applications have been applied one or several times, with second applications made 1 to 2 weeks after complete subsidence of the delayed hypersensitivity reaction to the preceding treatment.

In eight of these 14 patients complete remissions of clinical disease has been achieved with this treatment alone. In most cases, however, lesions have reappeared on the skin within a few months, though in one patient, in the tumor stage (stage III) of her disease, no evidence of disease has been detected now for over a 2-year period during which time no therapy at all has been administered (Figures 3 and 4).

As the efficacy of 5-FU on epidermal cancer has discouraged ex-

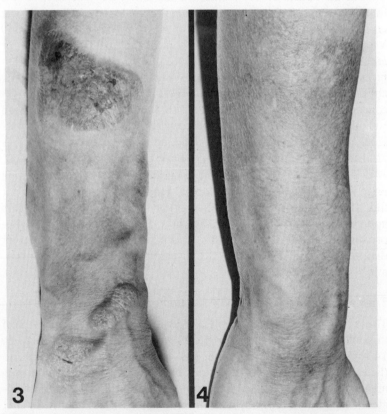

Figure 3. Tumor-plaque lesions of MF in patient topically allergic to HN2. Figure 4. Three months later, following several topical immunotherapeutic treatments with HN2, lesions have resolved. Complete remissions has been sustained without further treatment now for 2 years.

tensive exploration of therapeutic potential of topical immunotherapy, so has the efficacy of HN2 on early MF, in the absence of allergic sensitization, discouraged greater exploration of therapeutic potential of immunotherapy in this disease. A major difficulty in pursuing immunotherapy of late stage disease, which to date has not been reversible or controllable with other therapy, is the diminished immunologic reactivity encountered as the disease progresses (Van Scott and Kalmanson, 1973). Therefore, since topical immunotherapy has been shown to affect substantially the disease in its earlier stages, perhaps immunotherapeutic procedures should be routinely performed on all patients as part of initial therapy of early disease.

In summary, topical immunotherapeutic procedures of both epidermal cancer and cutaneous lymphoma have been demonstrated to have distinct beneficial effects in earlier stages of these diseases. More extensive explorations of immunotherapy of these types of cancers have been discouraged by the fact that topical chemotherapy has also been therapeutically effective. There is a need to pursue further investigations for immunotherapy for prevention or control of progressive disease.

REFERENCES

Block, J. P., J. Edgcomb, A. Eisen, and E. J. Van Scott. 1963. Mycosis fungoides. Natural history and aspects of its relationship to other malignant lymphomas. Amer. J. Med. 34:228–235.

Dillaha, C. J., G. T. Jansen, W. M. Honeycutt, and A. C. Bradford. 1963. Selective cytotoxic effect of topical 5-fluorouracil. Arch. Dermatol. 88:247.

Epstein, E. H., Jr., D. L. Levin, J. D. Croft, Jr., and M. A. Lutzner. 1972. Mycosis fungoides. Survival, prognostic features, response to therapy and autopsy findings. Medicine 15:61–72.

Haserick, J. R., J. H. Richardson, and D. J. Grant. 1959. Remission of lesions in mycosis fungoides following topical application of nitrogen mustard. Cleve. Clin. Q. 26:144–147.

Klein, E., H. Milgrom, F. Helm, J. Ambrus, H. L. Traenkle, and H. L. Stoll, Jr. 1962. Tumors of the skin. I. Effects of local use of cytostatic agents. Skin 1:81.

Ratner, A. C., D. S. Waldorf, and E. J. Van Scott. 1968. Alterations of lesions of mycosis fungoides lymphoma by direct imposition of delayed hypersensitivity reactions. Cancer 21:83–88.

Sipos, K., and G. Jasko. 1956. A mustárnirogen helyi alkamazása nehany börbetegségben. Bórgyögyászati és Venerologiai Szemle 32:198–203.

Van Scott, E. J., and J. D. Kalmanson. 1973. Complete remissions of mycosis fungoides lymphoma induced by topical nitrogen mustard. Control of delayed hypersensitivity to HN2 by desensitization and by induction of specific immunologic tolerance. Cancer 32:18–30.

Van Scott, E. J., and P. L. Winters. 1970. Responses of mycosis fungoides to intensive external treatment with nitrogen mustard. Arch. Dermatol. 102:507–514.

Van Scott, E. J., and R. J. Yu. 1974. Antimitotic, antigenic and structural relationships of nitrogen mustard and its homologues. J. Invest. Dermatol. 62:378–383.

Vonderheid, E. C., D. A. Grekin, and E. J. Van Scott. Intermediate-term results with topical nitrogen mustard therapy of mycosis fungoides. In preparation.

Williams, A. C., and E. Klein. 1970. Experiences with local chemotherapy and immunotherapy in premalignant and malignant skin lesions. Cancer 25:450–462.

New Concepts
in Testicular Cancer

B. J. Kennedy, M.D., F.A.C.P.

Carcinoma of the testis ranks first in incidence for males 20 to 34 years of age and accounts for 11.4% of all cancer deaths in the 24 to 34 age group (National Cancer Institute, 1974). As such, it has a significant impact on the social, economic, and psychic status of this young population. That this type of cancer has not been publicly emphasized in cancer education is a factor in the tragic delay before a definitive diagnosis is made and treatment begun.

The mode of presentation of testicular neoplasms is consistent. Symptoms referrable to the testis include a history of trauma, pain, or a lump. These symptoms may be intermittent, which often accounts for the delay in consulting a physician. Other symptoms, not referrable to the testis, include gynecomastia. The physician may mistake the early signs as due to an inflammatory process. In any circumstance where a young man consults a physician about testicular problems, careful follow-up examination should be continued until absolutely no residual sign of the original complaint exists. Persistence of any sign or symptom should be reviewed as a possible indication of cancer.

This research was supported by Research Grants CA-08101, CA-05158, and CA-08832 from the National Cancer Institute of the United States Public Health Service, the Minnesota Medical Foundation, and the Masonic Memorial Hospital Fund, Inc.

Patients with suspected testicular cancer should undergo inguinal orchiectomy with ligation of the cord at the internal ring. Transcrotal biopsy is absolutely contraindicated since implantation occurs allowing tumor access to the inguinal lymphatics. Multiple serial sections should be made from the primary tumor in order to gain a true impression of the possible multiple histologic types of tumor that may be present.

Once a diagnosis of testicular cancer is established, staging is undertaken to determine the extent of the disease as a guide to the selection of definitive therapy. The minimum studies include a complete physical examination, chest roentgenogram and whole lung tomograms, intravenous pyelogram, lymphangiogram, quantitation of urinary gonadotropins, and liver function studies. Other tests might include α-fetoproteins and serum gonadotropins. On the basis of these findings, the patients are classified into three categories according to the Walter Reed staging system (Table 1). The final staging is accomplished only after surgical resection of retroperitoneal nodes. The extent of the disease is correlated with the histologic tumor type, an important factor in comparative analysis of therapeutic results.

The current histologic classification of testicular tumors, referred to as the Armed Forces Institute of Pathology Classification, is the tentative World Health Organization Classification (Mostofi, 1973). Of the two general categories, nongerminal and germinal, the latter constitute 95% of all tumors of the testes. A pure cell type is present in 60%, but 40% show more than one histologic pattern. Five clinicopathologic groups are recognized (Table 2). That the histologic type is important is indicated by the mortality rate of 2 years.

Table 1. Walter Reed staging system for testicular neoplasms

Stage IA	Tumor confined to testis
Stage IB	Tumor in testis with histologic spread to retroperitoneal nodes
Stage II	Clinical or radiographic evidence of nodal metastases below the diaphragm; no demonstrable metastases above the diaphragm or to visceral organs
Stage III	Clinical or radiographic evidences of metastases above the diaphragm or other distant metastases to body organs

PRIMARY TREATMENT

The initial treatment is inguinal orchiectomy to establish the histology of the primary lesion. This alone is not a definitive therapy. The subsequent management depends on the histologic type.

Seminoma

The accepted therapy for pure seminoma includes inguinal orchiectomy followed by irradiation of the lymph node-bearing areas. There is disagreement as to the extent of irradiation necessary. Some regard treating the subdiaphragmatic paraaortic and iliac nodes bilaterally as sufficient. Others advocate treating the mediastinum and left supraclavicular area in addition. If a retroperitoneal node dissection has been done, radiotherapy to that region is not necessary.

Radiotherapy is also effective in treating recurrent or disseminated seminoma. Occasional cures occur even in the presence of widespread hematogenous metastases. Those patients who survive 2 years after initial therapy without recurrence approach the survival of normal males (Nefzger and Mostofi, 1972). Overall 5-year survival rates for seminoma have reached 91%.

Nonseminoma

The management of nonseminomatous germinal cell neoplasms involves surgery and radiotherapy. Their exact role has not been clearly defined. With the improvement of surgical techniques retro-

Table 2. Classifications of testicular tumors

Group	Pathologic type	Distribution (%)	% Dying at 2 years
I	Seminoma, pure	40	6
II	Embryonal carcinoma ± seminoma	30	59
III	Teratoma ± seminoma	9	
IV	Teratoma ± embryonal cell and/or choriocarcinoma ± seminoma	20	26
V	Choriocarcinoma ± seminoma and/or embryonal cell	1	83

peritoneal node dissection has become an important component of patient management. A thorough dissection is required. The procedure results in data of the histologic type and extent of nodal metastases. In more recent reports there has been a 65% 5-year survival (Skinner and Leadbetter, 1971). In stage I and II lesions retroperitoneal dissection alone has produced 86% and 70% 5-year survival, respectively. Other data are more difficult to assess, because of the use of postoperative radiotherapy. Whether radiotherapy contributes significantly to this program is not clear. Certainly the combination of surgery and radiotherapy involves long-term complications which must be considered.

CHEMOTHERAPY

Chemotherapy is administered to patients with stage III testicular neoplasms. The selection of agents is dependent on the histology of the neoplasm. Cure of advanced disease has been accomplished.

As the many agents have produced an increasing number of objective regressions, it has become apparent that distinction of the type of response is necessary. Many agents produce partial remissions, meaning > 50% regression, but many of these are of short duration. The complete response rate is of greater significance because with its occurrence comes the possibility of cure. Remissions maintained more than 2 years without maintenance therapy are probably cures. This certainly seems true after 5 years. Hence, measurement of effectiveness of agents should be assessed on the complete remission rate, and preferably those of greater than 1 year.

The first major advance in chemotherapy was the combination of actinomycin D, methotrexate, and chlorambucil with complete response rates of up to 12%. Subsequently actinomycin D alone was regarded as the effective agent in a series with 20% complete regressions (Mackenzie, 1966). This agent has been effective in choriocarcinoma, teratocarcinoma, and embryonal cell carcinoma.

Mithramycin was demonstrated to be specifically effective in embryonal cell carcinoma with complete responses in 29%. Initially this agent was regarded as very toxic with hemorrhage, renal, and hepatic toxicity. A high mortality was reported initially (Brown and Kennedy, 1965). The use of this agent by an alternate day regimen has avoided the serious toxicity and eliminated the mortality (Kennedy, 1970). Nevertheless, many investigators have not employed this agent, yet cures have occurred. Patients who have not responded to actinomycin D have responded to mithramycin.

The use of other single agents producing tumor regressions included methotrexate, vinblastine, and adriamycin. However, the complete response rates have been low and of short duration.

More recently combinations of chemotherapy employing vinblastine and bleomycin have been reported with enthusiasm (Table 3). The partial plus complete response rates range around 70 to 80%, with the complete responses at the 40% level. Still within these reports some of the complete responses are of short duration. This may reflect incomplete induction therapy or a need for maintenance therapy. The use of bleomycin by 24-hr continuous infusion has improved the complete remission rate (Samuels, 1975).

More recently, platinum compounds have been employed. As a single agent, this has not been rewarding, but in combination with adriamycin striking regressions have occurred. Development of appropriate dosage schedules is in progress (Twito and Kennedy, 1975).

The chemotherapy of disseminated seminoma is less well defined, because of the small number of patients treated. The alkylating agents seem to be effective as have the more recent combinations.

The use of adjuvant chemotherapy is under study. This tumor system provides another unique opportunity to develop this concept of management.

Table 3. Combination chemotherapy with vinblastine and bleomycin

Investigator	Agent[a]	No. of patients	% Complete remission
Samuels[b]	V + B	90	40
Spigel[c]	V + B infusion	40	47
Samuels[b]	V + B	11	45
Krakoff[d]	V + Act + B	37	40
Blom[e]	V + Act + B	35	26

[a]V, vinblastine; B, bleomycin; ACT, actinomycin D.
[b]Samuels, 1975.
[c]Spigel and Coltman, 1974.
[d]Critkovic et al., 1975.
[e]Blom and Brodovsky, 1975.

SUMMARY

The management of testis cancer is a multidisciplinary function involving surgery, radiotherapy, and medical oncology. Already it has been demonstrated that early detection and surgery can cure this disease. For disseminated disease chemotherapy has also cured some patients. With improved public education to encourage early diagnosis, the use of chemicals as adjuvant chemotherapy, and the improvement in the selected use of one or more agents in advanced testicular cancer, a high rate of cure of the disease can be envisioned.

REFERENCES

Blom, J., and H. S. Brodovsky. 1975. Comparison of the treatment of metastatic testicular tumors with actinomycin-D or actinomycin-D, bleomycin, and vincristine. Proc. Amer. Soc. Clin. Oncol. 16:247.

Brown, J. H., and B. J. Kennedy. 1965. Mithramycin in the treatment of disseminated testicular neoplasms. New Eng. J. Med. 272:111–118.

Critkovic, E., R. Wittes, R. Golby, and I. Krakoff. 1975. Primary combination chemotherapy (VABII) for metastatic or unresectable germ cell tissues. Proc. Amer. Assoc. Cancer Res. 16:174.

Kennedy, B. J. 1970. Mithramycin therapy in advanced testicular neoplasms. Cancer 26:755–766.

Mackenzie, A. R. 1966. Chemotherapy of metastatic testis cancer. Results in 154 patients. Cancer 19:1369–1376.

Mostofi, F. K. 1973. Testicular tumors. Epidemiologic, etiologic and pathologic features. Cancer 32:1186–1201.

National Cancer Institute, National Institutes of Health. 1974. Third National Cancer Survey, Advance Three Report, 1969-1971 Incidence (Dept. HEW Publication No. (NIH) 74-637).

Nefzger, M. D., and F. K. Mostofi. 1972. Survival after surgery for germinal malignancies of the testis. Cancer 30:1225–1232.

Samuels, M. L. 1975. Continuous intravenous bleomycin therapy with vinblastine in testicular and extragonadal germinal tumors. Proc. Amer. Assoc. Cancer Res. 16:112.

Skinner, D. A., and W. F. Leadbetter. 1971. The surgical management of testis tumors. J. Urol. 106:84–93.

Spigel, S. C., and C. A. Coltman, Jr. 1974. Vinblastine (NSC-49042) and Bleomycin (NSC-125066) therapy for disseminated testicular tumors. Cancer Chemother. Rep. 58:213–216.

Twito, D. I., and B. J. Kennedy. 1975. Treatment of testicular cancer. Annu. Rev. Med. 26:235–243.

Cancer of the Lung

Ronald I. Cantor, M.D.,
and Arthur J. Weiss, M.D., F.A.C.P.

Lung cancer, the second most common but singularly most lethal malignancy of mankind, will find 80,000 new victims in 1976 and will cause 70,000 deaths in the U.S. alone. This will represent close to 20% of all cancer deaths and 30% of cancer deaths in the male. Five-year survival will continue to remain at less than 10%, showing essentially no change in the past 30 years, and median survival from diagnosis will not exceed 6 months. Despite these disheartening statistics there is, however, reason for a modicum of both hope and scientific enthusiasm. This is due to our broadened understanding of etiology and biology, improved methods of diagnosis, and modest recent advances in therapy.

ETIOLOGY

There exists a multiplicity of factors which can both singly and jointly act to cause neoplasia of the bronchopulmonary tree. These can act both directly at the epithelial level and indirectly by diminishing normal pulmonary cleansing via alterations in mucous production, depression of the ciliary mechanism, and diminution of local macrophage defense activities. In the environment the retention of particulate matter is maximal at the 1.0 μm diameter and occurs mainly at the level of the segmental bronchi and distally. Various studies have documented that there exists a statistically significant correlation among the index of atmospheric deposits, the smoke index, the population density, and the incidence of bronchogenic carcinoma (Ackerman and del Regato, 1970).

The role of cigarette smoking seems indisputable. The Surgeon General's Report of 1964 develops in great detail a considerable argument which extends beyond even its apparently incontrovertible epidemiologic evidence as it clearly documents the presence of 3,4-benzpyrene and multiple other carcinogenic and cocarcinogenic compounds in the combustion products of tobacco, and the association of premalignant changes in the bronchial epothelium of heavy smokers. One must also be impressed with the relative paucity of lung cancers in nonsmokers, particularly in view of the fact that their most common cell type is adenocarcinoma, accounting for better than 50%, relative to the unlikelihood of epidermoid carcinoma in the nonsmoker. Harris (1973), in noting this disparity reinterprets Kreyberg's data (1969) to suggest that 95% of all epidermoid carcinomas in Norway are attributable to cigarette smoking, as well as 90% of all small cell cancers. In the instance of tobacco-related lung cancer, the hazard increases proportionately with the intensity and duration of exposure. This hazard, however, can be appreciably diminished by terminating the exposure, with reversal of epithelial atypia in greater than 90% of instances.

Unfortunately, this is not the case for occupational induction of lung cancer. Here, termination of exposure does not seem to reduce appreciably the later incidence of cancer, although it prevents further increments in the hazard of carcinogenesis. This is well documented in the case of asbestos-induced mesothelioma where a latent period of about 35 years exists between exposure and tumor recognition. Asbestos also acts synergistically with cigarette smoke to produce bronchogenic cancer (Selikoff, Hammond, and Chung, 1968). Other known carcinogens include radioactive materials, particularly uranium and fluorspar, arsenic derivatives, nickel, iron oxides, chromates, mustard gases, and the methyl ether compounds. Both chloromethyl methyl ether and bischloromethyl ether are known carcinogens for rats and mice. They are widely used chemical intermediates in organic synthesis and in the preparation of ion exchange resins. Clinical suspicion in man was first suggested in six suspected cases involvng exposure to chloromethyl methyl ether in California in 1972 (editorial, 1972). Figueroa, Raszkowski, and Weiss in 1973 then reported 14 additional cases in chemical workers with considerable exposure to chloromethyl methyl ether fumes. Thirteen of the 14 developed small cell carcinoma, which was fatal within 20 months. Most were in their 4th and 5th decades and had a duration of exposure of 3 to 14 years. Eleven were cigarette smokers.

There is also now some specific evidence of altered immune function secondary to carcinogen exposure. Colten and Borsos (1974) have shown that macrophage synthesis of the various components of complement can be measured in an in vitro system. After exposure to several known carcinogens they demonstrated distinct depression of macrophage synthesis of C_2 and C_4 without notable effect on the morphology or survival of the cells. Therefore, it is possible that some carcinogens may act by not only inducing malignant transformations, but also may interfere with immune function and induce immune permissiveness.

At the present, there exists no proof of a role for biologic agents in the induction of pulmonary cancer. There is, however, a suggestive animal model in sheep, pulmonary adenomatosis or Jaagsiekte, which is caused by a transmittable, ultrafilterable agent. This produces a progressive bilateral lung disease which metastasizes to bronchial lymph nodes and pathologically is quite similar to bronchoalveolar carcinoma of man.

Thus, the bulk of evidence at present is that carcinogenesis in man is a chemical phenomena. Most oncogenic chemicals either form electrophilic reactants and/or bind to DNA. In many instances these compounds undergo spontaneous or enzymatic activation. One possible explanation for differences in susceptibility is that genetic differences might account for a differential ability of various organ tissues to activate for inactivate oncogens. One such system currently under scrutiny is the enzyme, aryl hydrocarbon hydroxylase. This enzyme has been found in high quantity in the blood lymphocytes of smokers with lung cancer but not in nonsmokers or patients with pulmonary diseases other than lung cancer (Kellermann, Shaw, and Luyten-Kellermann, 1973). It is a potent enhancer of the polycyclic aromatic hydrocarbons producing epoxides which form reactive intermediates and bind DNA, thus producing mutations and malignant transformations. Prospective data is still forthcoming, but the implications are exciting.

From an epidemiologic standpoint various interventions might then be anticipated in the near future. One might develop screening procedures to identify individuals at high risk, that is, those persons with either a greater than normal ability to activate occupational or tobacco-produced carcinogens or a subnormal ability to inactivate these oncogens. One might then reduce the exposure, develop agents to either diminish activation or enhance inactivation, or perhaps, attempt to reverse the preneoplastic epithelial process with an agent such as vitamin A (Cowe and Nettesheim, 1973).

CLASSIFICATION

Differences in the classification of lung cancers have led to great difficulty in interpreting therapeutic data. Thus, in 1967, the World Health Organization Histological Classification of Lung Tumors was adopted. This schema provided an accurate means of designation for about 95% of all primary lung cancers. This was modified 6 years later by the Pathology Panel of the Working Party for Therapy of Lung Cancer because of fear that the WHO classification might allow for the overlapping of patterns of differentiation in both epidermoid and adenocarcinoma which might blur measurable variations in behavior and therapeutic responses from critical observation by the clinician, statistician, and pathologist. Table 1 compares the two systems.

CLINICAL MANIFESTATIONS

Lung cancer may first manifest via either the local effects of the tumor, symptoms attributable to invasion of adjacent thoracic structures, extrathoracic metastases, or systemic manifestations unrelated to tumor location. Local symptoms or symptoms due to intrathoracic invasion are most often associated with epidermoid carcinoma, and less often but not uncommonly with large cell and adenocarcinoma. These patients will most often complain of cough, symptoms secondary to atalectasis, hemotysis, dyspnea, or chest pain which can be due to local rib involvement or the invasion of nerve trunks. Less often they may present with hoarseness, dysphagia secondary to esophageal compression, phrenic nerve paralysis, vena caval obstruction, or pericardial invasion. Although any type may present with symptoms due to extrathoracic disease, this is most characteristic of small cell carcinoma. Symptoms may vary from specific complaints related to involvement of the central nervous systems, mass effect or obstruction with intra-abdominal disease, organ failure, or rarely

Table 1. Comparison of the World Health Organization classification and modifications suggested by the Pathology Panel of the Working Party for Therapy of Lung Cancer (WP-L)

WHO Classification	WP-L Modifications
I. Epidermoid carcinoma	10. Epidermoid carcinoma 11. Well-differentiated 12. Moderately differentiated 13. Poorly differentiated

II. Small cell anaplastic carcinoma
  1. Fusiform
  2. Polygonal
  3. Lymphocyte-like
  4. Others
	20. Small cell anaplastic carcinoma
	21. Lymphocyte-like (oat cell)
	22. Intermediate cell (fusiform, polygonal, others)

III. Adenocarcinoma
  1. Bronchogenic
    a. Acinar
    b. Papillary
  2. Bronchioloalveolar
	30. Adenocarcinoma
	31. Well differentiated
	32. Moderately differentiated
	33. Poorly differentiated
	34. Bronchioloalveolar/ papillary

IV. Large cell carcinoma
  1. Solid tumors with mucin
  2. Solid tumors without mucin
  3. Giant cell
  4. Clear cell
	40. Large cell carcinoma (40/30) with mucin production (40/30) with stratification
	41. Giant cell
	42. Clear cell

skeletal complaints, to nonspecific host effects related to both the endocrine and non-endocrine paraneoplastic syndromes.

DIAGNOSTIC ADJUVANTS

Cytology

Vast refinements of technique have increased the yield in cytologic examination from an initial 42.8, first reported by Liebow, Lindskog, and Bloomer, in 1948, to greater than 95% confirmed positives today with perhaps no false positives. Most workers in the field still recommend examination of five properly collected samples for maximum accuracy. The most significant change in recent years has been the increasing accuracy of histologic diagnosis, with a greater than 70% confirmation reported in one recent study (Lukeman, 1973).

Bronchoscopy

Adequate experience with fiberoptics has been gained at many centers. This technique has greatly enhanced the yield when one is dealing with peripheral lesions, upper lobe examination, small hilar tumors, or where one is interested in detailed study of the segments such as in the localization of hemoptysis or the work-up of a patient whose cytologic exam is positive in the presence of a normal x-ray. The rigid scope with its larger lumen still provides better space for both biopsy and aspiration, and remains the instrument of choice in obtaining differential cytologies.

Mediastinoscopy

Past studies have documented that close to 50% of all patients who have thoracotomy for lung cancer are found to be inoperable on the table. This figure is no doubt higher, for it does not allow for evaluation of the contralateral mediastinal nodes which may be involved in about 10% of instances due to the bilateral crossover of the lymphatic drainage. This low yield, in light of a probable 10% mortality rate and 20% incidence of serious morbidity, further emphasizes the need for better preoperative evaluation. Bilateral examination of the mediastinum via the mediastinoscope has been documented to increase resectability to 90% when the mediastinum is free of tumor (Reynders, 1964), and this interpreted in the light of published reports of close to 50% 4-year survivals in patients with negative mediastinoscopes prior to thoracotomy further underscores the great value of this procedure (Bergh and Schersten, 1965).

Other Studies

Knowledge of the natural history of lung cancer requires one to pursue the possibility of occult hematogenous metastases before considering a curative procedure. Evaluation for bony metastatic disease should include a skeletal survey, bone scan, and marrow evaluation. The bone marrow may be involved on presentation in as many as 43% of patients with small cell carcinoma (Hansen, Muggia, and Selawry, 1971). The incidence of positive marrows for adenocarcinoma and large cell may exceed 15%, while epidermoid is quite low (2.6%) (Muggia and Chervu, 1974). The skeletal survey is generally of low yield and is rarely positive even in the presence of known marrow involvement. The lesions of small cell and adenocarcinoma which are characteristically osteoblastic will not be visualized until larger than 1 cm in diameter. Likewise, the lytic lesions usually seen in epidermoid cancers cannot be seen on the radiograph until there is at least 50% decalcification. The bone scan though can discriminate more subtle changes, has a high incidence of correlation with the marrow biopsy, and may further add an additional 10 to 20% increase in yield (Hansen and Muggia, 1972).

Liver scanning is generally of higher yield than examination of the liver chemistries, although of only small yield in the absence of clinical suspicion. Prethoracotomy min-laparotomy is associated with a reported 14% incidence of liver metastases and an additional 5.7% incidence of other sites of intra-abdominal metastases (Yashar, 1966; Bell, 1968). The role of prethoracotomy peritoneoscopy with liver biopsy is still inadequately documented. The incidence of central nervous system metastatic disease varies from 20 to 40% of all patients at autopsy. As many as 40% of these may be found during the initial staging (Newman and Hansen, in press), although this most often occurs in the setting of clinical suspicion.

Other procedures currently being investigated for use in the staging of lung cancer are adrenal photoscanning, abdominal ultrasound, echocardiography of the brain, and a variety of newer scanning techniques using tumor-seeking markers. These include radioactive elements such as gallium, labeled anti-tumor compounds such as bleomycin, and investigation of labeled tumor-specific antibodies. The role of ordinary lung scanning has not yet been adequately exploited, as significant vascular obstruction has correlated well with later unresectability.

TUMOR MARKERS

Research in the variety of hormonal compounds produced by the lung cancers, their clinical sequelae and utility as measures of disease activity are detailed in the chapter on paraneoplastic syndromes. Fetoproteins may as well be present. Here too, their presence is probably due to derepression of a previously non-expressed fetal genome. The carcinoembryonic antigen, though nonspecific, has been noted to be positive in as high as 75% of patients with bronchogenic cancer and may aid in follow-up. α-Fetoprotein, though decidedly less common (7%), is a valuable assay as positivity is probably associated with the presence of hepatic metastases (Carlin and Tompkins, 1972).

RADIATION THERAPY

Attempts for cure using radiation therapy should be limited to those instances where the disease process does not exceed involvement of more than one hemithorax with mediastinal and ipsilateral supraclavicular involvement. Within such limits a 5-year survival of 5 to 10% is achievable. However, for lesser stages of disease there is no evidence of enhanced survival except in small numbers of patients with small cell carcinoma (MRC, 1966), and this modality may even diminish survival for epidermoid carcinoma (Morrison, Deeley, and Cleland, 1963). Likewise, there is neither benefit with preoperative radiotherapy, except for selected patients with superior sulcus tumors with direct extrapulmonary extention but negative nodes, nor postoperative therapy.

There is also little utility for adjuvant chemotherapy with radiation therapy excepting in small cell carcinoma. Some studies have suggested advantage, but in the majority of instances it appears at best ineffective, and in some deleterious. The role of adjuvant polychemotherapy has not yet been adequately evaluated. There is, however, clear evidence of enhanced survival with even single agent adjuvant therapy in small cell carcinoma. The role of aggressive prophylactic radiation therapy in small cell carcinoma is as yet unclear, but many studies are underway evaluating the role of this modality in sterilizing micrometastases of the brain, regional lymph nodes, and the upper abdomen in conjunction with polychemotherapy.

SURGERY

One cannot consider the role of curative surgery in lung cancer without being reminded that of every 100 lung cancer patients presenting for diagnosis, only 50 will be selected for thoracotomy. Fifteen of the remaining 50 will have a biopsy only, and five will undergo palliative surgery. Of the remaining 30 patients three will die of the attempt, and only seven or eight will survive 5 years. These data have been quite stable for many years and it seems that the role of surgery for cure will likewise remain stable until our epidemiologic and diagnostic tools are considerably improved. It is thus imperative before a decision is made to pursue a curative procedure that the patient be evaluated in light of not only his physiologic qualifications, but also with knowledge of those biologic factors predictive of a poor outcome. These are: 1) the presence of undifferentiated small cell carcinoma (which is a systemic disease), 2) the presence of hilar or mediastinal adenopathy, 3) direct mediastinal extension, 4) the presence of a pleural effusion, especially if malignant cells can be identified, and 5) metastatic disease to any area beyond the primarily involved hemithorax (Mountain, 1974). One should also be cautious of advising surgery in the instance of involvement of the stem bronchi as the 5-year survival rate is minimal and the mortality rate is quite high (Stoloff, 1974).

As noted earlier, there is little to recommend pre- or postoperative radiation therapy excepting in the circumstance of locally invasive superior sulcus tumor. The use of chemotherapy as an adjunct to surgery is attractive. Here one might attempt to make circulating tumor cells nonviable, eradicate known residual disease, or eliminate occult micrometastases. The data to date, excepting small cell carcinoma, have been unimpressive; but study designs have not been uniform, only a few drugs have been considered (usually mechlorethamine or cyclophosphamide), and these have usually been used in ineffective schema. Clearly, the role of adjunctive chemotherapy needs better study, and hopefully, this will involve the evaluation of both single and combined agents.

CHEMOTHERAPY

The physician's goal in dealing with the cancer patient is ideally to achieve for his patient a normal life span. At present this is not tenable when dealing with the bronchogenic carcinomas. So for the present we should be oriented to improving both the quantity and quality of survival. Clearly, this is now possible in the majority of patients with small cell carcinoma and in increasing numbers of patients with both epidermoid and adenocarcinoma. The chemotherapy of lung cancer by both single agents and combination therapy has recently been reviewed in great detail by Selawry (1974), who reviewed drug trials in more than 15,000 patients. The following discussion is based extensively on his review, except where otherwise noted.

Single Agent Therapy

The data relative to the monochemotherapy of lung cancer require interpretation in light of differences in cell type, stage of disease, performance status, underlying immune defenses, and perhaps even variability of administration as evidence continues to accumulate implicating immune suppression with continuous daily therapy in the instance of cyclophosphamide versus enhanced immune reactivity with high dose cyclical administration. Table 2 summarizes much of Selawry's review. Clearly, there are many instances where the data are insufficient but nowhere is this more marked than in the lack of data available for the antimetabolites 5-fluorouracil, hydroxyurea, and cytosine arabinoside; the anti-tumor antibiotics actinomycin D and mithramycin; and for the use of L-asparaginase.

The Central Oncology Group (Wilson et al., in press) has recently compared the use of dibromodulcitol versus hexamethylmelamine in patients with either recurrent disease following a curative procedure or patients amenable to only palliative resection. They followed 250 patients for survival, using the literature for control. Median survival historically ranges from 7 to 13 weeks (Wolf et al., 1960; Green et al., 1969). For epidermoid carcinoma they found a median survival of 31 weeks in the hexamethylmelamine-treated group versus 22 weeks for dibromodulcitol. These were essentially reversed in the instance of adenocarcinoma with a 34.7 median survival using dibromodulcitol versus 21.5 for hexamethylmelamine. These differences are statistically significant at the 5% level.

Combination Chemotherapy

Theoretically, polychemotherapy is derived from the use of combinations of effective single agents with divergent toxicities capable of producing different biochemical lesions in the biosynthetic pathways. This may be effected by either sequential blockade, concurrent inhibition, or complementary inhibition. The success of this kind of approach can be no better illustrated than in the instance of acute lymphocytic leukemia of childhood where the induction of complete remissions has improved from 22% with methotrexate alone to virtually 100% with combination therapy. To date, there are insufficient randomized prospective reports to assess adequately the potential of this modality in all but small cell carcinomas. The combination of procarbazine, cyclophosphamide, methotrexate, and vincristine has

Table 2. Response of bronchogenic carcinoma to monochemotherapy by cell type

Drug	Epidermoid		Small cell		Aderocarcinoma		Large cell	
	Patients	Response (%)	Patients	Response (%)	Patients	Response (%)	Patients	Response (%)
Alkylating agents								
Mechlorethamine	111	33	51	39	80	29	129	27
Cyclophosphamide	183	19	208	33	12	17	22	23
Dibromodulcitol	39	23						
CCNU[a]	35	30	18	17	26	23	23	17
Methyl-CCNU[a]	19	11	8	25	23	35		
BCNU[b]	34	6	19	21	22	0	22	9
1-Me-1-Nitrosoinea	13	15	18	78				
Hexamethylmelamine	68	12	44	32	39	15	39	18
Antibiotics								
Adriamycin	70	19	48	25	53	15	28	25
Bleomycin	251	13	27	0	30	13		
Mitomycin C	22	0	11	9	11	27	2	50
Antimetabolites								
Methotrexate	140	25	79	34	25	32	23	17
Plant alkaloids								
Vinblastine	20	16	9	33	6	16	2	100
Vincristine			6	33				
Uncertain								
Procarbazine	30	20	19	47	16	19	17	35

[a]CCNU, 1-(2-chloroethyl)-3-(4-methylcyclohexyl)-1-nitrosourea.
[b]BCNU, 1,3-bis(2-chloroethyl)-1-nitrosourea.

been shown to produce a response rate of 62% for evaluable patients with small cell cancer (Alberto, 1973). If one selects out those patients with early disease, responses exceed 75%. Likewise, in small cell carcinomas, the addition of methyl-1-(2-chloroethyl)-3-(4-methyl-cyclohexyl)-1-nitrosourea (methyl-CCNU) as a probable synergist with cyclophosphamide and methotrexate is reported to have a 57% response rate (Selawry et al., 1974). With increasing reports of prolonged complete remission in patients with small cell carcinoma it may soon be tenable to regard this as a potentially curable cancer.

The combination of procarbazine and fluorouracil looks useful in preliminary data in small numbers of patients with epidermoid carcinoma. Alberto's data (1973) showed a 39% response rate for simultaneous procarbazine, cyclophosphamide, methotrexate, and vincristine in 18 patients with epidermoid carcinoma, and enhanced survival. However, this decreased to 28% when nonrandomized patients were added. Thus, this combination is not superior to single agent therapy. Likewise, the use of cyclophosphamide with a nitrosourea, cyclophosphamide with methotrexate alone, or methotrexate and CCNU did not show evidence of increased utility.

For adenocarcinoma two clinically efficacious combinations have been reported. Selawry et al. (1974) have noted a 30% response rate with cyclophosphamide, methotrexate, and CCNU with a doubling in survival time when compared to cyclophosphamide and methotrexate alone. Bonadonna et al. (1969) have reported responses in five of six patients using the combination of procarbazine and fluorouracil. Only in the instance of large cell carcinoma is there yet no evidence of a combination regimen with superiority over single agent therapy.

IMMUNOTHERAPY

Recent advances in clinical immunology, tumor immunology, and immunotherapy lend themselves to the development of a rational immunotherapeutic approach to lung cancer. This approach is based on a variety of well accepted concepts. First, one is concerned for the role of general immunocompetence. Here cell-mediated immunity is of greater importance than humoral, both in the establishment of the neoplastic process and its progression. The association of purified protein derivative (PPD) negativity or the lack of immune blasto-genesis with a poor prognosis despite the stage of disease is now well accepted. More direct evidence has recently come from Stewart's work (Stewart, 1969) demonstrating in vivo delayed hypersensitivity response to lung cancer extracts. Whereas, there is little evidence of alteration in the humoral system until the disease process is far advanced.

The role of immunosuppression in carcinogenesis is less clear and further work is needed. However, the possibility of worsening cellular immune function with other therapies is quite disturbing. Knowledge of the timing and frequency of immune therapy as an adjuvant to chemotherapy or radiation is vague at present. Some workers suggest that concurrent immunotherapy should be applied, while others believe that the immune adjuvant should be saved until the period of postsuppression rebound. Last, the role of serum blocking factors is still not satisfactorily resolved. It has been shown that this material is probably circulating antigen or antigen-antibody complexes, which are capable of inhibiting immune lymphocyte function, and this has been demonstrated to be present in the sera of lung cancer patients (Hellström et al., 1971).

Therapeutically, one's goals should then be reversal of immuno-incompetence, or enhancement, or both, of already existent tumor immunity, prevention of prolonged iatrogenic immunosuppression, and diminution of serum blocking factors. To date, we are unable to find in the literature an adequately controlled randomized prospective study with sufficient patient numbers documenting clinical utility of either active or passive immunotherapy either as a single modality for prophylaxis or as an adjuvant in the management of metastatic brochogenic cancer. Appropriate studies are in progress, and as our reagents become more specific and we gain greater knowledge of appropriate timing, frequency, and sites of administration, hopefully our clinical armamentarium will be augmented.

REFERENCES

Ackerman, L. V., and J. A. del Regato. 1970. Cancer: Diagnosis, Treatment, and Prognosis. C. V. Mosby Co., St. Louis, Mo.

Alberto, P. 1973. Remission rates, survival and prognostic factors in combination chemotherapy for bronchogenic carcinoma. Cancer Chemother. Rep. 4:199–206.

Bell, J. W. 1968. Abdominal exploration in 100 lung cancer suspects prior to thoracotomy. Ann. Surg. 167:199–203.

Bergh, N. P., and T. Schersten. 1965. Bronchogenic carcinoma: A follow-up study of a surgically treated series with special reference to a prognostic significance of lymph node metastases. Acta Chir. Scan. (Suppl.) 347.

Bonadonna, G., S. Monfardini, S. Oldini, et al. 1969. Clinical studies of procarbazine and fluorouracil in advanced lung cancer. Tumori 52:277.

Colten, H.R., and T. Borsos. 1974. Biosynthesis of the second and fourth components of complement: Inhibition in vitro by chemical carcinogens. J. Immunol. 112:1107–1114.

Corlin, R. F., and R. K. Tompkins. 1972. Serum alpha-fetoglobulin in a patient with hepatic metastases from bronchogenic carcinoma. Digest Dis. 17:553–555.

Cowe, M. V., and P. Nettesheim, 1973. Effects of vitamin A on 3-methyl-cholanthrene-induced squamous metaplasias and early tumors in the respiratory tract of rats. J. Natl. Cancer Inst. 50:1599–1606.

Editorial. 1972. Chemical suspected in six cases of lung cancer. Occup. Health Saf. Lett. 2:6.

Figueroa, W. G., R. Raszkowski, and W. Weiss. 1973. Lung cancer in chloromethyl methyl ether workers. New Eng. J. Med. 288:1096–1097.

Green, R. A., E. Humphrey, H. Close, and M. E. Patno. 1969. Alkylating agents in bronchogenic carcinoma. Amer. J. Med. 46:516.

Hansen, M. H., and F. M. Muggia. 1972. Staging of inoperable patients with bronchogenic carcinoma with special reference to bone marrow examination and peritoneoscopy. Cancer 30:1395–1401.

Hansen, M. H., F. M. Muggia, and O. S. Selawry. 1971. Bone marrow examination in 100 consecutive patients with bronchogenic carcinoma. Lancet 2(7722):443–445.

Harris, C. C. 1973. The epidemiology of different histologic types of bronchogenic carcinoma. Cancer Chemother. Rep. 4(2):59–61.

Hellström, I., H. O. Sjogren, G. Warner, et al. 1971. Blocking of cell mediated tumor immunity by sera from patients with growing neoplasms. J. Natl. Cancer Inst. 7:226–237.

Kellermann, G., C. R. Shaw, and M. Luyten-Kellermann. 1973. Aryl hydrocarbon hydroxylase inducibility and bronchogenic carcinoma. New Eng. J. Med. 289:934–937.

Kreyberg, L. 1969. Aetiology of Lung Cancer, pp. 83–87. Universitets Forlaget, Oslo.

Liebow, A. A., G. E. Lindskog, and W. E. Bloomer. 1948. Cytological studies of sputum and bronchial secretions in the diagnosis of cancer of the lung. Cancer 1:223–233.

Lukeman, J. M. 1973. Reliability of cytologic diagnosis in cancer of the lung. Cancer Chemother. Rep. 4(3):79–93.

Medical Research Council. 1966. Comparative trial of surgery and radiotherapy for primary treatment of small-celled carcinoma of the bronchus. Lancet 2:979–986.

Morrison, R., T. J. Deeley, and W. P. Cleland. 1963. The treatment of carcinoma of the bronchus: A clinical trial to compare surgery and supravoltage radiotherapy. Lancet 1:683–689.

Mountain, C. F. 1974. Surgical therapy in lung cancer: Biologic, physiologic, and technical determinants. Semin. Oncol. 1:253–258.

Muggia, F. M., and L. R. Chervu. 1974. Lung cancer: Diagnosis in metastatic sites. Semin. Oncol. 1:217–228.

Newman, S. J., and M. H. Hansen. Frequency, diagnosis and treatment of brain metastases in 247 consecutive patients with bronchogenic carcinoma. Cancer. In press.

Reynders, H. 1964. Mediastinoscopy in bronchogenic cancer. Dis. Chest 45:605–612.

Selawry, O. S. 1974. The role of chemotherapy in the treatment of lung cancer. Semin. Oncol. 1:259–272.

Selawry, O., H. Hansen, D. Can, et al. 1974. Improved chemotherapy for advanced bronchogenic carcinoma. Proc. Am. Assoc. Cancer Res. 15: 118.

Selikoff, I. F., E. C. Hammond, and J. Chung. 1968. Asbestos exposure, smoking, and neoplasia. JAMA 204:106–112.

Stewart, T. H. M. 1969. The presence of delayed hypersensitivity reactions in patients toward cellular extracts of their malignant tumors. Cancer 23:1380–1387.

Stoloff, I. L. 1974. The prognostic value of bronchoscopy in primary lung cancer. JAMA 227:299–301.

Wilson, W., J. VanRyzin, A. J. Weiss, R. W. Froelich, and S. E. Moss. A Phase II study in lung carcinoma comparing hexamethylmelamine to dibromodulcitol. In press.

Wolf, J., P. Spaer, R. Yeswer, and M. E. Patno. 1960. Nitrogen mustard and steroid hormones in the treatment of inoperable bronchogenic carcinoma. Amer. J. Med. 29:1003.

Yashar, J. 1966. Transdiaphragmatic exploration of the upper abdomen during surgery for bronchogenic carcinoma. J. Thorac. Cardiovasc. Surg. 52:599–603.

The Impact of Cancer Staging on Cancer Management in the Community Hospital

Paul F. Engstrom, M.D., F.A.C.P.

Most physicians demonstrate little interest or expertise in the histo-logic or clinical classification of cancer. Simply establishing the presence of cancer in a patient is not adequate for a complete diag-nosis. Obviously, much more must be known about the patient and his cancer before treatment can be planned, or an estimate can be made of his chance of cure, or of his chance of surviving 1 to 5 years.

The accepted strategy in the treatment of malignant tumors includes the following steps:

1. Detecting the presence of a neoplasm.
2. Characterizing the histologic nature of the tumor.
3. Determining the extent of the disease process.
4. Staging the tumor according to established criteria.
5. Planning for total management including rehabilitation.
6. Conducting a clinical trial of therapy.
7. Evaluating the results of the treatment program.

This work was supported by National Cancer Institute Contract NO1-CN-45055 from the National Institutes of Health.

125

One can see that careful staging with histologic and clinical classification is an important prerequisite to embarking on the therapy of a malignant condition.

The objectives of a classification system for cancer are well stated by the International Union Against Cancer (UICC) (Rubin, 1973), and include:

A. Aiding the clinician in planning treatment.
B. Giving some indication of prognosis.
C. Assisting in the evaluation of end results.
D. Facilitating the exchange of information between treatment centers.
E. Assisting in the continuing investigation of cancer.

Each cancer has a number of characteristics influencing the natural history of that cancer and a particular host. Among these characteristics are the anatomic extent of the malignancy at the time of the diagnosis and the various systems that have been involved by anatomic extent of the disease. Increasingly sophisticated diagnostic techniques and more intensive study of each patient have enabled us to determine the extent of each cancer. Further developments may alter the amount and character of this information, and therefore result in revision of the classification system.

To achieve the objectives of a classification system, it is essential to develop a common language acceptable to the physician and useful in the treatment of his patient. The following general rules have been proposed:

1. The TNM system provides the basis for categorizing the extent of disease and when appropriate should be used. T represents the primary tumor with appropriate subscripts to determine increasing sizes of the tumor and/or involvement by direct extension. The letter N represents the regional lymph node involvement wtih appropriate subscript to describe the absence of involvement or increasing degrees of such involvement. The letter M represents distant metastases with appropriate subscripts to describe the degree of involvement. The various categories of T, N, and M may be grouped into appropriate combinations to create a small number of stages for each organ system.

2. For cancer at certain accessible sites, especially those that can be treated in appropriate manner by more than one treatment modality, the extent of the cancer should be determined and recorded before

definitive treatment is carried out. This provides a clinical classification and makes it possible to compare the results of different modalities. This is especially true of treatments for lesions such as carcinoma of the cervix, larynx, or oral cavity.

3. For cancer at sites inaccessible to clinical evaluation such as carcinoma of the ovaries, stomach, colon, or kidney, information obtained by surgical exploration and/or histopathologic studies of removed specimens may be used in describing the extent of disease. Thus, definitive treatment should be based on this surgical/evaluative classification, or on a postsurgical treatment classification where the specimen has been completely resected.

4. For cancers at some sites, it may be desirable to record a clinical classification, a surgical evaluative classification, and a postsurgical treatment classification.

5. Once the extent of disease has been established according to any classification, that classification should not be changed thereafter. The subsequent course of the neoplasm does not alter the original description of the extent of tumor or stage classification. Thus, recurrent cases cannot be grouped with primarily staged patients when comparing results.

6. Histologic or cytologic verification of the cancer is necessary Frequently a histologic classification may be useful in addition to the anatomic classification mentioned above.

The information that has been obtained from the retrospective staging of breast cancer patients illustrates the relationship of anatomic classification to prognosis and survival. The American Joint Committee for Cancer Staging and End Results Reporting (AJC) (Cutler, 1974) analyzed over 2,500 records of patients with newly diagnosed cancer managed with radical mastectomy. Figure 1 describes the TNM categories as applied to breast cancer. Although innumerable combinations of T, N, and M were noted, Table 1 summarizes data and shows survival of patients according to TNM categories and stages.

A discussion of classification systems would not be complete without referring to Philip Rubin's (1973) proposed modifications termed "Symbolic Oncotaxonomy." He has defined a single set of criteria in a cancer paradigm that is applicable to all cancers independent of site of origin. The interested reader should refer to his monograph on the subject.

Figure 1. AJC definition of TNM categories as applied to carcinoma of the breast (Cutler, 1974).

T—Primary Tumor

TIS   Pre-invasive carcinoma (carcinoma in situ), noninfiltrating intra-ductal carcinoma or Paget's disease of the nipple with no demonstrable tumor.

   NOTE: Paget's disease associated with a demonstrable tumor is classified according to the size of the tumor.

T0   No demonstrable tumor in the breast.

T1   Tumor of 2 cm or less in its greatest dimension.*

   $T1_A$ With no fixation to underlying pectoral fascia and/or muscle.
   $T1_B$ With fixation to underlying pectoral fascia and/or muscle.

T2   *Tumor more than 2 cm but not more than 5 cm in its greatest dimension.**

   $T2_A$ With no fixation to underlying pectoral fascia and/or muscle.
   $T2_B$ With fixation to underlying pectoral fascia and/or muscle.

T3   *Tumor more than 5 cm in its greatest dimension.**

   $T3_A$ With no fixation to underlying pectoral fascia and/or muscle.
   $T3_B$ With fixation to underlying pectoral fascia and/or muscle.

T4   *Tumor of any size with direct extension to chest wall or skin.*

   NOTE: Chest wall includes ribs, intercostal muscles, and serratus anterior muscle but not pectoral muscle.

   $T4_A$ With fixation to chest wall.
   $T4_B$ With edema (including peau d'orange), ulceration of skin of breast, or satellite skin nodules confined to the same breast.
   $T4_C$ Both of above.

N—Regional Lymph Nodes

N0   No palpable homolateral axillary nodes.

N1   Movable homolateral axillary nodes.

   $N1_A$ Nodes not considered to contain growth.
   $N2_A$ Nodes considered to contain growth.

N2   Homolateral axillary nodes considered to contain growth and fixed to one another or to other structures.

N3   Homolateral supraclavicular or infraclavicular nodes considered to contain growth, *or* edema of the arm.

   NOTE: Edema of the arm may be caused by lymphatic obstruction; lymph nodes may not then be palpable.

Figure 1. *continued*

M—Distant Metastasis

M0   No evidence of distant metastasis.

M1   Distant metastasis present including skin involvement beyond the
      breast area.

---

*Dimpling of the skin, nipple retraction, or any other skin changes except
those in $T4_B$ may occur in T1, T2, or T3 without affecting the classification.

In order to translate cancer management measures from a cancer
center to a community hospital, we have emphasized careful cancer
staging and classification in the overall treatment program. We have
initiated a Breast Cancer Control Program in a network of community
hospitals in Bucks County, Pennsylvania, and Mercer County, New
Jersey. The management program is based on an accurate but utilizable cancer classification system. The implementation plan of this
breast cancer program is as follows:

1. The TNM anatomic classification system provides useful criteria
for staging breast cancer. The examining physician should clinically
determine the extent of disease prior to definitive surgery. Figure 2
shows the simplified clinical reporting sheet that we ask attending
physicians to complete on each suspected case of breast cancer. The
standard or Patey modification of the standard mastectomy is advocated for each stage 1 and stage 2 patient. Because a postsurgical
stage is necessary to further manage patients (adjuvant chemotherapy,
postoperative radiotherapy, etc.), a pathologic reporting form has
been prepared (Figure 3). Close cooperation between the surgeon
and the pathologist is necessary to label and identify the level and
location of involved nodes.

2. Medical audit criteria have been developed for the initial management of breast cancer. The Joint Commission on Accreditation of
Hospitals (Porterfield and Jacobs, 1973) has disseminated a format
for developing a process audit of hospital care. Table 2 contains the
elements important in monitoring the adequacy of pretreatment evaluation of breast cancer. A clerical assistant should be able to evaluate
retrospectively patient care in an ongoing manner from data collected on this form.

Table 1. Survival of patient with breast cancer according to TNM categories and stage from AJC retrospective evaluation of 2,500 patients (Cutler, 1974)[a]

Stage	TNM category		Number of cases	Five-year survival by TNM category	Number of cases	Percent of total	Five-year survival
I	T1a N0		346	0.85			
	T1a N1a	M0	16	0.94			
	T1b N0		39	0.82	402	17%	85%
II	T1a N1b		160	0.74			
	T1b N1b		20	0.65			
	T2a N0		595	0.71			
	T2a N1a	M0	29	0.66			
	T2a N1b		335	0.58			
	T2b N0		64	0.65			
	T2b N1b		81	0.47	1287	53%	66%

III	T2a N2		15			0.52
	T2a N3		24			0.58
	T3a N0		122			0.52
	T3a N1b		116			0.43
	T3a N3		11			0.55
	T3b N0	M0	10			0.80
	T3b N1b		25			0.28
	T4a N1b		12			0.33
	T4b N0		76			0.53
	T4b N1b		157			0.32
	T4b N2		14			0.07
	T4b N3		30			0.20
				673	28%	41%
IV	Any T Any N	M1	62			0.10
				62	2%	10%

aIndividual categories with less than 10 patients are not shown but have been included in the appropriate summary stages. *Note:* The patients with carcinoma of the breast of unusual histologic types, such as medullary, papillary, lobular, colloid or mucinous, or comedocarcinoma, have not been included in the data presented in this table. Survival analysis for these 217 patients, using the proposed staging system, was carried out. The conclusions of this analysis were: 1) that a greater percentage of the unusual histologic types was in Stage I; and 2) that survival experience by stage for these patients is somewhat better than for those with the common histologic types. Further studies are needed to substantiate these conclusions.

<u>B R E A S T   C A N C E R   N E T W O R K</u>

<u>CLINICAL STAGING</u>

NAME_____CHART #_____DATE OF EXAMINATION_____

AGE_____G___P___AB___MENOPAUSE___Yes___No DATE OF LMP_____

<u>TO BE COMPLETED</u> <u>AT TIME OF ADMISSION</u>
SIZE OF PRIMARY_____cm

          FIXATION TO UNDERLYING MUSCLE OR FASCIA
          FIXATION TO SKIN
          ULCERATION
          EDEMA<1/3 Breast Skin
          EDEMA>1/3 Breast Skin
          ERYTHEMA
          PEAU D'ORANGE
          SATELLITE NODULES OF SAME BREAST

          NONE

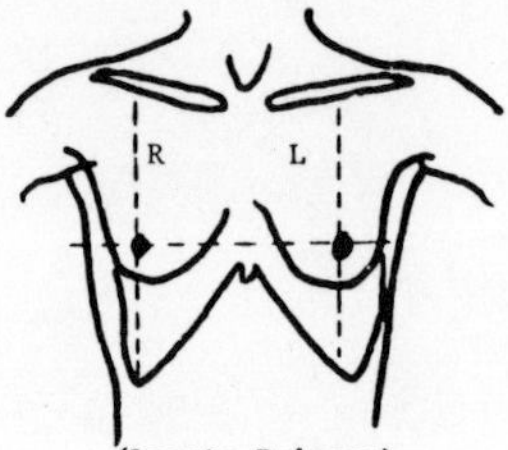

          (Locate Primary)

<u>NODES</u> <u>(CLINICAL)</u>

          PALPABLE AXILLARY NODES? R   L ___Yes___No   SIZE_____cm

          FIXATION TO CHEST WALL?   ___Yes___No   SIZE_____cm

          FIXED TO ONE ANOTHER?   ___Yes___No

          PALPABLE SUPRACLAVICULAR NODES? ___Yes___No   SIZE_____cm

          PALPABLE HOMOLATERAL AXILLARY OR INFRACLAVICULAR LYMPH NODES FIXED
                TO ONE ANOTHER OR TO OTHER STRUCTURES?_____Yes____No

<u>TO BE COMPLETED</u> <u>FOR THOSE</u> <u>STUDIES WHICH ARE NECESSARY</u>
<u>METASTASES</u>

CLINICAL AND RADIOGRAPHIC EVIDENCE OF METASTASIS?___Yes___No

          CHEST X-RAY   (+)____(-)____   BONE SCAN   (+)____(-)____

          LIVER FUNCTION TESTS (+)____(-)____ BONE SURVEY (+)____(-)____

          LIVER SCAN   (+)____(-)____   BRAIN SCAN   (+)____(-)____

COMMENTS:_____

_____

_____

_____

          Signature   Date

STAGING

T____N____M

STAGE_____

Figure 2. The Breast Cancer Network clinical staging form.

3. The community hospital executive board is asked to appoint staff members or consultants to a Multidisciplinary Tumor Review Committee. This committee should consist of an interested and qualified surgeon, radiologist, pathologist, internist, and physiatrist. This group

B R E A S T   C A N C E R   N E T W O R K

PATHOLOGY **REPORT**

SURGICAL PATH # _____

NAME_____CHART #_____DATE_____
   (Last)   (First)

TYPE OF SURGICAL PROCEDURE_____

                              RIGHT_____ LEFT_____
LOCATION OF TUMOR_____(SEE DIAGRAM BELOW)

SIZE OF TUMOR_____cm x_____cm x_____cm

HISTOLOGIC TYPE_____

GRADE: WELL DIFF._____MODERATELY DIFF._____POORLY DIFF._____

SKIN INVOLVEMENT   YES_____NO_____

LYMPHATIC PERMEATION   YES_____NO_____

MUSCLE INVOLVEMENT   YES_____NO_____

LYMPH NODES:

      LEVEL   I   (+) #_____OUT OF #_____

            II   (+) #_____OUT OF #_____

          III (+) #_____OUT OF #_____

     TOTAL   (+) #_____OUT OF #_____

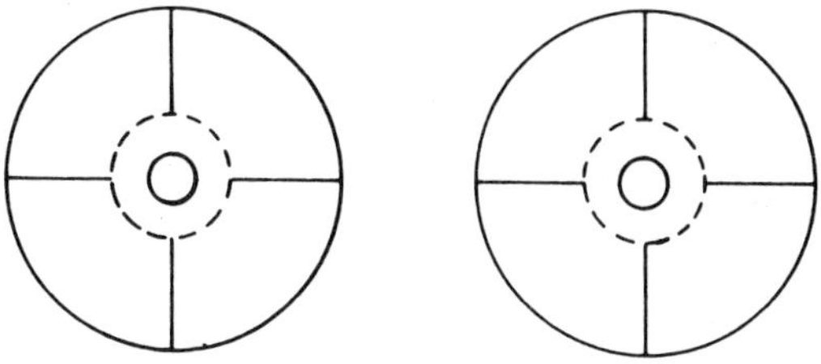

        RIGHT   LEFT

251-1   Signature   Date

Figure 3. The Breast Cancer Network pathologic staging form.

should meet frequently enough to review tumor cases; based on the accuracy of the clinical and pathologic stage, it can comment on the appropriateness of therapy and the adequacy of the patient's rehabilitation plans. It can serve as a consultative forum for difficult

Table 2. The medical audit elements utilizing the JCAH format

Audit topic elements	Initial management of breast cancer		Committee: Tumor board special instructions
	Standard	Exceptions	
	100 0		
1. Suspected breast cancer	x	Prior biopsy-proven breast cancer	Clinical history, physical exam, staging forms
2. Size and location of breast mass	x	None	
3. Description of regional nodes	x	None	
4. Definition of menopausal status	x	None	History, vaginal smear
5. Mammography positive	x	None	
6. Normal chest x-ray	x	None	
7. Bone scan	x	Clinical stage I tumor (lesion $<$ 2 cm) Nodes negative Absence of bone pain and normal alk. phos.	

8. X-ray bone survey	x	Negative bone scan
9. Liver function tests	x	None
10. Liver scan	x	Normal liver function studies Normal size and shape of liver on x-ray No complaints referrable to liver
11. Breast biopsy	x	None
12. Standard or modified radical mastectomy	x	Biopsy-proven distant metastases in bone, liver, or supraclavicular node
13. Radiotherapy consultation	x	Biopsy-proven dermal lymphatic involvement (inflammatory cancer) Stage I cancer ($<$ 22 cm lesion) No lymph nodes involved
14. Medical oncology consultation	x	Cancer $<$ 2.0 cm $<$ 4 nodes $+$ for cancer No metastatic cancer

(Note: Normal bili, alk. phos., SGOT, liver not palpable below costal margin, no jaundice, RUQ pain)

From Porterfield and Jacobs, (1973).

or complicated cases. This committee should stimulate the Tumor Registry Secretary to provide useful information in cancer patient follow-up and treatment efficacy. Through meetings with the professional staff, the Multidisciplinary Tumor Review Committee can function in a cancer education role for the hospital.

4. A plan for the sequential management of breast cancer has been developed based on the initial tumor classification (see Figure 4). As mentioned above, the initial treatment is based on clinical staging.

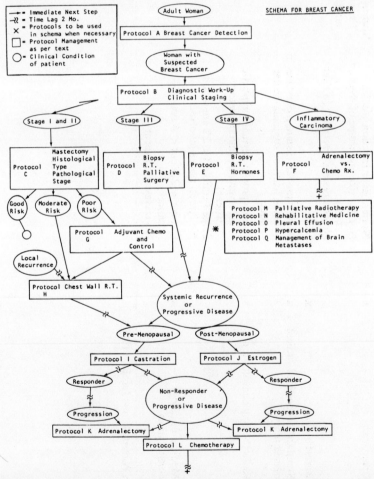

Figure 4. The Breast Cancer Network proposed management schema which is based on initial disease classification and anticipated complications.

The pathologic (postmastectomy) stage determines which patients are poor risk and require additional treatment. Women with four or more positive lymph nodes and/or anaplastic tumors who have all disease grossly resected should receive adjuvant chemotherapy with melphalan or combination cyclophosphamide, fluorouracil, and methotrexate. Patients with extranodal disease or chest wall infiltration require postoperative radiotherapy. Additional treatment protocols can be distributed in the community hospital for other unusual presentations of the disease or complications in the patient population. 5. The data generated in the Breast Cancer Control Program is collected on a data form. The initial staging, demographic, and treatment data are entered onto the forms for possible computerization. The Multidisciplinary Tumor Review Committee is encouraged to utilize the updated reports from the registry to monitor and improve the community hospital's management program.

In conclusion, the author has discussed the background and rationale for a formal cancer classification system. Using breast cancer as an illustration, staging criteria are detailed and related to prognosis. The classification system is further utilized as the basis for a cancer control program in the community hospital. This program can stimulate the hospital to utilize a Multidisciplinary Tumor Review Committee, to institute an ongoing medical audit of hospitalized cancer patients and to upgrade the tumor registry.

REFERENCES

Cutler, S. 1974. Classification of extent of disease in breast cancer. Semin. Oncol. 1:91–96.
Porterfield, J. D., and C. M. Jacobs. 1973. Medical audit team seminars. Joint Commission on Accreditation of Hospitals.
Rubin, P. 1973. A unified classification of cancers: An oncotaxonomy with symbols. Cancer 31:963–982.

M edical Management of Breast Cancer

Richard H. Creech, M.D., F.A.C.P.

The carefully planned staging and treatment of breast cancer are medically important because it is one of the most common cancers in women, occurring at an average age of 50. Even when metastatic, prolonged periods of regression are often attainable with sequentially applied systemic therapies. Dr. Carbone, in his chapter "Rationale for Combination Modality Therapy: Breast Cancer," has summarized the recent advances in tumor cell markers, estrogen receptor assays, postoperative adjuvant chemotherapy, and chemotherapeutic management of metastatic disease. This chapter focuses on the individualization and sequencing of radiation, hormonal, and chemotherapeutic management of patients with metastatic breast cancer.

STAGING AND SUBSEQUENT DEVELOPMENT OF METASTASES

Although any prediction of breast cancer recurrence after mastectomy is not possible for an individual patient, the statistical likelihood of recurrence and subsequent death from breast cancer can be estimated from a knowledge of a breast cancer's stage at the time of

This work was supported by United States Public Health Service Contract NO1-CN-45055 and Grant RR-05539 from the National Institutes of Health and by an appropriation from the Commonwealth of Pennsylvania.

initial diagnosis. Several staging procedures are currently in use. When evaluating reports in the literature, it is important to determine whether the staging under discussion is based on clinical findings, on surgical evaluation, or on postoperative data. Clinical staging includes historical information, physical examination, mammography, thermography, and xeroradiography, as well as laboratory and radiologic evaluations for metastatic disease. Surgical evaluative staging is determined from information obtained from clinical staging and pathologic results after standardized preoperative biopsies have been obtained. Postsurgical staging is based on all clinical, surgical evaluative, and postmastectomy pathologic data.

The American Joint Committee for Cancer Staging and End Results Reporting (1973) has correlated clinical staging with 5-year survival (Table 1). The 17% of patients presenting with stage I breast cancers measuring less than 2 cm in diameter and unassociated with malignant axillary adenopathy have an 85% 5-year survival. The 53% of patients with stage II carcinomas measuring less than 5 cm in diameter with clinically malignant axillary adenopathy have a 66% 5-year survival. Twenty-eight percent of patients present with stage III disease consisting of tumors greater than 5 cm in diameter or with supraclavicular, infraclavicular, or fixed axillary nodes. These patients have a 41% 5-year survival. The 2% of patients with distant metastases (stage IV disease) have a 5-year survival of 10%.

Table 1. Relationship of clinical stage to survival

	Primary	Nodes	Metastases	% of total	5-yr survival (%)
Stage I	< 2 cm	No	No	17	85
Stage II	< 5 cm	Yes	No	53	66
Stage III	> 5 cm		No	28	41
		Fixed axillary, supraclavicular, or intraclavicular	No		
Stage IV			Yes	2	10

American Joint Committee for Cancer Staging and End Results Reporting, 1973

Fisher et al. (1970), reporting for the National Surgical Adjuvant Breast Project (NSABP), have correlated the number of pathologically involved nodes at the time of radical mastectomy with 5-year recurrence rates and survival (Table 2). This postsurgical correlation refines the prognostic evaluation in clinical stage I and II patients by eliminating clinical discrepancies encountered when measuring primary tumor size and evaluating metastatic involvement of axillary nodes. The recurrence rates of 58% for one to three pathologically involved axillary nodes and 78% for four or more positive nodes 5 years after radical mastectomy serve as the historical background for utilization of postoperative adjuvant chemotherapy, as described in Carbone's chapter.

Fisher et al. (1970), when comparing radiotherapy of the internal mammary nodes, apex of the axilla, and supraclavicular area after radical mastectomy versus no postoperative therapy, found that radiation therapy decreased the incidence of chest wall recurrences in patients with four or more positive axillary nodes from 28% to 9% and in the one-to-three positive node patients from 21% to 5% (Table 3). The incidence of distant metastases in the radiotherapy-treated group appeared to be slightly higher than the control group. The 5-year survival for all patients correlated well with the degree of initial axillary node involvement, but appeared to be unaffected by the administration of postoperative radiotherapy. From these data it becomes evident that local control of breast cancer by mastectomy and radiation therapy often does not control the subsequent development of distant metastases, particularly in patients with pathologically proved axillary nodal metastases. Hopefully, postoperative adjuvant chemotherapy will prove effective in reducing the incidence of distant metastases and improving survival rates in these patients.

Table 2. Five-year recurrence and survival rates after radical mastectomy

No. positive nodes	Recurrence (%)	Survival (%)
None	29	77
1–3	58	65
≥ 4	78	31

Fisher et al., 1970

Table 3. Disease status 5 years after radical mastectomy

Disease status (%)	Radiotherapy			Control		
	Positive nodes			Positive nodes		
	0	1–3	≧4	0	1–3	≧4
No recurrence	78.6	49.1	28.4	71.2	42.4	21.9
Recurrence						
Chest wall	8.9	5.3	9.0	3.8	21.2	28.1
Regional nodes	0	0	1.5	3.8	3.0	3.1
Distant	12.5	43.9	59.7	21.2	33.3	46.9
Survival (%)	74	59	38	80	65	31

Fisher et al., 1970

DETECTION, EVALUATION, AND SPECIFIC TREATMENT OF METASTASES

Of those patients who had recurrence within 5 years of radical mastectomy, Fisher et al. (1970) found that 30.5% had their first recurrence on the chest wall, 6.8% in the supraclavicular nodes, and 62.7% in distant sites, particularly bone (28.8%) and lung (22%). Myelophthisis, distant nodal, hepatic, and central nervous system metastases accounted for 11.9% of initial recurrences (Table 4).

Table 4. First area of recurrence within 5 years after radical mastectomy

	%
Local	30.5
Chest wall	10.2
Scar	20.3
Regional	6.8
Supraclavicular nodes	6.8
Distant	62.7
Bone	28.8
Lung	22.0
Hemic and lymph	5.1
Gastrointestinal	5.1
Nervous	1.7

Fisher et al., 1970

Since 67% of all patients with axillary nodal metastases will develop recurrence within 5 years of mastectomy (Fisher, 1972), careful follow-up of breast cancer patients is necessary.

In patients who have previously not had metastases, suspected recurrence of breast carcinoma should be carefully documented, preferably by biopsy. It is important to remember that breast cancer patients often survive for long periods of time and have the same likelihood as the rest of the general population of developing other illnesses, including second primary cancers. It also should be realized that breast cancer patients may develop recurrence many years after their mastectomy and that seemingly nonspecific complaints may represent metastatic disease.

Chest wall, nodal, opposite breast, and subcutaneous recurrences can easily be documented by biopsy. At the time of recurrence, evaluation for other areas of metastases is necessary in order to design an optimal treatment program for each patient. This should include a careful history; physical examination with particular attention to the chest wall, opposite breast, subcutaneous tissue, lungs, liver, and Blumer's shelf; laboratory evaluation of the blood count and peripheral blood smear, liver functions, alkaline phosphatase, and calcium; chest x-ray; and liver and bone scans. Brain scans and bone surveys are not worthwhile screening procedures in asymptomatic patients. By performing this baseline evaluation, the detection of other clinically unsuspected areas of metastases is significant and often greatly influences decisions regarding oncologic management.

Development of bone pain in the patient who has previously had a mastectomy is often difficult to attribute initially to bony metastases because of the high incidence of osteoporosis, osteoarthritis, and the low back syndrome in the general population. At the time of presentation, bone scans and surveys may be normal. The bone scan may subsequently become abnormal and, after approximately 50% of the bony structure has been replaced by tumor, the bone survey will show lytic or blastic lesions. If the scan and survey are negative initially and the patient is quite symptomatic, a bone marrow aspiration and biopsy may document metastatic disease. Radiotherapy to areas of bony metastases is symptomatically gratifying.

Hypercalcemia occurs in breast cancer patients with bony metastases as a result of immobilization, dehydration, or initiation of additive systemic hormonal therapy. It should be suspected in any patient who develops behavioral changes, polyuria, polydipsia, somnolence, or loss of consciousness. It is important to determine whether loss of consciousness is due to hypercalcemia, hepatic failure, or brain metastases because hypercalcemia may be rapidly reversed by hydration, and corticosteroid or mithramycin administration. Although ectopic hormone production may cause hypercalcemia in other malignancies, it is almost never seen in breast cancer patients.

Myelophthisis caused by bone marrow infiltration should be suspected if a patient is anemic, leukopenic, or thrombocytopenic, and on peripheral blood smear has tear drop cells, nucleated red blood cells, immature white blood cells, or large platelets. This syndrome can be documented by aspiration and biopsy of the bone marrow. Since it represents bone marrow infiltration by metastatic cancer cells, it is not necessarily associated with abnormal bone scans and surveys. Myelophthisis can be improved by the administration of androgens to stimulate erythropoiesis, and occasionally by corticosteroids. Although patients with bony metastases may also have poor bone marrow reserve, the cause of their cytopenias can be explained by the extent of their bony metastases associated with radiation and chemotherapeutic damage of normal marrow elements.

Pulmonary recurrence often presents symptomatically as dyspnea and cough. Pleural effusions secondary to pleural metastases may be documented by laboratory evaluation of fluid removed by thoracentesis. Exudative fluid with cytologic evidence of malignant cells or a pleural biopsy consistent with metastatic breast cancer indicates recurrence. If no other areas of metastases are evident, it is important to rule out other causes of pleural effusions before instituting antineoplastic therapy. Pleural fluid accumulation may be controlled by thoracentesis and systemic therapy. If the fluid reaccumulates rapidly, closed tube thoracostomy with prolonged suction is usually effective in preventing reaccumulation of fluid. Although sclerosing agents may also be used, they probably add little to the stimulation of adhesions between the parietal and visceral pleural surfaces.

Mediastinal adenopathy may cause pulmonary symptoms by compression of the tracheo-bronchial tree. These symptoms may be relieved by mediastinal irradiation. Pulmonary nodular disease, even though extensive on chest x-ray, may be asymptomatic, whereas lymphangitic metastases are often clinically devastating without much radiographic evidence of disease. Corticosteroid administration can be used to improve symptomatically patients with lymphangitic disease.

Hepatic enlargement may represent nonmalignant conditions or metastatic breast cancer. Hepatic metastases result in a poor prognosis if they are extensive (Nemoto and Dao, 1966). Liver scans, although unreliable for detecting metastases less than 2 cm in diameter, may show metastatic disease, particularly if multiple filling defects are evident. If clinically suspected, liver metastases should be documented pathologically in order to determine an optimal therapeutic regimen. Since hepatic metastases are relatively unresponsive to hormonal therapy, combination chemotherapy should be instituted at the time of diagnosis. Massive hepatic metastases unassociated with liver function abnormalities may respond well to combination chemotherapy, with mean survivals of 16 months. On the other hand, metastases causing abnormal liver function tests may respond transiently to chemotherapy, but result in death from hepatic failure within 4 months of instituting chemotherapy (Creech et al., 1975).

Brain metastases account for only 1.7% of the sites of initial recurrence, but are becoming more common as the effectiveness of systemic control of metastases improves. Patients with brain metastases may present with persistent headaches, unexplained nausea and vomiting, behavioral changes, and a variety of neurologic syndromes. Documentation of brain metastases is often difficult initially when brain scans, electroencephalograms, lumbar punctures, and contrast studies are normal. The introduction of computerized axial tomography, however, has recently improved our ability to diagnose suspected brain lesions.

Brain irradiation should be the primary form of treatment in patients with brain metastases unassociated with life-threatening systemic metastases. Corticosteroids may also be used acutely to improve neurologic symptoms caused by the edema surrounding brain metastases. In patients with limited life expectances or recurrence after radiation therapy, corticosteroids may be used effectively to reverse neurologic dysfunction.

Spinal cord compression should be suspected in any patient with severe localized back or radicular pain, especially if associated with sensory changes or motor weakness. Since continued neurologic function is paramount in the management of patients with cord compression, a high index of suspicion, neurosurgical consultation, and myelography will lead to early diagnosis and appropriate radiotherapy or surgical decompression of symptomatic epidural metastases. Successful preservation of lower extremity, bowel, and bladder function is extremely rewarding for the patient who might otherwise be paraplegic.

SYSTEMIC THERAPY OF METASTATIC BREAST CANCER

Although radiation therapy can control local recurrences, systemic therapy should be instituted in an attempt at prolonged control of multiple metastases. The choice of systemic therapy is based on the extent, location, and growth rate of metastases, as well as the menopausal status of the patient. If the metastases are not causing life-threatening infiltration of the lungs, liver, or brain, the primary form of systemic management should be hormonal therapy. If at all possible, areas of metastatic disease should be evaluable for response after hormonal therapy is instituted. A patient with multiple chest wall recurrences and an abnormal bone scan requires documentation of recurrence by biopsy of one skin lesion; the other lesions should be left for evaluation of therapeutic response. If all known areas of metastatic disease are surgically or radiotherapeutically removed, evaluation of hormonal responsiveness is difficult to determine. Since hormonal responsiveness is an important clinical prerequisite for secondary adrenal or hypophyseal ablations, careful documentation of hormonal responsiveness may predict a prolonged beneficial response in the hormonally responsive patient and obviate a major ineffective surgical procedure in an unresponsive patient.

Primary Hormonal Therapy

Patients with systemic metastases are best treated initially with hormonal manipulation, consisting of oophorectomy in the premenopausal patient and estrogen administration in the postmenopausal patient (Table 5). In the premenopausal patient, oophorectomy causes regressions in 35% of patients for 9 to 18 months with lymph node, soft tissue, pulmonary, and bony metastases being most responsive. Liver metastases and inflammatory carcinoma respond in only 20% of patients, whereas brain metastases are responsive only to radiation and corticosteroid therapy (Fracchia et al., 1969).

Kennedy (1974) has summarized the results of several studies of estrogen and androgen therapy for metastatic breast cancer in postmenopausal patients. Estrogens cause regression in approximately 35% of patients with 40% of soft tissue and 25% of skeletal metastases responding, whereas androgens cause regressions in 20% of

Table 5. Primary hormonal therapy of metastatic breast cancer

	Response (%)	Duration (months)
Premenopausal		
Oophorectomy	35	9–18
Nodes	50	
Soft tissue, lung, bone	40	
Inflammatory, liver	20	
Brain	0	
Postmenopausal		
Estrogens	35	6–18
Soft tissue	40	
Skeletal	25	
Androgens	20	6–15
Soft tissue	16	
Skeletal	19	

patients with 16% soft tissue and 19% skeletal responses. The duration of response to these additive hormone therapies ranges from 6 to 18 months. The estrogenic compound diethylstilbesterol may be administered orally at night, starting at a 5-mg dose and gradually increasing to 15 mg per day. Patients are often initially nauseous, but may lose this symptom with continued therapy. Occasionally nausea or phlebitis obviates continuation of estrogens. Patients should be warned of the possible side effects of areolar hyperpigmentation, breast tenderness, vaginal discharge, urinary urgency, and uterine bleeding. Hypercalcemia may be precipitated by estrogen administration. This does not necessarily indicate exacerbation of disease, and can be associated with prolonged hormonal response, provided the hypercalcemia is well controlled by hydration and corticosteroid administration.

Androgens may be administered parenterally as testosterone enanthate or orally as fluoxymesterone (Halotestin), 10 mg, twice per day. The side effects include deepening of the voice, hirsutism, fluid retention, hypercalcemia, and, with fluoxymesterone, cholestatic jaundice. Testolactone (Teslac), although less effective, may be substituted for the preceding androgens if virilizing side effects are unacceptable.

The appropriate hormonal therapy should be continued as long as there is no evidence of disease progression. Most patients who are going to have objective regressions have some response by 2 months, although their maximal response may not occur for many months.

Decisions regarding primary systemic therapy in the perimenopausal age group are often difficult. The likelihood of response to castration in a patient who is more than 1 year postmenopausal is small. On the other hand, response to additive hormone therapy within 4 years after menopause is less than 10%. Therefore, patients with seemingly indolent disease may be started on androgen therapy initially; if responsive, they should be considered for secondary hormonal ablation at the time of recurrence. Patients with rapidly progressive disease or unresponsiveness to androgen therapy should be started on systemic chemotherapy.

Secondary Hormonal Therapy

Patients responding to primary hormonal therapy have a 40% chance of responding to subsequent adrenalectomy or hypophysectomy, whereas castration failures have only a 15 to 20% chance of response (Table 6) (Fracchia, Randall, and Farrow, 1967). Since the secondary form of hormonal therapy involves major surgery, which may possibly be ineffective, careful consideration must be given to all aspects of a patient's disease process before either adrenalectomy or hypophysectomy is recommended. Harris and Spratt (1969) and Fracchia et al. (1967) found that the best responses to adrenalectomy occurred in patients with a 24-month latent period between mastectomy and initial recurrence, with predominant soft tissue and bony metastases, and with a previous therapeutic response to oophorectomy. They also felt that patients with central nervous system metastases, pulmonary insufficiency, hepatic metastases, and rapidly progressive bony metastases were not benefited and should be excluded from these procedures. Since patients lacking estrogen receptors in their tumor tissue have only an 8% probability of response to hormonal therapy, these patients should also be excluded from endocrine ablative procedures (McGuire, 1975).

The duration of response to either bilateral adrenalectomy or hypophysectomy ranges between 12 and 24 months. The adrenalectomy patients are maintained on cortisone acetate at a dose of 50 mg per day. They may require, especially during the summer, mineralo-

Table 6. Secondary hormonal therapy for metastatic breast cancer

	Response (%)	Duration (months)
Adrenalectomy		
Previous hormonal response	40	12–24
Previous castration failure	15	
Soft tissue, skeletal, inflammatory	35	
Lung	20	
Liver, anemia	10	
Brain	0	
Hypophysectomy		
Unselected	40	12–24
Hormonal responders	60	
Castration failures	20	
Androgens (Indolent disease)	20	4–8
Corticosteroids	20	4–8
Progestins (Postmenopausal)	20	6–12

corticoid replacement in the form of fludrocortisone acetate (Florinef), 0.1 mg, two or three times weekly. Hypophysectomy patients require cortisone acetate (50 mg per day) and thyroid replacement (2 grains per day); they may also require maintenance vasopressin nasal spray if they have symptomatic diabetes insipidus. The choice between adrenalectomy and hypophysectomy is usually determined by the interest and expertise of each hospital's surgical subspecialists.

Patients who are not surgical candidates may be treated with androgens, corticosteroids, or adrenal suppression by aminoglutethimide, dexamethasone, and fludrocortisone acetate (Lipton and Santen, 1974). The response rates are 20% and the responses last about 6 months. Progestins, such as megesterol acctate (Megace), may be effective in postmenopausal patients who cannot tolerate or have become resistant to estrogens (Muggia et al., 1968; Ahmann, Hahn, and Bisel, 1972; Ansfield et al., 1974).

Single Agent Chemotherapy

In patients who have exhausted or who are unresponsive to hormonal therapy, or who present with life-threatening involvement of the lungs or liver, chemotherapy should be instituted as the next form of systemic treatment. Single drugs found to be effective in the control of metastatic cancer include the alkylating agents cyclophosphamide, 1-phenylalanine mustard, chlorambucil, and thio-TEPA; the anti-metabolites 5-fluorouracil and methotrexate; the mitotic inhibitors vincristine and vinblastine; and the anti-tumor antibiotic Adriamycin (Table 7). Carter (1974a, 1974b) has summarized the response rates for these single agents. Adriamycin has been found to be the most effective single agent with responses in 35% of patients. The other drugs cause responses in 20 to 35% of patients. Using 1-phenylala-nine mustard, the Eastern Cooperative Oncology Group found 5% complete responses and 14% partial responses with a 4-month median duration of regression (Taylor et al., 1974).

Combination Chemotherapy

After single agents were found to have significant anti-breast cancer activity of brief duration, Greenspan (1966) introduced the concept of multi-agent breast cancer chemotherapy in an attempt to increase the regression induction rate and duration. He found an 81% re-sponse using a combination of cyclophosphamide, methotrexate, 5-fluorouracil, prednisone, and testosterone. Cooper (1969) later cor-roborated the effectiveness of multi-agent chemotherapy, finding a

Table 7. Single drug treatment of metastatic breast cancer

	Response (%)
Alkylators	
Cyclophosphamide	35
1-Phenylalanine Mustard	35
Chlorambucil	20
Thio-TEPA	30
Antimetabolites	
5-Fluorouracil	25
Methotrexate	35
Mitotic inhibitors	
Vincristine	20
Vinblastine	20
Antibiotics	
Adriamycin	35

Carter, 1974a, 1974b

90% response rate in 60 patients treated with cyclophosphamide, 5-fluorouracil, methotrexate, prednisone, and vincristine. Carter (1974b) has reviewed and summarized the published literature of combination chemotherapy of breast cancer (Table 8). "Cooper-like" 5-drug, "Cooper-like" 4-drug without prednisone, Adriamycin-vincristine (DeLena et al., 1975), Adriamycin-cyclophosphamide-5-fluorouracil (DeJager et al., 1975; Smalley, Bornstein, and the Southeastern Cancer Study Group, 1975), cyclophosphamide-5-fluorouracil-vincristine (Baker et al., 1974), and 5-fluorouracil-prednisone-vincristine (Leone and Rege, 1973) combinations have been found to cause complete and partial regressions in approximately 50% of patients. Jones, Durie, and Salmon (1975), using Adriamycin and cyclophosphamide, and Blumenschein et al. (1974), using cyclophosphamide-Adriamycin-5-fluorouracil, report partial and complete regressions in 80% and 72% of patients, respectively.

Cross comparison of response rates and toxicities among various treatment regimens published in the literature is often quite difficult because of the nonuniformity of response criteria. These problems are minimized in a comparison of three reports on the use of combination cyclophosphamide, methotrexate, and 5-fluorouracil (CMF) therapy, in which the schedules, response criteria, and toxicity evaluations are all uniform (Taylor et al., 1974; Eastern Cooperative Oncology Group Progress Report, May 1971–May 1974; Bonadonna et al., 1974; DeLena et al., 1975; Creech et al., 1974, 1975). In these reports, complete regression means complete disappearance of all lesions and the recalcification of osteolytic metastases; partial regression means a greater than 50% decrease in the product of the two longest perpendicular diameters of all measurable lesions and a partial recalcification of osteolytic metastases; stabilization indicates subjective clinical improvement without objective change in tumor measurements or appearance of new metastases; and progression indicates a 25% increase in the sum of perpendicular tumor measurements or the subjective impression of clinical deterioration.

Table 9 compares the drug dosages, response rates, and the toxicities in these three studies. In each study, cyclophosphamide was administered orally for the first 14 days of each 28-day cycle, while methotrexate and 5-fluorouracil were given intravenously on days 1 and 8 of each cycle. The drug dosages in the low dose regimen were approximately one-half of the high dose regimens. The 10 to 15% complete and 33 to 38% partial response rates were essentially

Table 8. Multi-agent therapy of metastatic breast cancer

ADRIA	CTX	5FU	MTX	PRED	VCR	Response (%)	Duration (months)
	X	X	X	X	X	50 (29–70)	5–8
	X	X	X		X	57 (45–100)	
X					X	48	
X	X	X				70	
X	X	X				55 (23–72)	
	X	X			X	44	
		X		X	X	42	
	X	X	X (High dose)			48, 53	9
	X	X	X (Low dose)			46	10

[a]ADRIA, Adriamycin; CTX, cyclophosphamide; 5FU, 5-Fluorouracil; MTX, methiotrexate; PRED, prednisone; VCR, vincristine.

Table 9. Comparison of high versus low dose CMF

Drugs	E.C.O.G. (1974) (High dose CMF)			DeLena et al. (1975) (High dose CMF)			Creech et al. (1975) (Low dose CMF)		
Dosages (mg/m²)	CTX	MTX	5FU	CTX	MTX	5FU	CTX	MTX	5FU
	100	60	600	100	40	600	40	16	34
Responses (%)									
Complete		15			10			13	
Partial		38			38			33	
Stable					22			26	
Progression					30			28	
Toxicity (%)									
WBC < 3000/mm³		74			68			26	
Stomatitis		28			25			2	
Cystitis		8			20			0	
Alopecia		17			53			0	

identical in each study, but the toxicities were commensurate with drug dosages. As of August 1975, the low dose CMF response durations and survivals are 11.5 and 18.2 months, respectively, for the complete responders; 9.2 and 16.2 months for the partial responders; 7.4 and 13.5 months for the stabilized patients; and a 4.9-month survival for the patients progressing on this regimen. Of these low dose CMF patients, 63% were considered poor risks for high dose chemotherapy because of compromised bone marrow reserve, extensive liver metastases, or poor performance status. Clinically beneficial complete, partial, and stable responses occurred in 72% of these patients, whereas the remaining 28% who had progressed on therapy showed a poor survival rate.

Upon analysis of the responses by metastatic disease sites, the data of DeLena et al. (1975) and Creech et al. (1975) demonstrate that soft tissue metastases, including breast and nodes, are most responsive with 60 to 85% complete and partial regressions (Table 10). Pulmonary metastases are responsive in two-thirds of patients treated with CMF, but only in 11% of Adriamycin-vincristine-treated patients. Liver metastases are also more responsive to CMF than Adriamycin-vincristine, particularly in those patients with normal liver functions at the initiation of therapy. Low dose CMF appears to be inferior to high dose CMF and to Adriamycin-vincristine for patients with skin and osteolytic metastases.

Table 10. Objective response rates of metastases by site

	DeLana et al. (1975)		Creech et al. (1975)
	Adriamycin-vincristine (%)	High dose CMF (%)	Low dose CMF (%)
Breast	52	82	71
Skin	55	61	36
Nodes	73	85	60
Lung	11	67	66
Pleura	50	100	28
Liver	0	20	46
Bone	25	24	0

After reviewing the published literature on combination chemotherapy of breast cancer, it becomes apparent that combinations of 2 to 5 active agents result in approximately 50% complete and partial regressions of 8 to 12 months duration. This is obviously an improvement over the single drug-induced 25% responses of 4 months duration.

SUMMARY

Despite aggressive surgery and local radiotherapy, two-thirds of all breast cancer patients with pathologic axillary metastases documented at the time of mastectomy eventually develop metastatic disease. Hopefully, postoperative adjuvant chemotherapy, which has recently been found to reduce the incidence of early recurrences, will also be shown to reduce the recurrence rate permanently and thereby improve survival.

Thorough evaluation of disease extent and development of individualized sequential treatment programs can significantly improve the productive longevity of patients with metastatic disease. Locally painful or obstructing metastases can be successfully treated with local radiation therapy, but systemic forms of therapy are necessary for prolonged control of metastases (Table 11). The primary form of systemic therapy should be oophorectomy in premenopausal patients and additive estrogen therapy in postmenopausal patients. Approximately one-third of these hormonally treated patients have 9- to 18-month regressions. Unfortunately, androgen therapy in the perimenopausal patients is less effective than the primary hormonal therapies of the young and elderly.

Patients who have good regressions to their primary hormonal therapy are also good candidates for secondary hormonal therapy involving ablation of the adrenal glands or hypophysis, which produces a 40 to 60% response rate for 12 to 24 months.

Patients who are hormonally unresponsive, who have exhausted all hormonal therapies, or who present with hepatic or symptomatic pulmonary metastases should be treated with tolerable 2 to 5 drug combinations of the effective anti-breast cancer drugs, Adriamycin, cyclophosphamide, 5-fluorouracil, methotrexate, prednisone, and vincristine. The complete and partial response rates are approximately 50%, with another 25% deriving clinically beneficial disease stabilization. The duration of these responses ranges from 6 to 12 months.

Table 11. Summary of sequential therapy of metastatic breast cancer

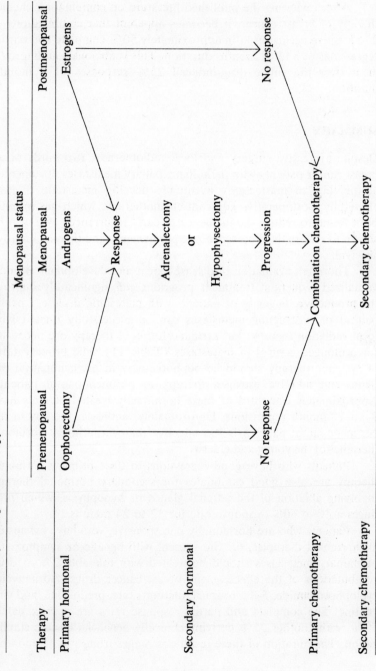

At the time of progression, other combinations of previously unused chemotherapeutic agents may be used to induce additional regressions.

Since metastatic breast cancer patients may have prolonged antineoplastic responses to several hormonal and chemotherapeutic regimens, their lives can frequently be beneficially extended by the period of time spent in systemically induced regressions.

REFERENCES

Ahmann, D. L., R. G. Hahn, and H. F. Bisel. 1972. Disseminated breast cancer: evaluation of hormonal therapy utilizing stilbesterol and medrogestone (AY-62022) singly and in combination. Cancer 30:651–653.

American Joint Committee for Cancer Staging and End Results Reporting. 1973. Clinical staging system for carcinoma of the breast (revision). 23 pp.

Ansfield, F. J., H. L. Davis, R. A. Ellerby, and G. Ramirez. 1974. A clinical trial of megestrol acetate in advanced breast cancer. Cancer 33: 907–910.

Baker, L. H., C. B. Vaughn, M. Al-Sarraf, M. L. Reed, and V. K. Vaitkevicius. 1974. Evaluation of combination vs. sequential cytotoxic chemotherapy in the treatment of advanced breast cancer. Cancer 33: 513–518.

Blumenschein, R., J. O. Cardenas, E. J. Freiereich, and J. A. Gottlieb. 1974. FAC chemotherapy for breast cancer. Proc. Amer. Assoc. Cancer Res., Amer. Soc. Clin. Oncol. 15:193.

Bonadonna, G., C. Brambilla, M. DeLena, and U. Veronesi. 1974. Controlled study with multiple drug combination in advanced breast carcinoma. Proc. Amer. Assoc. Cancer Res., Amer. Soc. Clin. Oncol. 15: 176.

Carter, S. K. 1974a. Some thoughts on combination chemotherapy of breast cancer. In Maurice Staguet (ed.), The Design of Clinical Trials in Cancer Therapy, pp. 336–358. Futura, New York.

Carter, S. K. 1974b. The chemical therapy of breast cancer. Semin. Oncol. 1(2):131–144.

Cooper, R. G. 1969. Combination chemotherapy in hormone resistant breast cancer. Proc. Amer. Assoc. Cancer Res. 10:15.

Creech, R. H., R. Catalano, M. Mastrangelo, and P. Engstrom. 1974. An effective low dose 3 drug treatment for metastatic breast cancer. Proc. Amer. Assoc. Cancer Res., Amer. Soc. Clin. Oncol. 15:179.

Creech, R. H., R. B. Catalano, M. J. Mastrangelo, and P. F. Engstrom. 1975. An effective low-dose intermittent cyclophosphamide, methotrexate, and 5-fluorouracil treatment regimen for metastatic breast cancer. Cancer 35:1101–1107.

DeJager, R., R. Kaufman, M. Ochoa, and I. H. Krakoff. 1975. Chemotherapy of advanced breast cancer with a combination of cytoxan, Adriamycin, and 5-FU (CAF). Proc. Amer. Assoc. Cancer Res., Amer. Soc. Clin. Oncol. 16:273.

158   Creech

DeLena, M., C. Brambilla, A. Morabito, and G. Bonadonna. 1975. Adriamycin plus vincristine compared to and combined with cyclophosphamide, methotrexate, and 5-fluorouracil for advanced breast cancer. Cancer 35:1108–1115.

Eastern Cooperative Oncology Group Progress Report. May 1971–May 1974. pp. 91–125.

Fisher, B., N. H. Slack, P. J. Cavanaugh, B. Gardner, R. G. Ravdin, and cooperating investigators. 1970. Postoperative radiotherapy in the treatment of breast cancer: results of the NSABP clinical trial. Ann. Surg. 172(4):711–732.

Fisher, B. 1972. Surgical adjuvant therapy for breast cancer. Cancer 30: 1556–1564.

Fisher, B., P. Carbone, S. Economou, R. Frelick, A. Glass, H. Lerner, C. Redmond, M. Zelen, P. Band, D. Katrych, N. Wolmark, and E. Fisher. 1975. 1-Phenylalanine mustard (L-PAM) in the management of primary breast cancer. New Eng. J. Med. 292:117–122.

Fracchia, A. A., H. T. Randall, and J. H. Farrow. 1967. The results of adrenalectomy in advanced breast cancer in 500 consecutive patients. Surg. Gynecol. Obstet. 125:747–756.

Fracchia, A. A., J. H. Farrow, A. J. DePalo, D. P. Connolly, and A. G. Huvos. 1969. Castration for primary inoperable or recurrent breast carcinoma. Surg. Gynec. Obstet. 128:1226–1234.

Greenspan, E. M. 1966. Combination cytotoxic chemotherapy in advanced disseminated breast cancer. Mt. Sinai J. Med. N.Y. 33:1–27.

Harris, H. S., and J. S. Spratt. 1969. Bilateral adrenalectomy in metastatic mammary cancer. Cancer 23:145–151.

Jones, S. E., B. G. Durie, and S. E. Salmon. 1975. Combination chemotherapy with Adriamycin and cyclophosphamide for advanced breast cancer. Cancer 36:90–97.

Kennedy, B. J. 1974. Hormonal therapies in breast cancer. Semin. Oncol. 1(2):119–130.

Leone, L. A., and V. Rege. 1973. Treatment of metastatic, recurrent or inoperable carcinoma of breast with VCR/PRED/5-FU/MTX/CYCLO (REG I) vs. VCR/PRED/5-FU (REG II). Proc. Amer. Assoc. Cancer Res. 14:125.

Lipton, A., and R. J. Santen. 1974. Medical Adrenalectomy using aminoglutethimide and dexamethasone in advanced breast cancer. Cancer 33: 503–512.

McGuire, W. L. 1975. Current status of estrogen receptors in human breast cancer. Cancer 36:638–644.

Muggia, F., P. Cassileth, M. Ochoa, F. Flatlow, A. Gellhorn, and G. Hyman. 1968. Treatment of breast cancer with medroxyprogesteron acetate. Ann. Intern. Med. 68:328–337.

Nemoto, T., and T. L. Dao. 1966. Significance of liver metastases in women with disseminated breast cancer undergoing endocrine ablative surgery. Cancer 19:421–427.

Smalley, R., and R. Bornstein for the Southeastern Cancer Study Group. 1975. C-A-F treatment of metastatic breast cancer. Proc. Amer. Assoc. Cancer Res., Amer. Soc. Clin. Oncol. 16:265.

Taylor, S. G., G. P. Canellos, P. Band, and S. Pocock. 1974. Combination chemotherapy for advanced breast cancer: randomized comparison with single drug therapy. Proc. Amer. Assoc. Cancer Res., Amer. Soc. Clin. Oncol. 15:175.

Rationale for Combination Modality Therapy: Breast Cancer

Paul P. Carbone, M.D., F.A.C.P.

Breast cancer is the most common cancer in women and accounts for 28% of all malignancies. More than 50% of women developing breast cancer will die of their disease in 10 years. The mortality for breast cancer has not changed in the last 4 decades. While most patients seen by medical oncologists have metastatic disease, at the time of diagnosis 90% of patients present with regional or localized disease (Axtell and Myers, 1975).

TREATMENT APPROACHES

The classic approach to primary therapy has been surgery, an operation devised by Halsted over 80 years ago (Halsted, 1894–1895). The operation is based on the premise that breast cancer starts as a localized process, spreads contiguuouosly, and invades the local muscular and lymph node structures before disseminating via the blood stream. Doubting this concept, several investigators have advocated using less surgery or substituting radiotherapy for the more radical procedures (Crile, 1975; Hayward, 1974). Currently, the operative options range from simple excision of the tumor or removal of the breast only to the extreme of doing an internal mammary node dissection with resection of part of the chest wall. Since radiotherapy can be added to each of the varied surgical procedures, one has twice as many possibilities. As yet no firm data are available to select the best approach that has the least morbidity and produces the best cosmetic result.

The primary treatment problem can be approached as one of treatment technique, that is, one surgical procedure versus another. However, the same therapeutic dilemma can be approached as cancer biologic questions.

Thus, if breast cancer is a locally spreading process, then obviously the more surgery, the better the results. The facts indicate:

1. Procedures less than a radical mastectomy are equivalent to a radical mastectomy (Atkins et al., 1972).
2. The enlarged extended radical mastectomy procedures are no better than a radical mastectomy (Caceres, 1967).
3. The addition of postoperative radiotherapy to a radical mastectomy does not add to the results of a radical mastectomy (Fisher et al., 1970).

Moreover, a simple mastectomy that leaves in axillary nodes when compared to a radical mastectomy produces equivalent results (Atkins et al., 1972). Since we know that clinical negative nodes have a finite probability (30 to 40%) (Wallace and Champion, 1972) of containing microscopic cancer, these same studies clearly indicate that resection of the nodes does not improve the results and that failure to cure results from blood-borne metastases. Thus we must conclude that breast cancer is not a localized disease in most patients that should be treated with localized methods only. This new concept of breast cancer clearly mandates the use of systemic treatments as well as good local surgical and/or radiotherapy approaches and is known as the combined modality approach.

Chemotherapy has accomplished dramatic results in children with acute lymphocytic leukemia, Burkitt's tumor, and in advanced Hodgkin's disease (Zubrod, 1972). Yet in the solid tumors, regressions when they occur are less than complete and are transient, persisting for only a few months. One can also examine the effectiveness of chemotherapy in breast cancer as biologic questions. Is it a problem of drug resistance or one of kinetic/high volume resistance? Drug resistance implies an intensive search for new agents and/or better ways to use our current drugs. Since the screening program of the National Cancer Institute has involved the annual evaluation of 10,000 to 40,000 compounds per year for the last 20 years, the hypothesis that the failure to control solid tumors is a function of drug resistance implies a very pessimistic outlook for the future. Many more years of screening would be required. On the other hand the theory that failure to affect solid tumors is one of a high volume (large tumor load) and unfavorable growth kinetics of the advanced disease offers an optimistic possibility. The implications are that the drugs we currently use are active but that the clinical situation in which they have been used has been unfavorable.

If we examine the experimental data we find that: 1) tumor cells grow rapidly initially and then slow down drastically when they reach large volumes; 2) chemotherapy is much less effective against the gross tumor deposits than the small foci of rapidly dividing cells; and 3) surgery and chemotherapy are very effective in animal tumor systems for controlling the large primary and small metastatic foci (Schabel, 1975; Stolfi, Martin, and Fugmann, 1971). Most importantly, chemotherapy that is relatively ineffective against the large primary tumor can often effectively cure the small metastatic disease deposits when applied after surgery. Thus the combined modality approach of surgery and chemotherapy offers the best chance of cure in the clinical situation.

The population of breast cancer patients most likely to benefit from this combined approach are those with positive lymph nodes (Table 1). Dr. Fisher has recently reported on the 10-year follow-up of patients treated by radical mastectomy (Fisher et al., 1975a). Clearly those patients with positive lymph nodes have a poor prognosis with only a 25% chance at 10 years of being disease free.

Table 1. Axillary node involvement and survival

Nodal status	Recurrence (%)		Survival (%)	
	5 years	10 years	5 years	10 years
Negative	21	24	76	65
Positive	67	76	46	25
1–3 Positive	53	65	62	38
$\geq$ 4 Positive	80	86	31	13

Data from Fisher (1975a).

Particularly dire results are achieved when four or more lymph nodes are involved.

CHEMOTHERAPY

A variety of single agents (Carter, 1974) have been reported to cause tumor regressions in patients with breast cancer. In order to increase the effectiveness of these single agents combination chemotherapy programs have been developed (Broder and Tormey, 1974). The basic principles of combination chemotherapy programs include the use of several agents with nonoverlapping toxicities and mechanisms of action. This allows the utilization of drugs at almost full doses. Another important attribute of the combinations has been the use of these drugs in intermittent schedules to allow for recovery of host toxicities and immune response. The effectiveness of combinations has increased the proportion of responses as well as the complete response rate. Several studies have clearly indicated the value of combinations over single agents used alone or in sequential fashion (Smalley et al., 1973; Hoogstraten and George, 1974). Despite these excellent response rates of 50% to 70% (Broder and Tormey, 1974), the duration of remissions and survival benefit are measured in months.

Since the purpose of this presentation is to present the rationale of the combined modality approach, the question of the relative effectiveness of chemotherapeutic regimens in the postoperative (adjuvant) situation and the advanced disease patient is relevant. The Eastern Group recently reported the results of a randomized study comparing L-phenylalanine mustard (L-PAM) and cyclophosphamide, methotrexate, and 5-fluorouracil (CMF) (Canellos et al., in press). The results are shown in Table 2. Using L-PAM 20% of the patients achieved a complete and/or partial response, a relatively weak effect. CMF treatment resulted in a 53% complete plus partial response rate ($p < 0.01$). Both of these regimens have also been used in the adjuvant situation and are commented on later.

Adriamycin is one of the most active single agents used in breast cancer chemotherapy with a tumor regression rate of about 40% (Hoogstraten and George, 1974; Carter, 1974). In combination chemotherapy trials Adriamycin added to cyclophosphamide, or cyclophosphamide, 5-fluorouracil, prednisone, and/or vincristine has had substantial improvement in complete and partial response rate

Table 2. Eastern Cooperative Oncology Group Study 0971

	CMF	L-PAM
Number of patients	93	91
Complete regression	15%	5%
≧ 50% Regression	38%	15%
Total response rates	53%	20%[a]

Data from Canellos et al. (in press).

[a]$p < 0.01$

(Blumenschein et al., 1975; Lloyd, Jones, and Salman, 1975; Bull et al., 1975). The most current approaches involve the use of all of the active drugs in three or four drug combinations used sequentially or alternating treatments (DeLena et al., 1975). The value of this approach has not been fully evaluated.

COMBINED MODALITY APPROACH

We have discussed the excellent results of treatment of murine tumors using surgery and chemotherapy (Schabel, 1975). Clinically there have been at least two studies done almost 10 years ago that have attempted to combine surgery and radiotherapy. Dr. Nissen-Meyer of the Scandinavian Breast Cancer Therapy Group employed cyclophosphamide postoperative for 5 days in stage I and II breast cancer. At 4, 5, and 6 years postoperatively there was a significant increase in survival (Nissen-Meyer, Kjellgren, and Marson, 1971). Another study done by the NSABP in the U.S.A., utilized thio-TEPA for 3 days postoperatively. Overall, there was no difference in disease-free survival and/or overall survival. However, in patients who were premenopausal and with ≧ 4 positive nodes there was a significant decrease in recurrences and an improvement in survival at 5 and 10 years (Fisher et al., 1975a). The basic concept behind these studies was that tumor cells were disseminated in showers into the vascular system via the manipulation of the primary tumor by the surgeon. Therefore, the chemotherapy was administered in a bolus perioperatively to kill off tumor cells before they started to grow as microscopic foci. We know that these studies were based on an erroneous concept of tumor cell growth. The kinetics of breast cancer growth indicate that these metastatic foci had been present prior to the initial diagnosis. Moreover, the minimal amount of chemotherapy administered was inadequate and failed to take into account the first order kinetics of cell kill by drugs (Wilcox, 1966). Longer term administration of chemotherapy seems to be indicated as well as the combinations of drugs to ensure a higher cell kill.

Modern adjuvant therapy began with a collaborative trial by the NSABP, Eastern Cooperative Oncology Group (ECOG), and the COG with the use of L-phenylalanine mustard (L-PAM) (Fisher et al., 1975b). In this trial patients were randomized to L-PAM or a placebo. All patients had positive nodes microscopically following a radical or modified radical mastectomy. The preliminary results indicated that a significant decrease in the recurrence rate occurred for patients receiving L-PAM. Particularly impressive were the results with patients who were premenopausal where there was only a 3% recurrence rate compared to a 30% failure rate in control surgery alone patients.

The choice of L-PAM as the agent for this trial was based on several premises. First, most patients with primary breast cancer are seen and treated by surgeons usually in smaller or primary care hospitals. Therefore, in this first trial it was important to select a drug that had known activity and relatively mild side effects. Second, the agent should, if possible, be easily administered, preferably by the oral route. Third, based on theoretical considerations of drug action, an alkylating agent or noncycle-sensitive agent would be preferable to a cell cycle-specific drug since in the latter situation more intensive and prolonged treatment needed to be given. For these reasons, L-PAM was chosen as the initial agent for trial in preference to other treatments. It was clearly appreciated by the investigators planning the trial that the strategy was to be one of building up an effective combination rather than to start off with a three or more drug trial. Since this trial involved many hospitals and was done primarily through surgeons, it was agreed that an intensive multidrug program was not feasible as a starting program.

Moreover, this study was part of an overall National Cancer Institute Breast Cancer Task Force treatment program that involved several integrated trials looking at various other options of treatment (Carbone, 1975). L-PAM was also tested almost simultaneously in advanced disease patients in the ECOG and produced a 20% response rate (Canellos et al., in press). The three-drug program involving cyclophosphamide, methotrexate, and 5-fluorouracil (CMF), the other arm of the ECOG study, was being tested in a similarly designed trial by Dr. G. Bonadonna in Milan (Bonadonna et al., 1975). The results in the adjuvant trial using this combination which achieved 53% response rate in advanced disease patients are particularly impressive. A 3% overall failure rate was achieved with CMF as compared to 30% in surgery alone controls. Table 3 compares the two trials by nodal and menopausal status. One can clearly see a striking correspondence between the two studies in terms of their relapse rates for surgery alone patients. The L-PAM treatment was clearly effective. The CMF treatment is obviously more effective than the single agent. However, the effect of L-PAM and CMF clearly supports the experimental data that effective treatment of early disease is a much more achievable goal than treatment of advanced disease.

ENDOCRINE THERAPY

The beneficial role of hormonal approaches to therapy have long been recognized in breast cancer. The use of additive hormonal therapy or ablative endocrine procedures clearly results in achieving tumor regressions in 20 to 30% of patients. Since the side effects were relatively mild and much has been learned about selection of patients for various treatment attempts, endocrine maneuvers are frequently applied as first approaches to managment of metastatic disease. The details of treatment and results have been summarized numerous times. In this paper, two relatively new concepts are stressed.

First, hormonally dependent cells, both normal and malignant, have been shown to possess a cytoplasmic receptor, estrogen receptor (ER). The cytoplasmic receptor specifically binds estrogens and transforms to enter the nucleus and then binds to nuclear chromatin. At a recent workshop several interesting aspects to the ER assay in breast cancer were appreciated (McGuire, Carbone, and Vollmer, 1975). The proportion of patients with breast cancer that are ER positive was about 60%. There was little relationship between clinical features of tumor size, node involvement, disease-free interval, and the ER assay. However, ER positivity was associated with a 56% response rate whereas the absence of the ER was associated with only a 5% probability of response. Thus, the absence of the ER assay in the tumor appears to be able to eliminate patients from the

Table 3. Recurrence rates for L-PAM and CMF adjuvant trials

	Positive nodes				Menopausal status			
	No. patients	1–3	No. patients	≥ 4	No. patients	Pre	No. patients	Post
Surgery alone								
Fisher (1975b)	74	8%	74	31%	54	24%	85	18%
Bonadonna (1975)	92	10%	36	33%	42	17%	86	16%
Surgery and chemotherapy								
Fisher	75	3%	73	16%	50	10%	86	10%
Bonadonna	70	1.4%	33	3%	48	0%	55	4%

Data as of February 1975.

hormone track and spare them from undergoing the morbidity and delay of endocrine treatment. More recently McGuire (unpublished data) has suggested that measurement of the progesterone receptor in the tumor cells clearly never occurs in the absence of the estrogen receptor and interestingly correlates with an endocrine response more often than the ER test.

A second new aspect to hormone therapy is the realization that chemotherapy and hormone therapy may be ideal candidates for combinations. Since, theoretically, removal of estrogens may slow down tumor growth, simple addition of the two treatments may result in antagonistic effects. The chemotherapy may be less responsive in the slower growing tumors. Adding estrogens to stimulate tumor growth and then giving chemotherapy has been tried empirically and has not been shown to be additive (Taylor et al., in press). Several trials are currently underway in the United States that attempt to combine chemotherapy and endocrine therapies (Carbone, 1975). These trials are being done in such a way to look at simultaneous and delayed combined approaches.

SELECTION OF THERAPIES

The use of tumor cell markers such as HCG, α-fetoprotein, and CEA is well known. These markers, while not necessarily cancer specific or diagnostic, can be used to follow the course of the disease following either primary or secondary treatments. Recently, Tormey and his collaborators (1975) have examined the relative incidence of several markers in patients with breast cancer. They have reported the presence of CEA, HCG, and a methylated tRNA to be increased in the blood or urine of 97% of 64 patients with metastatic breast cancer. In unpublished results, the level of these markers has correlated with the progression and regression of disease state as well as the extent of disease. Other markers will undoubtedly be developed that will be useful to follow the course of the disease, and may form a basis as to when treatment will be started and how long it will be continued.

The ER assay represents a major advance in the goal of cancer treatment to be specific. As yet the ability to decide which of the several chemotherapeutic agents should be given to maximize effect and decrease toxicity is not available. However, with the study of breast cancer cell lines derived from patients and the ability to allo-transplant human tumors into athymic mice, one can easily visualize the possibility of developing in vitro or in vivo test systems to delineate the appropriate assay system (Giovanella, Stehlin, and Williams, 1974).

SUMMARY

In this presentation, the author has attempted to show how human breast cancer, a common solid tumor, has become an important model system for asking important biologic questions. The many approaches to local treatment with surgery and radiotherapy have not shown marked differences in long-term therapeutic effectiveness, mainly because they all presume that breast cancer is a localized process. In reality most patients eventually die of their cancer despite local cure and therefore failure is a direct manifestation of micrometastatic disease at the time of initial treatment. Chemotherapy, likewise, when utilized as a last ditch effort rarely produces long-term benefit. Animal studies have shown us that curability of the solid tumor can be achieved readily only when the combination of local and systemic treatments is applied. Early attempts in combining chemotherapy and surgery in breast cancer involved too little systemic treatment. Modern day adjuvant trials have already shown dramatic effects on disease-free survival. The hormone-receptor assay for estrogen has proven to be effective in selecting specific therapy for individual patients. Other tumor markers are being examined.

Most important, however, is the feeling that while new basic advances in cancer research will undoubtedly produce new approaches, the current tools available for effective treatment of breast cancer when applied appropriately are capable of changing the natural history of breast cancer mortality. This idea is still only anticipatory but, using combination chemotherapy program and surgery, a dramatic effect on recurrence has already been seen. The application of these principles of combined modality treatment to other solid tumors will also prove to be effective, thus developing an increasing optimism for cancer victims.

REFERENCES

Atkins, H., J. L. Hayward, D. J. Klugman, and A. B. Wayte. 1972. Treatment of early breast cancer, a report after 10 years of a clinical trial. Brit. Med. J. 2:423–429.

Axtell, L. M., and M. H. Myers. 1975. Recent trends in survival of cancer patients 1960–1971. End Results in Cancer Report No. 4, DHEW Publication (NIH) No. 767.

Blumenschein, G. R., J. O. Cardenos, R. B. Livingston, L. H. Einhorn, E. J. Freireich, and J. A. Gottlieb. 1975. 5-fluorouracil, adriamycin and cyclophosphamide combination chemotherapy for metastatic breast cancer. Clin. Res. 23:336 (Abstr).

Bonadonna, G., E. Brusamolino, P. Valagussa, and U. Veronesi. 1975. Adjuvant therapy with combination chemotherapy in operable breast cancer. Proc. Amer. Assoc. Cancer Res. 16:254 (Abstr).

Broder, L. E., and D. C. Tormey. 1974. Combination chemotherapy of carcinoma of the breast. Cancer Treat. Rev. 1:183–203.

Bull, J., D. Tormey, G. Falkson et al. 1975. A comparison of cyclophosphamide, adriamycin and 5-fluorouracil versus cyclophosphamide, methotrexate and 5-fluorouracil in metastatic breast cancer. Proc. Amer. Assoc. Cancer Res. 16:246 (Abstr).

Caceres, E. 1967. An evaluation of radical mastectomy and extended radical mastectomy for cancer of the breast. Surg. Gynecol. Obstet. 125:337–341.

Canellos, G. P., S. J. Pocock, S. G. Taylor, III, M. E. Sears, D. J. Klasen, and P. R. Band. Combination chemotherapy for metastatic breast carcinoma: Prospective comparison of multiple drug therapy with L-phenylalanine mustard. Lancet. In press.

Carbone, P. P. 1975. The role of chemotherapy in treatment for breast cancer. In Cancer Chemotherapy—Fundamental Concepts and Recent Advances, pp. 311–322. Year Book Medical Publishers, Inc., Chicago, Ill.

Carter, S. K. 1974. The chemical therapy of breast cancer. Semin. Oncol. 1:131–144.

Crile, G. 1975. Results of conservative treatment of breast cancer at ten and fifteen years. Ann. Surg. 181:26–30.

DeLena, M., C. Brambilla, A. Morabito, and G. Bonadonna. 1975. Adriamycin plus vincristine compared to and combined with cyclophosphamide, methotrexate, and 5 fluoracil for advanced breast cancer. Cancer 35:1108–1115.

Fisher, B., N. H. Slack, P. J. Cavanaugh, B. Gardner, R. G. Ravdin, et al. 1970. Postoperative radiotherapy in the treatment of breast cancer: Results of the NSABP clinical trial. Ann. Surg. 172:711–732.

Fisher, B., N. Slack, D. Katrych, and N. Wolmark. 1975a. Ten year followup results of patients with carcinoma of the breast in a cooperative clinical trial evaluating surgical adjuvant therapy. Surg. Gynecol. Obstet. 140:528–534.

Fisher, B., P. Carbone, S. G. Economou, et al. 1975b. l-phenylalanine mustard (L-PAM) in the management of primary breast cancer; a report of early findings. New Eng. J. Med. 292:117–122.

Giovanella, B. C., J. S. Stëhlin, and L. J. Williams, Jr. 1974. Heterotransplantation of human malignant tumor in nude thymusless mice. II.

Malignant tumors induced by injection of cell cultures derived from human solid tumors. J. Natl. Cancer Inst. 52:921–930.

Halsted, W. S. 1894–1895. The results of operations for the cure of cancer of the breast performed at the Johns Hopkins Hospital from June 1889 to January 1894. Johns Hopkins Hosp. Rep. 4:297–350.

Hayward, J. 1974. The conservative treatment of early breast cancer. Cancer 33:593–599.

Hoogstraten, B., and S. George. 1974. Adriamycin and combination chemotherapy in breast cancer. Abstr. XI Internatl. Cancer Cong. 3:595 (Abstr).

Lloyd, R. E., S. E. Jones, and S. E. Salman. 1975. Phase II trial of adriamycin and cyclophosphamide; a Southwest Oncology Group pilot study. Proc. Amer. Assoc. Cancer Res. 16:265 (Abstr).

McGuire, W. L., P. P. Carbone, and E. P. Vollmer. 1975. Estrogen Receptors in Breast Cancer. Raven Press, New York. 284 pp.

Nissen-Meyer, R., K. Kjellgren, and B. Marson. 1971. Preliminary report from the Scandinavian Adjuvant Chemotherapy Study Group. Cancer Chemother. Rep. 55:561–566.

Schabel, F. M. 1975. Concepts for systemic treatment of micrometastases. Cancer 35:15–24.

Smalley, R. V., S. Murphy, Y. K. Chan, and C. M. Huguley. 1973. Comparison of two five drug regimens versus sequential chemotherapy in metastatic breast cancer. Cancer Chemother. Rep. 57:110 (Abstr).

Stolfi, R. L., D. S. Martin, and R. A. Fugmann. 1971. Spontaneous murine mammary adenocarcinoma: model system for evaluation of combined methods of therapy. Cancer Chemother. Rep. 55:239–249.

Taylor, S. G., III, S. J. Pocock, B. I. Shnider, J. Colsky, and T. C. Hall. Clinical studies of 5-fluorouracil + premarin in the treatment of breast cancer. Med. Pediatr. Oncol. In press.

Tormey, D. C., T. P. Waalkes, D. Ahmann, C. W. Gehrke, R. W. Zumwatt, J. Snyder, and H. Hansen. 1975. Biological markers in breast cancer. I. Incidence of abnormalities of CEA, HCG, three polyamines and three minor nucleosides. Cancer 35:1095–1100.

Wallace, I. J., and H. R. Champion. 1972. Axillary nodes in breast cancer. Lancet 1:217–218.

Wilcox, W. S. 1966. The last surviving cancer cell: the chances of killing it. Cancer Chemother. Rep. 50:541–542.

Zubrod, G. 1972. The basis for progress in chemotherapy. Cancer 30:1474–1479.

$\mathbf{M}$anagement
of Acute Leukemia

Richard H. Creech, M.D., F.A.C.P.

During the past 28 years, the progress in the treatment of acute lymphocytic leukemia (ALL) of childhood has been impressive. Before the discovery that aminopterin had antileukemic activity (Farber et al., 1948), these children survived less than 3 months. Gradually other effective drugs were found. Eventually, combinations of prednisone with vincristine, methotrexate, or 6-mercaptopurine induced complete remissions in 90% of cases. Next, remission durations were prolonged by using combinations of drugs including methotrexate and 6-mercaptopurine. More recently, prophylactic cranial radiation and administration of intrathecal methotrexate have greatly reduced the incidence of meningeal leukemia. These advances in antileukemic therapy as well as intensive support with new antibiotics and red cell, granulocyte, and platelet transfusions have resulted in a 50% 5-year survival. We now expect that many of these 5-year survivors will be cured of their leukemia.

Unfortunately, the same degree of progress has not been made in the treatment of adults with acute myelogenous leukemia (AML). Although the chemotherapy regimens in these patients are becoming more and more effective, and we can more effectively support patients through prolonged periods of pancytopenia, the majority of adults

This work was supported by Grant RR-05539 from the National Institutes of Health, and by an appropriation from the Commonwealth of Pennsylvania.

173

with this disease still die within 3 months of their initial diagnosis. At this time, successful remission induction offers the best opportunity for prolonged survival.

The aims of this discussion are: 1) to review the presenting symptoms and signs of acute leukemia; 2) to define the criteria for diagnosing acute leukemia; 3) to review specific clinical problems associated with this disease; 4) to review the development of chemotherapeutic regimens and prophylactic cranial irradiation and intrathecal methotrexate administration; and 5) to discuss the investigational techniques of laminar air flow rooms and oral nonabsorbable antibiotics, immunotherapy, and bone marrow transplantation.

PRESENTING SYMPTOMS AND SIGNS

The majority of acute leukemia patients present initially to their physicians with symptoms related to anemia, granulocytopenia, or thrombocytopenia. Anemia causes dyspnea and fatigue and, much less commonly, congestive heart failure. A wide spectrum of symptoms may be associated with granulocytopenia. In children, low-grade fever may be associated with a sore throat and minimal cervical adenopathy. The adult with acute myelogenous leukemia, on the other hand, often does not present with such a clinically benign picture. He may present with a perirectal abscess, severe bacterial pneumonia, periappendiceal inflammation simulating appendicitis, or sepsis. Thrombocytopenia-associated problems include petechiae, gingival bleeding, and gastrointestinal, intrapulmonary, or subarachnoid hemorrhage.

Patients with skeletal pain, sometimes associated with normal circulating blood counts, may be found to have acute leukemia at the time a bone marrow aspiration is performed. Although this type of presentation is rare, a hyperactive bone marrow should be suspected in any patient with symptomatic but poorly understood musculoskeletal syndromes.

It is important to remember that acute leukemia not only invades the bone marrow, but may infiltrate almost any area of the body and, if strategically located, may cause symptoms. Perhaps the most clinically devastating syndrome is intracranial hemorrhage associated with peripheral blast counts greater than 100,000/mm^3, cerebrovascular leukostasis, and intracerebral leukemic nodules (Moore et al., 1960). Since this rapidly fatal intracerebral hemorrhage is not often seen in patients with blast counts less than 100,000/mm³, immediate reduction of the circulating blast cell population is imperative.

Meningeal leukemia, before the advent of prophylactic cranial radiation therapy and intrathecal administration of methotrexate, occurred in approximately two-thirds of the patients entering prolonged systemic remissions. This syndrome includes nausea, vomiting, headaches, and lethargy in the early stages and papilledema, cranial nerve palsies, and convulsions in the more advanced stages. The diagnosis can be confirmed by lumbar puncture which reveals an increase in the opening pressure, opalescent fluid, an increase in the protein content, and a decrease in the glucose concentration due to its consumption by the great numbers of leukemic cells seen on cytologic examination. Cultures should be done to rule out bacterial and fungal causes of meningitis. Meningeal leukemia may be present at the time of initial diagnosis, particularly if the patient has an aggressive leukemia, often manifesting clinically with a circulating blast count of greater than 100,000/mm³. The symptoms and signs of this syndrome are caused by leukemic cell infiltration of the arachnoid, resulting in obstruction of cerebrospinal fluid flow (Moore et al., 1960).

Although dural infiltration by leukemic cells approaches 70% at autopsy, local symptomatic compression of the brain or spinal cord is extremely uncommon. Infiltration of cranial nerve sheaths and epidural deposits may occasionally cause clinical problems.

Patients with testicular masses, especially when associated with cytopenias, should be suspected of having acute leukemia. Although this complication is more common during the later phases of the disease, it may be an initial presenting complaint. Ovarian infiltration also occurs, but is much less frequent.

Gingival hypertrophy, similar clinically to Dilantin-induced hypertrophy, is often associated with acute monocytic or acute myelomonocytic leukemia.

DIAGNOSIS

Acute lymphocytic leukemia (ALL) accounts for 82% of all cases of acute leukemia occurring during childhood, with a peak incidence in the 3- and 4-year age group. Acute myelogenous leukemia (AML), on the other hand, occurs equally frequently in all age groups and accounts for 87% of all cases of adult acute leukemia (Hayhoe,

1968). AML is often called acute nonlymphocytic leukemia so that
the subclassifications of AML (63%), acute progranulocytic leukemia (4%), acute myelomonocytic leukemia (28%), and DiGugliel-
mo's erthroleukemia (5%) may be combined as one general category
in contrast to ALL (Ellison, 1973). Hereafter, for convenience, the
myelogenous subclassifications are collectively referred to as AML.

The previously described symptoms and signs should be evaluated by performing a hemoglobin, white blood cell count, platelet
count, peripheral blood smear, and bone marrow aspiration and
biopsy. In acute leukemia, the hemoglobin and platelet counts are
often subnormal while the white blood cell counts may be subnormal,
normal, or elevated. The peripheral blood smear with circulating
blast cells is often the first indicator of acute leukemia. This suspicion
must be confirmed by finding the bone marrow aspirate infiltrated with
acute leukemia cells. If no marrow can be aspirated, a bone marrow
biopsy must be performed to distinguish among aplastic anemia, marrow fibrosis, metastatic cancer, and acute leukemia. On examination
of the marrow aspirate, the diagnosis of acute leukemia can be made
relatively easily because of the monotonous infiltration by leukemic
cells.

Most cases can be classified morphologically as ALL or AML.
There are, however, a small percentage of patients with acute leukemia that is difficult to categorize. Special strains are often helpful
in evaluating these cases. Table 1 summarizes some of the morphologic features that help differentiate ALL from AML. The nuclei of
the ALL cells are dense and generally do not contain nucleoli,
whereas the cytoplasm is relatively scant and devoid of inclusion
bodies. A positive periodic acid-Schiff (PAS) stain for glycogen and
mucopolysaccharides is also helpful in identifying these cells. On the
other hand, there is moderate pleomorphism of the AML cells, the
nuclear chromatin stains lightly and the more abundant cytoplasm
contains inclusions, particularly the characteristic Auer rods. Cyto-
chemically the AML cells have peroxidase activity and the lipids
found in the mitochondria and cytoplasmic granules of these cells
stain with Sudan black B.

On physical examination the ALL patients may have shotty
adenopathy and mild hepatosplenomegaly whereas the AML patients
rarely have these findings. Gingival hypertrophy is most often associated with the monocytic leukemias. Patients with high circulating
blast counts or acute progranulocytic leukemia may develop intra-

Table 1. Morphologic differentiation of acute leukemias

	ALL	Malignant lymphoma with marrow involvement	AML
Degree of pleomorphism	Minimal	Moderate	Moderate
Staining of nuclear chromatin	Dark	Dark	Light
Number of nucleoli	Few	Several	Several
Amount of cytoplasm	Minimal	Minimal	Moderate
Cytoplasmic granules	Rare	Rare	Common (Esp. Progranulocytic)
Auer rods	No	No	Yes
Positive stains	PAS	PAS	Peroxidase Sudan black B

vascular coagulation, particularly after initiation of chemotherapy. Destruction of leukemic cells containing thromboplastin-like material can precipitate this clinical syndrome.

Patients presenting with marked adenopathy and pancytopenia may have bone marrow and peripheral blood involvement with non-Hodgkin's lymphoma. As can be seen in Table 1, their circulating cells have morphologic characteristics intermediate between ALL and AML cells. These cells have varying degrees of differentiation, darkly staining clefted nuclei containing several nucleoli, relatively small amounts of cytoplasm, and a positive PAS stain. The knowledge that the patient has marked adenopathy can be helpful when determining morphologically whether the patient has stage IV lymphoma with marrow involvement or acute leukemia.

Occasionally patients presenting with a pancytopenia are misdiagnosed as having acute undifferentiated leukemia. In reality, they have small cell carcinoma of the lung with bone marrow metastases. It is therefore important to evaluate carefully each patient's chest x-ray, particularly when the morphology of the "leukemic" cells is atypical.

ASSOCIATED CLINICAL PROBLEMS

During discussions of acute leukemia management, many physicians concentrate on the improved effectiveness of the most recently reported combinations of chemotherapeutic agents. Although these advances are important, it is perhaps even more important that these patients be cared for by physicians specializing in the treatment of these diseases. Continuous coverage by a well trained staff and facilities for aggressive support are necessary for optimal management. If the decision has been made to treat a patient with marrow hypoplasia-inducing regimens, the physicians must be prepared to support the patient during the periods of profound pancytopenia with its possible resulting complications of hemorrhage, infection, and emotional depression. The following problems should be anticipated in patients with acute leukemia and appropriate measures should be taken to minimize the possibilities of their causing morbidity.

Intracerebral Hemorrhage

As has been previously discussed, patients with circulating blast counts greater than $100,000/mm^3$ have an increased incidence of cerebrovascular leukostasis and intracerebral leukemic deposits associated with massive fatal intracerebral hemorrhage. This disastrous clinical syndrome can be obviated by quickly lowering the circulating blast count. This can be accomplished by initiation of specific antileukemic therapy or nonspecifically by the administration of intravenous cyclophosphamide at a dose of $1g/m^2$ of body surface area or by leukophoresis. Leukophoresis has the advantage of minimizing the circulating uric acid concentration caused by chemically induced cell destruction.

Uric Acid Nephropathy

Uric acid nephropathy due to accumulation of uric acid in the renal tubules and ureters can be prevented by ensuring that the patient's uric acid is normal before instituting chemotherapy. This can be achieved by adequate hydration and immediate institution of oral allopurinol therapy at a dose of 100 mg orally every 6 hours. With these measures, the uric acid can usually be reduced to the normal range within 24 to 48 hr. If a patient has good renal function and is not hyperuricemic at the time of chemotherapy-induced catabolism of purines to uric acid, the development of renal failure is unlikely.

Infection

At the National Cancer Institute, Levine et al. (1974) found in 450 autopsied patients having hematologic malignancies, that 69% died of infection, 11% of hemorrhage, 10% of infection and hemorrhage, and 10% of other causes. When the causes of systemic infection related to death were analyzed, septicemias were present in 53% of the patients and pneumonias in 43%. The etiologic agents associated with the septicemias and pneumonias were evenly divided among *Pseudomonas*, other gram-negative organisms, and the fungi. Pneumocystis Toxoplasma and viral agents accounted for only 6% of the lethal infections.

From these statistics it is obvious that infections, particularly sepsis and pneumonia, are the most prevalent life-threatening problems occurring during the treatment of patients with hematologic malignancies. The serious nature of these infections is magnified in these patients by the lack of host defenses, particularly granulocytes. Although there is often much discussion regarding the proper choice of antibiotics to cover the widest possible spectrum of possible infectious agents, it is more important that physicians attending these patients closely monitor patients' temperatures, do appropriate cultures soon after a temperature elevation becomes evident, and start wide-spectrum antibiotic coverage immediately, even though there is no evident source of infection or bacteriologic proof that the patient is infected. In granulocytopenic patients, especially those with less than 500 granulocytes/mm³, the time from temperature elevation through sepsis, shock, and death may be less than 12 hours. Because of the fulminant nature of sepsis in these patients, one cannot determine antibiotic coverage based on results of cultures and antibiotic sensitivities. Although this concept is initially difficult to accept, its importance is positively reinforced when a granulocytopenic patient becomes afebrile soon after immediate institution of antibiotic therapy and negatively reinforced when aggressive antibiotic coverage is begun only at the time a patient is in gram-negative shock. Nonleukemic patients in gram-negative shock are difficult enough to treat, but granulocytopenic patients in shock are almost impossible to save.

After appropriate cultures, newly febrile granulocytopenic patients should be started on maximum antibiotic coverage, assuming that the patient is septic and that any or several pathogens may be the etiologic agents. Carbenicillin and gentamicin are an effective combination against *Pseudomonas aeruginosa;* carbenicillin or clindamycin against *Bacteroides;* cephalothin or oxacillin against *Staphylococcus;* and combined cephalothin and gentamicin against most gram-negative bacteria. An effective wide-spectrum combination regimen consists of gentamicin (1 to 1.5 mg/kg, i.m., or slowly i.v., q. 8 hr), carbenicillin (5 g, i.v., q. 4 hr), and cephalothin (25 mg/kg, i.m., or carbenicillin (5 g, i.v., q. 4 hr), and cephalothin (25 mg/kg, i.v., q. 4 hr). These dosages are recommended for adults with normal renal function. Electrolytes should be followed closely because hyokalemia can be induced by the administration of large amounts of the sodium salt of carbenicillin. Intramuscular injections should be minimized in these patients because of the possibilities of thrombocytopenia-associated intramuscular hemorrhage, and subsequent granulocytopenia-related abscess formation. As soon as culture and sensitivity results become known, antibiotic coverage should be appropriately modified. Clindamycin (5 to 10 mg/kg, i.v., q. 6 hr) may be substituted for carbenicillin if the patient has a penicillin-resistant *Bacteroides* infection. Oxacillin (2 g, i.v., q. 4 hr) may be substituted for cephalothin if the patient has a penicillinase-producing *Staphylococcus* infection.

Besides sepsis, a particularly perplexing clinical problem in these patients is pneumonia. Without adequate circulating granulocytes, these infections are very difficult to diagnose and to control. The differential diagnoses of causative agents include *Pseudomonas*, gram-negative bacteria, gram-positive bacteria; the fungi, including *Candida, Aspergillus,* and *Mucor;* viruses including cytomegalovirus, varicella-zoster, Herpes simplex, vaccinia, measles; and protozoal infestations by Toxoplasma and Pneumocystis. Organisms cultured by routine bacteriologic techniques do not always correlate with subsequent autopsy-proved causes of pneumonia. It has therefore been necessary to resort to more aggressive diagnostic techniques, particularly in those patients with a rapidly progressive pneumonia which is not responding to maximal antibacterial therapy. Fiberoptic bronchial brushing has recently yielded positive diagnoses in patients with fungal and Pneumocystis pneumonias. The most certain method of making a correct diagnosis is by lung biopsy. This procedure may result in considerable morbidity, primarily because of the poor clinical condition of these patients. These patients often have severe hypoxia due to their extensive pneumonia and thrombocytopenia secondary to their leukemia or chemotherapy. An open lung biopsy preceded by platelet infusions in thrombocytopenia patients is preferred because the surgeon is in control of the lung at the time of the biopsy. If hemorrhage occurs, this can usually be controlled by local measures. A chest tube will facilitate re-expansion of the lung. On the other hand, percutaneous biopsy of involved lung is relatively simple to do and does not result in the morbidity of a limited thoracotomy. The disadvantage is that the surgeon does not have control of the biopsied lung if a pneumothorax or intrabronchial hemorrhage should occur. Although these procedures are formidable, the necessity for definitively diagnosing the etiologic agent in these pneumonias can be life-saving when specific therapy is given. Seriously ill patients with Pneumocystis pneumonia diagnosed pathologically on Gomori's methenamine silver stain can be effectively treated by the administration of pentamidine isethionate at a dose of 4 mg/kg/day intramuscularly for 10 to 14 days. This drug can be obtained from the Center for Disease Control in Atlanta, Georgia. Recently, pyrimethamine and sulfadizine have been advocated as an alternative form of therapy. Although this combination can effectively treat this disease, especially the more indolent cases, pentamidine is still favored as the most effective agent in patients with rapidly progressive pneumonia.

It is to be stressed that these patients should be evaluated and biopsied as quickly as possible because of the often rapid progression of the pneumonia. The pentamidine usually is not effective in reversing the clinical symptoms caused by Pneumocystis for 48 to 96 hr. It is therefore imperative that the patient have sufficient respiratory capacity and support to withstand worsening respiratory distress before clinical improvement occurs.

Some might argue that the patient should be treated for all possible causes of progressive pneumonia and avoid the morbidity of lung biopsy. Unfortunately, this would require the use of three nephrotoxic agents, including gentamicin, amphotericin B, and pentamidine. Combining these three drugs almost uniformly causes renal failure, a complication to be avoided in these critically ill patients. Walzer et al. (1974) reported a 46.8% morbidity rate from the administration of pentamidine. The toxicities include renal function impairment (23.5%), injection site reactions (18.3%), abnormal liver function tests (9.6%), immediate reactions (9.6%), hypoglycemia (6.2%), hematologic disturbances (4.2%), skin rashes (1.5%), and hypocalcemia (1.2%). Since this drug has major toxicity, it should not be used unless there is histologic or highly suggestive clinical evidence that a patient has Pneumocystis pneumonia.

If the lung biopsy shows a fungal infection, the treatment of choice is Amphotericin B, possibly in combination with 5-fluorocytosine. If Nocardia is identified, sulfadiazine should be used. Toxoplasmosis is treated with pyrimethamine and sulfadiazine. Folinic acid prevents host megaloblastosis induced by pyrimethamine without interfering with its toxic effect on the Toxoplasma. Viral infections are not influenced by any specific therapy. They often may be seen in association with other pathogens. We have recently successfully treated two patients with biopsy proved Pneumocystis and cytomegalovirus pneumonia by using pentamidine. We assume that the Cytomegalovirus component of the pneumonia was of less clinical significance than the Pneumocystis.

Hemorrhage

Hemorrhage is the second most common life-threatening problem in acute leukemia patients. It is generally associated with platelet counts less than 20,000/mm³. An individual's capillary integrity also significantly modifies the chance of spontaneous hemorrhage. Some patients with extremely low platelet counts may not have petechiae while others with platelet counts of greater than 50,000 may have massive hemorrhages. With the advent of platelet transfusions, the incidence of severe uncontrolled hemorrhage has been greatly reduced. Presently the indications for administration of platelets are variable. Some physicians will administer platelets to all patients with platelet counts less than 20,000/mm³ independent of physical signs of bleeding while others give platelets only to thrombocytopenic patients who are actively bleeding. Careful clinical evaluation of each thrombocytopenic patient, taking into consideration his platelet count and whether it has plateaued or is precipitously dropping, clinical evidence of bleeding, and knowledge of past hemorrhagic episodes as related to platelet counts, most often influences our decisions regarding the timing of platelet transfusions. If a thrombocytopenic patient is developing gingival bleeding, epistaxis, or progressive petechiae, platelets should be administered. If the platelet count is rapidly declining and the patient is beginning to develop petechiae, it can be assumed that the platelet count will continue to decline and that the patient will probably develop a more severe bleeding diathesis. In these examples, the administration of random donor platelets is likely to be of more benefit than the risk of sensitizing the patient to foreign platelet antigens. Since platelets carry HL-A antigens, repeated exposure to nonhistocompatible platelets will eventually result in transfusion reactions and refractoriness to random donor platelet transfusions.

One unit of platelets, containing an average of 7.5×10^{10} platelets, is obtained from the platelet-rich plasma of one 500-ml whole blood donation. Multiple units of platelets from random donors are concentrated and administered intravenously to thrombocytopenic patients as soon as possible after donation and preparation. Platelet increments per unit of platelets are determined at 1 and at 20 hr after transfusion. By following the increment in platelet count, the relative effectiveness of the transfusions can be determined. After the initial platelet transfusions the increments are maximal. After multiple transfusions, however, antibodies develop and cause refractoriness to subsequent platelet administration.

Yankee, Grumet, and Rogentine (1969) were able to circumvent the problem of refractoriness to random platelet donor transfusions by administering platelets from HL-A histocompatible siblings. By HL-A typing of lymphocytes of thrombocytopenic patients and family donors, they were able to correlate sustained platelet increments with HL-A histocompatibility of patient and donor. Since the results of histocompatibility testing are not readily available at most centers that treat leukemia patients, it is more practical to identify a histocompatible sibling by sequentially subjecting him to platelet phoresis and transfusing the individual sibling's platelets to the patient. By closely following the 1- and 20-hr post-transfusion platelet counts, the sibling's platelets causing a good increment, particularly at 20 hr, will later be found to be HL-A histocompatible. This sibling can support the thrombocytopenic patient with intermittent platelet donations for long periods of time.

More recently, Lohrmann et al. (1974), also working at the National Cancer Institute, have found that nonrelated, but HL-A histocompatible donors, can effectively support thrombocytopenic patients. Although thrombocytopenia is the most common underlying cause of hemorrhage in leukemic patients, local factors such as steroid-related or stress-induced gastrointestinal ulcers must also be carefully evaluated and treated.

In patients with markedly elevated circulating blast counts, the sudden lysis of cells after institution of chemotherapy may result in disseminated intravascular coagulation (DIC). The most well documented cases of DIC associated with leukemia, however, have occurred in patients with acute progranulocytic leukemia. It has been shown that these leukemic cells contain relatively large amounts of thromboplastic material which is presumed to initiate DIC. If these patients are closely monitored during the administration of chemotherapy, laboratory evidence of DIC can often be documented. Most of these patients, however, do not develop clinical evidence of DIC. For those who do develop a hemorrhagic diathesis secondary to ongoing DIC, heparin therapy can be beneficial despite the great risk of heparin-induced hemorrhage in a thrombocytopenic patient.

SPECIFIC ANTILEUKEMIC THERAPY

Chemotherapy

Since Farber first found aminopterin to be an effective antileukemic agent, the advances in the development of effective chemotherapeutic regimens for childhood ALL have been substantial. As can be seen in Table 2, single agent therapy for induction of complete remissions in childhood ALL ranges between 20 and 65%. Daunorubicin, vincristine, prednisone, and asparaginase are the most effective agents while cytosine arabinoside, cytoxan, 6-mercaptopurine, and metho-

Table 2. Complete remission induction in ALL

Drugs[a]	Children	Adults
ARA-C CTX 6MP MTX	20–30%	10–20%
DAUNO	45%	25%
VCR	55%	40%
PRED ASP	65%	45%
CTX + PRED 6MP + PRED MTX + PRED	80%	
VCR + PRED VCR + PRED + DAUNO VCR + PRED + 6MP + MTX	85–95%	50%
VCR + PRED + ASP		70%

[a]ARA-C, cytosine arabinoside; CTX, cytoxan; 6MP, 6-mercaptopurine; MTX, methotrexate; DAUNO, daunorubicin; VCR, vincristine; PRED, prednisone; ASP, asparaginase.

trexate are somewhat less effective. The combination of prednisone with cytoxan, 6-mercaptopurine, methotrexate, or vincristine improves the response rates to 80 to 85%. By adding daunorubicin or methotrexate and 6-mercaptopurine to the vincristine and prednisone regimen, the complete regressions in childhood ALL approach 95% (Henderson, 1969, 1973).

Adult ALL has not been found to be as responsive as childhood ALL. In Table 2 it can be seen that the adult complete regression rates for each regimen are approximately half those of the children (Henderson, 1969, 1973; Henderson and Glidewell, 1974).

As the remission rates improved, it became necessary to develop regimens for prolonging remissions. In Table 3, the median duration of remissions in childhood ALL is summarized. If patients receive no chemotherapy after remission induction, they relapse within 2 months. Maintenance with either vincristine or cytosine arabinoside does not prolong remissions whereas daunoribicin, asparaginase, or prednisone each prolongs remissions to 3 months. 6-Mercaptopurine

Table 3. Median remission duration—Childhood ALL

Drugs[a]	Months
None ⎱ ARA-C ⎰ VCR	2
DAUNO ⎱ ASP ⎰ PRED	3
6MP	3.5
6MP ⇌ VCR + PRED	7
MTX ⇌ 6MP ⎱ VCR + PRED + MTX + 6MP (POMP) ⎰	14
MTX (× 16)	10.5
MTX (× 16) ⇌ VCR + PRED	16
MTX (Schedule dependent—Holland, 1971)	5–36

[a]Abbreviations same as in Table 2; POMP, prednisone, vincristine, methotrexate, and 6-mercaptopurine.

prolongs remissions to 3.5 months, and if combined with intermittent reinduction courses of vincristine and prednisone extends remissions to 7 months. Alternating methotrexate and 6-mercaptopurine or intermittent vincristine, prednisone, methotrexate, and 6-mercaptopurine (POMP) therapy lengthens the median duration of remissions to 14 months (Henderson, 1973). The importance of intensive consolidation therapy after remission induction followed by prolonged maintenance therapy has been documented by Holland (1971). He found that 5-day courses of methotrexate given at 2-week intervals for 6 courses versus 16 courses resulted in remission durations of 5 and 10.5 months, respectively. If these consolidation courses were followed by maintenance biweekly methotrexate, the remissions could be extended to 20 and 36 months, respectively. He also found that intermittent reinduction with vincristine and prednisone during the 16-course consolidation could increase remission durations from 10.5 to 16 months.

In view of the preceding concepts, childhood ALL remissions are currently induced by vincristine and prednisone, which do not significantly affect the circulating normal red blood cells, granulocytes, or platelets. After three to six induction courses the marrow initially develops an intense erythroid hyperplasia followed by a normocellular marrow with less than 5% lymphoblasts present. This, along with normal circulating blood counts, constitutes a complete remission. A remission is then consolidated with intensive courses of therapy which usually include methotrexate and 6-mercaptopurine. After the intensive consolidation phase, the patients are started on a less intensive prolonged maintenance phase. The duration of maintenance therapy for patients with no evidence of active disease is variable. After 12 to 30 months of chemotherapy-induced and maintained complete remission, the likelihood of relapse if chemotherapy is discontinued is approximately 10%. With prolonged chemotherapy, however, the likelihood of developing chronic drug toxicity increases considerably. Since patients who relapse after chemotherapy is discontinued can usually be reinduced into a complete remission, serious consideration should be given to discontinuation of active chemotherapy in patients with prolonged disease control. The optimal time for discontinuation of therapy in disease-free children probably ranges between 1 and 3 years.

The treatment of adult AML is much more intensive than that of ALL. In these patients, the marrows have to be made hypoplastic, resulting in prolonged periods of great risk of developing life-threatening sepsis, pneumonia, and hemorrhage. The associated medical problems of the patients as well as their age greatly influence the outcome of chemotherapy. Often adult AML patients present initially with severe infections or hemorrhage which cannot be reversed despite maximum supportive therapy. If, however, the patient presents without complications and does not have significant medical problems, the chances of surviving intensive chemotherapeutic regimens are better. The importance of close observation, aggressive antibiotic therapy, and administration of blood products has been previously stressed.

The complete remission induction rates in AML are listed in Table 4. Childhood AML, although less responsive than childhood ALL, is more responsive than adult AML (Henderson, 1969). Methotrexate and 6-mercaptopurine have minimal remission induction activity. The two most effective agents against adult AML are cytosine arabinoside and daunorubicin. When used as single agents, they induce remissions in 30% of adults. POMP (prednisone, vincristine, methotrexate, and 6-mercaptopurine) induces 45% complete remissions in adults and 70% in children. Various combinations of thioguanine, daunorubicin, vincristine, prednisone, and cytoxan with

Table 4. Complete remission induction in AML

Drugs[a]	Children	Adults
6MP ⎫ MTX ⎭	10%	10%
ARA-C ⎫ DAUNO ⎭	50%	30%
6MP + MTX + PRED + VCR (POMP)	70%	45%
ARA-C + TG ⎫ ARA-C + DAUNO ⎪ ARA-C + DAUNO + VCR ⎬ ARA-C + DAUNO + VCR + PRED ⎪ ARA-C + CTX + VCR + PRED ⎭		45–65%
Intensive ARA-C + DAUNO		85%

[a]Abbreviations same as in Tables 2 and 3; TG, thioguanine.

cytosine arabinoside in the listed regimens result in 45 to 65% remission rates (Beard and Fairley, 1974). Most recently, preliminary reports show an intensive 7-day cytosine arabinoside infusion at 100 mg/m^2/day and 3 days of daunorubicin at 45 mg/m^2/day have induced 87.5% remissions in 16 patients treated (Henderson, personal communication, 1975). Corroboration of these results and expansion of this study will be necessary before this regimen can be accepted as the most effective regimen for adult AML patients under the age of 60. As in ALL, maintenance chemotherapy has been shown to be effective in prolonging remissions.

Because of the intensive nature of the AML treatment regimens designed to cause marrow hypoplasia, a physician must carefully evaluate the older patient. If a patient is physiologically old, managing him as an aplastic anemia patient is often preferable to intensive chemotherapy. Patients with preleukemia or smoldering acute leukemia are also best treated conservatively. Since patients in this latter group often have relative marrow hypoplasia and normally survive for longer periods than other AML patients, aggressive chemotherapy is often detrimental.

Radiotherapy

Although chemotherapy is the primary modality of therapy in acute leukemia patients, palliative radiotherapy can effectively relieve symptoms caused by local infiltration of cranial nerve sheaths, gonads, mucosa, and epidural areas. It is relatively ineffective in controlling established meningeal leukemia, but is very effective in preventing meningeal infiltration when administered prophylactically.

Prophylactic Central Nervous System Therapy

Since 1962, Simone et al. (1975) have studied methods for preventing the development of meningeal leukemia in children with ALL. Initially they found that 500 and 1,200 rads of prophylactic craniospinal irradiation were ineffective in reducing the incidence of meningeal leukemia. In study V, they found that 2,400 rads of cranial irradiation and intrathecal methotrexate prevented the development of meningeal leukemia in 90% of their patients. In study VI, they found that 2,400 rads of craniospinal irradiation prevented meningeal leukemia in 96% of treated patients while 67% of the control group receiving no prophylactic CNS therapy eventually developed meningeal leukemia. In study VII, 2,400 rads of cranial irradiation along with intrathecal methotrexate was compared with 2,400 rads of craniospinal irradiation. The incidence of meningeal leukemia in the combined modality group was 7% while in the craniospinal irradiated group it was 4% (Aur et al., 1973). Since the relapse rates were similar in the two groups and because irradiation of the spine as compared to intrathecal methotrexate caused more leukopenia necessitating interruption of chemotherapy, their present prophylactic CNS therapy includes 2,400 rads of cranial irradiation and intrathecal methotrexate. Although there have been occasional CNS complications with this therapy, the potential benefit of prolonged control of CNS leukemia outweighs the risks (Simone, 1973). Through the careful research of these investigators, prophylactic CNS therapy has added another dimension to the prolonged control of childhood ALL.

EXPERIMENTAL PROCEDURES

Laminar Air Flow Rooms and Prophylactic Antibiotics

Since serious infections associated with granulocytopenia have been the most serious problem in the treatment of patients with AML, several groups have studied the potential benefits of decreasing exogenous bacterial flora by isolation of patients in laminar air flow rooms as well as by reduction of endogenous bacteria through prophylactic administration of oral, nonabsorbable antibiotics. Levine et al.

(1973) found a 50% reduction in severe infections in laminar air flow room patients treated with oral antibiotics as compared to controls. Schimpff et al. (1975) and Yates and Holland (1973) also found that isolation and antibiotics reduced the number of severe infections. The efficacy of treatment with oral, nonabsorbable antibiotics without isolation is not clear. Levine et al. (1973) and Yates and Holland (1973) did not find any benefit from this therapy. On the other hand, Schimpff et al. (1975) found that infections were reduced in patients who continued to take the antibiotics, but that serious *Pseudomonas* infections occurred in 4 of 6 granulocytopenic patients who discontinued antibiotics.

Laminar air flow rooms and oral antibiotics, which suffer the disadvantages of expense, psychologic stress, and nausea, are impractical at present. These modalities of supportive therapy should therefore still be considered research techniques.

Granulocyte Transfusions

Granulocytes can be harvested from donors by single unit leukophoresis, continuous flow centrifugation, or continuous flow filtration. The single unit leukophoresis is time consuming and the cells collected are insufficient to improve circulating granulocyte counts unless chronic myelogenous leukemia donors with very high circulating granulocyte counts are used. The continuous flow NCI-IBM centrifuge can successfully harvest 1.5×10^{10} granulocytes from a normal donor during a 4-hr collection. These cells can increase the granulocyte count by $800/mm^3/m^2$ when transfused into a granulocytopenic patient. The chief disadvantage of this method is its expense (Levine et al., 1974). Continuous flow filtration takes advantage of the property of the granulocyte to adhere to nylon. Although up to 10^{11} granulocytes can be harvested by this technique, the increment is only one-fourth that of the cell separator. Therefore the actual number of "effective" granulocytes is similar for the two methods. The filtration method has the advantages of being less complex and more economical than the centrifuge (Boggs, 1974).

As was seen with platelet transfusions, HL-A compatibility is important in maximizing effective circulating granulocyte levels. Unlike platelets, the granulocytes have to be ABO matched. If the patient and sibling donor are HL-A and ABO matched, the average recovery of granulocytes 1 hr post-transfusion is 50%, whereas, with

ABO and increasing HL-A mismatching, the recovery rate approaches 5% (Graw et al., 1972).

Graw et al. (1972) compared the effectiveness of compatible granulocyte transfusions in 39 granulocytopenic septic patients with a matched group of 37 patients treated with similar antibiotic regimens. They found that 30% of the nontransfused patients survived their septic episodes as compared to 46% of the transfused patients. This study has been extended (Levine et al., 1974). The nontransfused patients' survival has remained stable, while the transfused patients' survival has increased to 75%. The median survival for the antibiotic group was 6 days and for the transfused and antibiotic group was 26 days.

Although this study suggests benefit from the administration of compatible granulocytes, results of prospective randomized trials are necessary before granulocyte transfusions can be considered other than a research technique.

Immunotherapy

Mathé et al. (1970) introduced the concept of immunotherapeutic maintenance of remission in ALL. In his initial 30 patient study, he found that BCG, allogeneic leukemic cells, or both prolonged remissions as compared to controls. This concept has not been corroborated by others (Medical Research Council, 1971; Leventhal et al., 1973; Heyn et al., 1973).

Powles et al. (1973) studied 45 AML patients who had been chemotherapeutically induced into complete remission. Nineteen received maintenance chemotherapy and 23 received chemotherapy and immunotherapy consisting of Heaf gun administered Glaxo BCG and intradermal irradiated allogeneic AML cells. Three patients were not included in the analysis. Maintenance chemotherapy was discontinued in all patients after 1 year of complete remission while immunotherapy was continued indefinitely. At the time of publication, 37% of the 19 patients receiving only maintenance chemotherapy were alive with a median survival of 303 days and 26% were in their first remission for a median duration of 188 days. Of the 23 patients allocated to chemoimmunotherapy, 70% were alive for a median of 545 days and 35% were in their first remission for a median of 312 days. The difference in survival between the two groups is statistically significant. If these findings are corroborated, the use of chemoimmunotherapy for maintenance of remissions in AML patients will be a valuable adjunct to our present AML treatment armamentarium.

Bone Marrow Transplantation

Bone marrow transplantation has been studied experimentally in patients with acute leukemia and aplastic anemia. The intent has been to repopulate the marrow with normal cells and perhaps induce an anti-tumor effect. All patients are immunosuppressed prior to transplantation from histocompatible siblings; Graw (Levine et al., 1974) has reviewed the data on 95 transplanted patients. Seventy-three percent of the transplants resulted in engraftment. Fifty-seven percent had graft versus host reactions despite HL-A matching and 37% died because of this problem. Another distressing finding has been the high incidence of fatal acute interstitial pneumonia. The median survival for all engrafted patients is in the 1- to 3-month range although approximately 10% of the AML patients have had prolonged unmaintained remissions. Because of the high mortality rate due to graft versus host reactions and post-transplant infections, this procedure should still be considered experimental.

SUMMARY

Acute leukemia presents to the physician as a combination of symptoms and signs related to anemia, granulocytopenia, thrombocytopenia, and local leukemic cell infiltration. The diagnosis is confirmed by obtaining blood counts, a peripheral smear, and bone marrow aspiration.

Although the chemotherapeutic regimens have been improved considerably since 1948, the life-threatening problems of infection and hemorrhage are still a complex clinical problem requiring intensive supportive care. Early and aggressive wide-spectrum antibiotic therapy in febrile granulocytopenic patients, aggressive diagnostic evaluations in patients with unresponsive pneumonias, and platelet transfusions have permitted many patients to survive long enough to enter complete remissions. The rapid reduction of elevated circulating blast counts and prevention of uric acid nephropathy have minimized morbidity.

Acute lymphocytic leukemia (ALL) of childhood has been more responsive to chemotherapy than adult acute myelogenous leukemia (AML). In ALL, combinations of vincristine and prednisone with or without asparaginase or daunorubicin have increased the complete remission rate to 95%. After remission induction, effective maintenance drugs, particularly methotrexate, have extended remission durations for several years. Most recently, prophylactic cranial irradiation and intrathecal methotrexate administration have reduced the incidence of meningeal leukemia from 67% to 4%. These advances have improved the 2-month prechemotherapy era survival to a 50% 5-year survival.

The advances in the management of adult AML have not been as great. Cytosine arabinoside and daunorubicin when used as single agents induce remissions in 30% of patients. When used with other agents, the remission rates increase to 50%. Recently intensive therapy with a combination of cytosine arabinoside and daunorubicin has further improved remission rates. Maintenance therapy, especially chemoimmunotherapy, has prolonged remissions.

At the present time laminar air flow rooms, nonabsorbable antibiotics, granulocyte transfusions, and bone marrow transplantation are still considered experimental techniques.

ACUTE LEUKEMIA WORKSHOP

Case A

A.B. is a 3-year-old boy who presented to his pediatrician with a 3-week history of cough and a temperature of 100°F. During the previous week his mother had noted several bruises caused by minor trauma. On physical examination the child had small cervical nodes, clear lungs, a slight tachycardia, a barely palpable liver and spleen, as well as numerous ecchymoses and petechiae. His temperature was 100.8°F.

A blood count showed a hemoglobin of 8, a white count of 250,000, and a platelet count of 22,000. The white cell differential showed 80% large lymphocytic-appearing cells with minimal cytoplasm, 10% normal mature lymphocytes, and 10% polies.

1. As the consultant, what is your differential diagnosis and what studies would you perform to establish a diagnosis?
2. After you have done these studies and made a diagnosis, what aspects of this child's clinical picture are most disturbing and how would you decrease the likelihood of life-threatening complications?
3. What therapy would you start for treatment of this child's primary disease process?

4. When do you think this therapy would result in an appreciable change in his primary disease process?
5. Provided the child had a beneficial response, what ancillary forms of therapy would you give in order to ensure the maximum possible prolonged benefit?

Fortunately the child had an unexpectedly good response to all of your therapeutic measures. After the sixth course of therapy, however, the child developed a temperature of 102°F. This was associated initially with a hacking cough and some dyspnea. The next morning the mother noted rapid shallow breathing, and duskiness of the nailbeds.

6. When the mother called you, what did you suggest she do to help you manage her child?
7. At the time you were able to evaluate the child, what studies did you perform?
8. What were your differential diagnoses?
9. After the diagnosis was confirmed histologically, what therapy did you start?
10. How long was it before your therapy proved to be effective?

Fortunately the child recovered from his acute respiratory distress and returned to normal activity.

The initially prescribed antileukemic therapy resulted in a complete regression which continued after 3 years of therapy.

11. What question regarding his therapy would you then ask yourself?

You made the correct decision because the patient is now doing well 8 years after the initial diagnosis.

Case B

Mr. C.D. is a 38-year-old airline pilot who suddenly developed excruciating rectal pain and saw his family physician. He noted that the patient looked pale and that his temperature was 103°F. The rest of the physical examination was normal except for tenesmus on rectal examination. Because of his rectal infection and pallor, he performed a blood count. It showed a hemoglobin of 7 g, white count of 500, and platelet count of 100,000. The differential was relatively normal, although there were a few atypical white cells.

1. Because of these findings, what should the family physician suggest to the patient regarding diagnostic work-up?

The patient agreed to this evaluation, was admitted to the hospital, and seen by a surgeon. The surgeon noted the tenesmus and could not feel any definite evidence of perirectal abscess. He stated that he would be willing to try to incise and drain the tender area.

   2. What did you decide?

Your hematologic consultant performed a bone marrow.

   3. What did it probably show?
   4. Which clinical problem was most disturbing?
   5. How did you evaluate and treat this patient?
   6. How should this patient's underlying condition be treated?
   7. What are the chances of a good result with this therapy and what special resources are necessary to ensure a maximally effective outcome?

Case C

Mrs. E.F. is a 78-year-old patient with severe emphysema and a history of a cerebrovascular accident 1 year before you saw her initially. She was referred to you by her family physician because of a mild anemia of 7.5 g %.

   1. In order to evaluate her anemia, what tests did you obtain?

The bone marrow showed a cellular marrow with erythrocytic hyperplasia. The white cell series was somewhat atypical because of the slight left shift and the mild megaloblastic changes in the erythrocytic and granulocytic series. The iron stain showed increased stores with many ringed sideroblasts.

   2. What studies did you then obtain?

These studies were not conclusive.

   3. Because of the bone marrow abnormalities, what did you tell the referring doctor regarding diagnosis, treatment, and prognosis?

The patient did relatively well on your prescribed therapy for 6 months. She then became progressively weak. At that time the physical examination had not changed. The hemoglobin, however, had fallen to 4.5 g % and the white count had increased to 15,000/mm^3.

   4. What did you do next?
   5. What did the bone marrow most likely show?

Your worst fears were realized.

   6. What alternative types of therapy did you consider and how did you arrive at your ultimate therapeutic decision?

ANSWERS TO ACUTE LEUKEMIA WORKSHOP QUESTIONS

Case A

Answer 1: The most likely diagnosis is acute lymphocytic leukemia because of the high circulating lymphoblast count and thrombocytopenia. In less pronounced cases, other causes of lymphocytosis such as pertussis, infectious lymphocytosis, and infectious mononucleosis should be carefully considered. The diagnosis is made on bone marrow aspiration.

Answer 2: The most disturbing problems are possible massive intracerebral hemorrhage associated with blast counts greater than $100,000/mm^3$, bleeding from thrombocytopenia, uric acid nephropathy, and sepsis. Morbidity can be decreased by lowering the blast count with chemotherapy or leukophoresis, administering platelets, hydrating the patient, beginning allopurinol and treating infection.

Answer 3: A combination of vincristine and prednisone is the most effective remission induction regimen.

Answer 4: He should start feeling better within 2 weeks and will probably be in a complete remission in 4 weeks.

Answer 5: In order to maintain the patient in a complete remission for as long a time as possible, he should receive intensive consolidation chemotherapy, less intensive maintenance chemotherapy, and prophylactic cranial irradiation and intrathecal methotrexate.

Answer 6: Bring him to the hospital *immediately*.

Answer 7: Chest x-ray, arterial blood gases, and routine bacteriologic cultures. If the chest x-ray showed a rapidly progressive interstitial pneumonia, the child should have fiberoptic bronchial brushings or a lung biopsy performed.

Answer 8: The differential diagnoses include bacterial, fungal, viral, and protozoal pneumonias.

Answer 9: The patient was proved to have Pneumocystis carinii pneumonia. He was started on pentamidine isethionate at a dose of 4 mg/kg/day intramuscularly for 10 days.

Answer 10: The patient continued to have progressive pulmonary insufficiency with anoxia for 48 hr before stabilizing and beginning to improve.

Answer 11: Am I potentially causing chronic toxicity which may be more detrimental than the small likelihood of the patient relapsing? Because only 10% of patients relapse within the 1st year after discontinuation of prolonged maintenance chemotherapy and the majority can be readily reinduced into remission, it was decided to stop therapy.

Case B

Answer 1: He should be admitted to the hospital immediately, cultures taken, and a bone marrow aspiration performed.

Answer 2:   You elected not to have any surgery performed because it would not be beneficial and most probably cause sepsis.

Answer 3:   Acute myelogenous leukemia.

Answer 4:   The perirectal abscess associated with granulocytopenia.

Answer 5:   The patient had cultures performed immediately after admission and was begun on intensive antibiotic therapy.

Answer 6:   After bacteriologic stabilization, this patient should receive intensive chemotherapy with a regimen including cytosine arabinoside and daunorubicin.

Answer 7:   If the patient initially survives his sepsis the chances of having a remission are approximately 50%. In order to ensure a beneficial outcome, the patient must be watched carefully and aggressively supported as problems develop.

Case C

Answer 1:   The patient should have a complete blood count, evaluation of the peripheral smear, and bone marrow aspiration.

Answer 2:   Folate and B_{12} levels and a Schilling test.

Answer 3:   Her primary diagnosis is sideroblastic anemia with some atypical changes in the bone marrow suggesting preleukemia. The patient can be treated with packed red cell transfusions, pyridoxine, and folic acid, assuming that she has secondary sideorblastic anemia. Her prognosis is related to whether or not she develops acute leukemia.

Answer 4:   Her platelets, peripheral smear, and bone marrow aspirate were re-evaluated.

Answer 5:   Acute myelogenous leukemia.

Answer 6:   Because of the patient's age and frailty due to previous medical problems, the toxicities of chemotherapy were thought to outweigh the potential of developing a remission. The patient was therefore treated with red cell transfusions and other conservative supportive measures.

REFERENCES

Aur, R., H. Hustu, M. Verzosa, A. Wood, and J. Simone. 1973. Comparison of two methods of preventing central nervous system leukemia. Blood 42:349–357.

Beard, M., and Fairley, G. 1974. Acute leukemia in adults. Semin. Hemat. 11:5–24.

Boggs, D. 1974. Transfusion of neutrophils as prevention or treatment of infection in patients with neutropenia. New Eng. J. Med. 290:1055–1062.

Ellison, R. R. 1973. Acute myelocytic leukemia. In J. F. Holland and E. Frei, III (eds.), Cancer Medicine, pp. 1199–1234. Lea and Febiger, Philadelphia.

Farber, S., L. Diamond, R. Mercer, R. Sylvester, and J. Wolff. 1948. Temporary remissions in acute leukemia in children produced by folic acid antagonist 4-aminopetroylglutamic acid (Aminopterin). New Eng. J. Med. 238:787–793.

Graw, R., G. Herzig, R. Perry, and E. Henderson. 1972. Normal granulocyte transfusion therapy. New Eng. J. Med. 287:367–371.

Hayhoe, F. G. J. 1968. Clinical and cytological recognition and differentiation of the leukemias. *In* C. J. D. Zarafonetis (ed.), Proceedings of the International Conference on Leukemia-Lymphoma, pp. 307–320. Lea and Febiger, Philadelphia.

Henderson, E. 1969. Treatment of acute leukemia. Semin. Hematol. 6: 271–319.

Henderson, E. S. 1973. Acute lymphocytic leukemia. *In* J. F. Holland and E. Frei, III (eds.), Cancer Medicine, pp. 1173–1199. Lea and Febiger, Philadelphia.

Henderson, E. S., and O. Glidewell. 1974. Combination therapy of adult patients with acute lymphocytic leukemia (ALL). Proc. Amer. Assoc. Cancer Res. 15:102.

Heyn, R., W. Borges, P. Joo, M. Karon, M. Nesbit, N. Shore, N. Breslow, and D. Hammond. 1973. BCG in the treatment of acute lymphocytic leukemia. Proc. Amer. Assoc. Cancer Res. 14:45.

Holland, J. F. 1971. E Pluribus Unum: presidential address. Cancer Res. 31:1319–1329.

Leventhal, B., A. LePourhiet, R. H. Halterman, E. S. Henderson, and R. B. Herberman. 1973. Immunotherapy in previously treated acute lymphatic leukemia. Natl. Cancer Inst. Monogr. 39:177–188.

Levine, A., S. Siegel, A. Schreiber, J. Hauser, H. Preisler, J. Goldstein, F. Seidler, R. Simon, S. Perry, J. Bennett, and E. Henderson. 1973. Protected environments and prophylactic antibiotics. New Eng. J. Med. 288:477–483.

Levine, A., S. Schimpff, R. Graw, and R. Young. 1974. Hematologic malignancies and other marrow failure states: Progress in the management of complicating infections. Semin. Hematol. 11:141–202.

Lohrmann, H-P., M. Bull, J. Decter, R. Yankee, and R. Graw. 1974. Platelet transfusions from HL-A compatible unrelated donors to alloimmunized patients. Ann. Intern. Med. 80:9–14.

Mathé, G., J. L. Amiel, L. Schwarzenberg, M. Schneider, A. Cattau, M. Hayat, F. deVassal, and J. R. Schlumberger. 1970. Strategy of the treatment of acute lymphoblastic leukemia: Chemotherapy and immunotherapy. Recent Results Cancer Res. 30:109–137.

Medical Research Council. 1971. Treatment of acute lymphoblastic leukaemia. Comparison of immunotherapy (BCG), intermitten methotrexate, and no therapy after a five-month intensive cytotoxic regimen (Concord Trial). Preliminary report to the Medical Research Council by the Leukaemic Committee and the Working Party on Leukaemia in Childhood. Brit. Med. J. 4:189–194.

Moore, E., L. Thomas, R. Shaw, and E. Freireich. 1960. The central nervous system in acute leukemia. Arch. Intern. Med. 105:451–468.

Powles, R., D. Crowther, C. Bateman, M. Beard, T. McElwain, J. Russell, T. Lister, J. Whitehouse, P. Wrigley, M. Pike, P. Alexander, and G.

Fairley. 1973. Immunotherapy for acute myelogenous leukemia. Brit. J. Cancer 28:365–376.

Schimpff, S., W. Greene, V. Young, C. Fortner, L. Jepsen, N. Cusack, J. Block, and P. Wiernik. 1975. Infection prevention in acute nonlymphocytic leukemia. Ann. Intern. Med. 82:351–358.

Simone, J. V. 1973. Preventive central-nervous-system therapy in acute leukemia. New Eng. J. Med. 289:1248–1249.

Simone, J. V., R. Aur, H. Hustu, M. Verzosa, and D. Pinkel. 1975. Combined modality therapy of acute lymphocytic leukemia. Cancer 35: 25–35.

Walzer, P., D. Perl, D. Krogstad, P. Rawson, and M. Schultz. 1974. Pneumocystis carinii pneumonia in the United States: epidemiologic, diagnostic, and clinical features. Ann. Inter. Med. 80:83–93.

Yankee, R., F. Grumet, and G. Rogentine. 1969. Platelet transfusion therapy. New Eng. J. Med. 281:1208–1212.

Yates, J., and J. Holland. 1973. A controlled study of isolation and endogenous microbial suppression in acute myelocytic leukemia patients. Cancer 32:1490–1498.

Brief Overviews of Management and Detection

Chronic Leukemia

S. Benham Kahn, M.D., F.A.C.P.

CHRONIC MYELOGENOUS LEUKEMIA (CML)

This disease has two phases, the chronic phase and the acute phase. Management of the acute phase is similar to and is discussed under the management of acute nonlymphoblastic leukemia. Problems that are likely to arise in the chronic phase of the disease are listed in Table 1.

Management

It is the usual practice to initiate therapy as soon as the diagnosis is established since the disease runs a fairly rapid course and the patient, even if asymptomatic, will soon develop clinical symptoms.

Reduction of Cellular Proliferation A number of chemotherapeutic agents are available but the most commonly used are: 1) busulfan, 2) melphalan, 3) hydroxyurea, and 4) radiation therapy.

Busulfan In many clinics, including ours, busulfan is the therapy of choice. Doses of 4 to 10 mg per day are customarily begun. The level of the initial dose is proportionate to the presenting white blood count (WBC). For example, for a WBC in excess of $100,000/\mu l$ a dosage of 10 mg daily is begun, while a dosage of 8 mg is given for a WBC between 75,000 and $100,000/\mu l$, 6 mg for a WBC between

Table 1. Problems in chronic myelogenous leukemia

Problem	Pathogenesis
Leukocytosis	Cellular proliferation
Anemia	Dilution (and some suppression)
Splenomegaly	Proliferation of cells
Hyperuricemia and increased LDH	Increased cellular turnover
Thrombocytosis and bruisability	Increased survival of abnormal platelets
Weight loss, weakness, and sweating	Hypermetabolism

50,000 and 75,000/μl, and 4 mg daily for a WBC less than 50,000/μl. The daily dose rate is not as important as is the total dosage. Generally speaking, about 125 to 250 mg of the drug are required to bring the WBC to a near normal level. In general, a rule of thumb states that, when the WBC halves, the daily dose rate should be halved. The patient should be checked weekly and a complete blood count (including platelets) should be performed. Maintenance therapy is usually begun when the WBC reaches 10,000/μl. At this time the spleen has regressed to almost normal size, the hemoglobin concentration has risen to above 12 g % and the platelet count is within the normal range. Dosages of 2 mg daily (or even less) may be all that is necessary to maintain the remission.

The most important dosage limitation is marrow depression. Thrombocytopenia may occur before the WBC reaches 10,000/μl and if the platelet count falls below 200,000/μl during therapy the drug should be stopped. Continued therapy may result in marrow aplasia. Unfortunately, the induction of aplasia has not resulted in prolonged survival even if the patient recovers from this toxic effect. Toxic side effects of busulfan include pulmonary fibrosis, hyperpigmentation of the skin, cataracts, and an Addisonian-like pucture. These toxicities are unusual and can be halted if dosage is reduced. Sterility and amenorrhea occur frequently during therapy but reproductive function may be restored if the drug is stopped.

Melphalan The dosage and management schedules are similar to busulfan. Marrow suppression, especially thrombocytopenia, occurs with the same frequency and at approximately the same dosage levels as with busulfan. Pulmonary changes and the Addisonian-like syndrome are less frequently seen. This drug is an excellent alternative if the patient shows intolerance to busulfan.

Hydroxyurea   This drug may be used in the initial therapy of the disease but because of expense and frequency of side effects (most commonly nausea), its use is not recommended. The initial dosage is 40 to 50 mg/kilo/day in divided doses or a single dose and maintenance therapy is 30 mg/kg/day.

Patients who fail to respond to busulfan may respond to hydroxyurea. Thus, the drug is an excellent back-up drug for use in those patients who are truly busulfan-resistant but who are not entering the blast crisis. An example of such a patient is one who develops thrombocytopenia (with busulfan) before the white count comes under control.

Marrow suppression during hydroxyurea therapy is easily corrected. This is an advantage over busulfan. However, nausea, vomiting, anorexia, alopecia, and skin rash occur with a much greater frequency with this drug than with busulfan.

Radiation Therapy   In the past, P-32 or irradiation to the spleen was recommended. However, data comparing irradiation to chemotherapy indicate that chemotherapy results in better survival than irradiation therapy. Therefore, irradiation therapy alone is no longer recommended.

Experimental Protocols   Despite the fact that more than 90% of all patients with CML may enter remission when chemotherapy is administered, overall life expectancy following diagnosis and successful induction of remission is less than 5 years. In an effort to improve these results and in consideration of the fact that the disease terminates as an acute leukemia, several investigative groups have initiated protocols utilizing drugs such as cytosine arabinoside and 6-thioguanine. Splenectomy after initial remission is also being evaluated. At the present time, no firm data concerning survival improvement are available but pilot projects attest to the usefulness of this approach in controlling cellular proliferation, and the safety of splenectomy early in the disease has been proved.

Hyperuricemia and Hyperuricosuria   Usually the serum uric acid level returns to normal when the remission occurs, but prevention of urate build-up may be achieved by the administration of Allopurinol, 300 to 600 mg/day. Renal stones may be prevented by adequate hydration and the use of the sodium bicarbonate to alkalinize the urine.

Hypermetabolism   The signs of hypermetabolism include fever, weight loss, and sweating. These signs are lessened as the proliferative phase of the disease is brought under control by chemotherapy. The use of Indomethacin may help control fever and an anabolic agent may be useful to control weight loss. The latter agents may be useful when the patient becomes resistant to chemotherapy.

Resistance to Therapy   A few patients fail on all standard forms of chemotherapy. In those patients who show resistance to chemotherapy (usually because of the thrombocytopenia) but who continue to have high granulocyte counts, leukophoresis may be useful. Some investigators have attempted to maintain all of their CML patients by means of leukophoresis with the rationale that this procedure maintains the patient in a symptom-free state and provides needed white cells to other patients with acute leukemia or aplasia of the marrow. As laudable as the latter goal is, it does not truly treat the patient except in a very superficial way. When one has little else to offer, however, leukophoresis may help lessen some symptoms of this disease. However, in our experience, leukophoresis has not been a useful method of controlling CML.

CHRONIC LYMPHOCYTIC LEUKEMIA (CLL)

This disease has a longer and more variable prognosis than does CML. Specific anti-leukemic therapy does not effect as complete control of the proliferative aspect of the disease as does busulfan in CML. Finally, the disease is much more indolent and less likely to produce symptoms than is CML. For these reasons, the clinician is faced not only with the problem of selecting an agent but also with the problem of deciding when to treat the patient.

The problems created by this disease are listed in Table 2.

Management

The patient with CLL may present with any one of a combination of the problems presented in Table 2. In many patients, the only abnormality found is lymphocytosis. Such patients need not be treated since many of them show no symptoms of illness for years, even if nothing is done. In such cases, the side effects of therapy are worse than the disease itself.

However, once a specific problem or set of problems such as those listed occurs, therapy is indicated. While the height of the

Table 2. Problems in chronic lymphocytic leukemia

Problem	Pathogenesis
Lymphocytosis	Cellular proliferation
Nodal enlargement, splenomegaly, and local pressure on adjacent organs	Cellular proliferation
Anemia	Marrow invasion and immune disturbance
Thrombocytopenia	Marrow invasion and immune disturbance
Granulocytopenia	Marrow invasion
Increased incidence of infection	Immune disturbance and granulocytopenia
Hypogammaglobulinemia	Block or defective production due to altered immune function
Weight loss, anorexia	Hypermetabolism
Skin lesions, including herpes zoster	"Allergic phenomena" and immune suppression

lymphocyte count is not in and of itself an indication of the need for therapy, once the count shows a tendency to rise, other problems usually follow. This is especially true when the lymphocyte count reaches 100,000/μl.

Reduction of Cellular Proliferation   The following agents are useful in reducing the tumor load in CLL: 1) alkylating agents (for example, cyclophosphamide and chlorambucil); 2) radiation therapy; and 3) corticosteroids.

Alkylating Agents   The backbone of almost all therapeutic programs in CLL involves the use of alkylating agents. Most often chlorambucil, 4 to 10 mg/day, is begun, with larger doses given to patients with higher WBC counts. As with most alkylating agent therapy, the total dose administered is more important than is the daily dose rate. A total dose of 3 to 6 mg/kg delivered over 30 to 60 days usually reduces the WBC and yields clinical improvement. If cyclophosphamide is chosen the total dose is 25 to 50 mg/kg over 1 to 2 months.

As the tumor bulk is reduced, anemia and thrombocytopenia usually lessen and lymph nodes and other tumor masses begin to shrink. At this time maintenance therapy is begun and continued on an indefinite basis.

Once therapy is begun the patient should be followed at weekly intervals for the first week and then every 2 weeks for several months. A complete blood count and platelet count should be done on each visit. Follow-up on a monthly basis when the patient is on maintenance therapy is the usual practice.

The chief dose-limiting side effect of alkylating agent therapy is marrow suppression. Further suppression of an already low red blood count (RBC), platelet, and granulocyte count may occur. This usually indicates a fair degree of resistance to therapy and suggests the need for other agents such as androgens and corticosteroids.

Alopecia, skin rash, or cystitis may occur following the use of these agents (especially cyclophosphamide). Fortunately, these toxicities are reversible if therapy is stopped.

Radiation Therapy P-32 therapy for CLL has been largely replaced by chemotherapy. P-32 is inconvenient and very difficult to titrate. However, external beam irradiation of tumor masses may be required in selected instances. For example, spinal epidural masses may require radiation therapy, chemotherapy, and surgery for management if paralysis is to be prevented. Groin, axillary, and mediastinal masses may require irradiation in addition to chemotherapy in order to relieve symptoms fully. Most tumor masses are very sensitive to rather moderate doses of irradiation, and if after chemotherapy the symptoms related to the presence of such masses persist, irradiation therapy as a supplement to chemotherapy should be ordered.

Corticosteroids These agents are rarely used alone in CLL, although they will reduce tumor bulk in about 50% of patients. These drugs, however, if used in combination with alkylating agents create a very effective combination. Usually, prednisone, 0.5 to 1 mg/kg, is given along with an alkylating agent. The dosage of prednisone is reduced to 0 over a 2- to 3-week period while the alkylating agent is continued. Alternate day schedules are not recommended. Short bursts of chemotherapy for 5 to 10 days may be useful periodically if tumor load seems to be increasing while maintenance alkylating agent chemotherapy is being administered.

Combination Chemotherapy At times patients with CLL will present a picture that is much more aggressive than the usual. Tumor load is rather large, as evidenced by large bulky lymph nodes and a very high WBC. The morphology of the lymphoid cells may show characteristics of immaturity (i.e., nucleoli and more finely reticulated chromatin). Such clinical pictures have even been called chronic lymphosarcoma cell leukemia. In these instances, periodic courses of intensive cyclic chemotherapy may be necessary to control the disease. A combination that is often used includes vincristine, 1 mg/m on day 1; cytoxan, 1,100 mg/m^2 on day 1; and prednisone, 50 to 100 mg/m^2 each day for 5 days. These cycles or cycles similar to these are repeated every 21 days. This therapy is very effective in the management of patients with lymphosarcoma and reticulum cell sarcoma and may be valid in patients who have the aggressive form of chronic lymphocytic leukemia. (N.B. The usefulness of intensive chemotherapy in early CLL is being evaluated by some groups.)

Control of Altered Immunity   About 20% of patients will develop immunohemolytic anemia, or a syndrome resembling ITP, or a skin rash (not caused by local invasion). These are instances of aberrant immune function.

Immunohemolytic Anemia   This anemia, whose main diagnostic characteristic is a positive direct Coombs' test, should be managed by the administration of large doses of corticosteroids. This complication may occur at any time during the course of CLL and indeed may be the presenting sign of CLL. After beginning corticoid therapy, in approximately 2 weeks the anemia will be brought under control. However, a minority of patients may fail to respond to this therapy and may actually enter a terminal state because of this complication. Splenectomy may be resorted to in such instances and in over 50% of such patients there will be control of the disease. Splenectomy may also convert a relatively high dose corticosteroid-dependent patient to a rather sensitive patient who can then be maintained on rather small doses of corticosteroids. No matter what therapy is needed, it is likely that the patient will require small doses of corticosteroids and frequent monitoring of the Coombs' test for the duration of his life. Blood transfusions are often impossible and even if a unit is found the risk of reaction is very high. Patients with hemolytic anemia should also be treated with alkylating agents to reduce tumor bulk.

ITP   A minority of patients with CLL will present with severe thrombocytopenia, no splenomegaly, and adequate numbers of megakaryocytes in the marrow. Were it not for the presence of the large number of lymphocytes, such patients would be diagnosed as having ITP. These patients also seem to respond to corticosteroids. However, more often than not splenectomy will bring this problem under control or at least will convert a resistant patient to a sensitive one. This syndrome must be differentiated from the thrombocytopenia that occurs as the disease affects the marrow. In the latter instance, bone marrow megakaryocytes are absent while in the ITP syndrome they are abundant.

Skin Rash Severe exfoliative erythroderma may be under unusual circumstances a presenting sign of CLL. It is axiomatic that any person presenting with an exfoliative erythroderma should be considered to have a lymphoma. This problem is very difficult to control without the use of corticosteroids. Administration of alkylating agents is indicated to reduce tumor bulk and corticosteroids are given to afford relief of the skin manifestations. However, the skin lesions tend to remain resistant and fairly chronic.

Improvement of Marrow Function and Correction of Cytopenias

Androgens Androgens are extremely useful in the management of patients with lymphoproliferative disease. Even without reduction of tumor bulk, androgens may raise the red cell mass by causing stimulation of red blood cell production in the marrow. A combination of androgens with appropriate treatment of the tumor bulk by the use of alkylating agents and corticosteroids in our hands is a very valid approach to the management of many patients with CLL. Side effects of the androgens include a tendency towards hyperuricemia, increased sweating, increased appetite, acne, some change in libido, and perhaps a slight change in prostatic size. Because CLL is a disease of elderly men, it is exceedingly important to evaluate these individuals for carcinoma of the prostate before therapy. In our experience we have not seen any patient develop carcinoma of the prostate on androgen therapy. In addition, we have noted, even in the absence of specific chemotherapy for CLL, an improvement in platelet count and granulocyte count suggesting that the androgens stimulate myeloid and megakaryocyte function as well as erythroid activity in the marrow.

Splenectomy Splenectomy may find its greatest use in CLL in the management of the ITP syndrome and in certain instances of resistant immunohemolytic anemia. However, in any instance in which the spleen enlarges and the marrow shows an attempt to produce normal cells while a pancytopenia persists, splenectomy may be indicated for hypersplenism. This is much more commonly seen in the lymphomas than it is in CLL.

Control of Infection   Hypogammaglobulinemia occurs very often in CLL. Because of the hypogammaglobulinemia, granulocytopenia, debility, weight loss, and altered organ function that is commonly seen in the elderly, these patients are exceedingly susceptible to infection. Pneumonia is the most common infection, although urinary tract infection and skin infection are fairly frequent. Vigilance in the detection of these infections is absolutely essential if the patient is to be helped. Cultures followed by aggressive antibiotic therapy are usually ordered. Hypogammaglobulinemia is not usually improved nor is infection prevented by the administration of parenteral γ-globulin. In rare instances, herpes zoster may become disseminated. Such an event may kill the patient. Zoster immune globulin, which is γ-globulin obtained from patients who have recovered from varicella, may be obtained (from the Cancer Detection Center on request and only if available) and can be helpful in controlling this infection. However, the usual patient with herpes zoster and CLL is managed by symptomatic remedies, perhaps coupled with the use of corticosteroids.

OTHER FORMS OF CHRONIC LEUKEMIA

Leukemic Picture as Part of Lymphoma

In the past, this entity was known as leukosarcoma, but it would be best called a leukemic picture associated with a lymphoma. This disease behaves in a different fasion than does CLL and usually requires combination intensive chemotherapy. Management is very similar, therefore, to lymphoma.

Leukemic Reticuloendotheliosis (Hairy Cell Leukemia)

This unusual form of lymphoma may present with a leukemic blood picture. This presentation may confuse the clinician initially and lead to the diagnosis of lymphatic leukemia. The cardinal sign of leukemic reticuloendotheliosis is a massive splenomegaly. Most patients present with pancytopenia, some have leukocytosis, but virtually all have splenomegaly. The diagnosis is established by morphologic characteristics of the cell. Management of this disease is emphasized since chemotherapy fails to control the disease. Rather, splenectomy may yield survivals that are measured in decades rather than in years.

SUMMARY

Lymphocytic leukemia has a rather long survival when compared to chronic myeloid leukemia (CML). However, available chemotherapy is not as effective in producing remission as is chemotherapy for CML. Alkylating agents, corticosteroids, androgens, and irradiation form the backbone of therapy. Splenectomy also may be indicated. Aggressive management of infection and control of immune complications are essential if maximum survival is to be realized. Aggressive therapy of early disease is being evaluated.

REFERENCES

Brodsky, I., and S. B. Kahn (eds.). Cancer Chemotherapy, Vol. II. Grune & Stratton.

DiPalma, J., B. Calesnick (eds.), S. B. Kahn and I. Brodsky (guest eds.). Seminars in Drug Therapy, Vol. 3, No. 1. 1973.

Hodgkin's Disease: Evaluation and Therapy Protocol

Peter A. Cassileth, M.D.

RATIONALE

In recent years, the therapy of Hodgkin's disease has become more successful than in the past in improving the patient's clinical course and in prolonging survival. These successes have led to more aggressive approaches in terms of the evaluation of the patient and with regard to treatment with radiotherapy and/or chemotherapy.

The crux of the argument in favor of extensive radical radiotherapy is based on the concept that in most patients with Hodgkin's disease the disease progresses in a sequential, predictable fashion extending contiguously from lymph node bearing area to lymph node bearing area (Rosenberg and Kaplan, 1966). Since radiotherapy is tumoricidal for Hodgkin's disease when administered appropriately in 96% of the radiated fields (Kaplan, 1966), the concept arose that radiation of extended lymph node bearing areas could yield cure even in advanced (nonvisceral) disease (Kaplan and Rosenberg, 1966). The early data in the 1950's of Vera Peters (1950) showed prolonged survival in patients treated with x-ray therapy to the areas of disease and the next adjacent areas. Kaplan and others proceeded to advocate what has come to be essentially total nodal radiotherapy for patients with even relatively limited disease.

It is clear from all of the data assembled that patients whose disease is confined above the diaphragm (after intensive staging) can be cured by radiotherapy in a high percentage of the cases (approaching 90%) (Rosenberg and Kaplan, 1970). It still remains to be proved that disease that has extended below the diaphragm is also amenable to cure. The critical issue is whether disease presenting in the chest extends below the diaphragm to involve the retroperitoneal nodes and/or the spleen by retrograde flow against the flow of lymph. It seems much more likely that disease that has reached the spleen and the abdominal nodes has done so by hematogenous dissemination (Aisenberg, 1972; Smithers, 1972). If this is true, then, as with almost all other disseminated neoplasms, cure of abdominal disease may not be attainable by extensive radiotherapy alone.

For disease that is more widespread than stages I and IIA, combination chemotherapy results now rival the effects of extensive radiotherapy with regard to induction of remission and remission duration and perhaps prolongation of life (Frei et al., 1973). In many instances of disseminated disease, chemotherapy may actually offer a substantial advantage over radiotherapy (Leavell, 1973).

Although controversy still exists as to the best mode(s) of therapy to employ for the different stages of Hodgkin's disease, therapy decisions are based on a determination of the extent of disease involvement. It is clear that the disease is curable when relatively limited in extent, and, with aggressive forms of therapy, complete remission and substantial prolongation of life are obtained even in advanced disease. For these reasons, much effort is expended to delimit precisely the location of all detectable disease.

INITIAL EVALUATION

1. Biopsy or review of outside slides.
2. Pertinent history—constitutional symptoms (fever, night sweats, weight loss).
3. Physical examination—record sites of involvement on a diagram.
4. Routine lab:
     CBC, platelets, reticulocytes, urinalysis, creatinine and BUN
     Bilirubin, direct and indirect, alkaline phophatase, SGOT, and
       prothrombin time
     Calcium, phosphorous, uric acid, protein electrophoresis
5. Anergy panel—mumps, tbc, etc.
6. Radiographic studief
     a. Chest x-ray
     b. Spleen and liver scan (primarily for size)
     c. Lymphangiogram (plus lymph node scan if available)
     d. Bone scan
     e. Intravenous pyelogram
7. Bone marrow biopsy (no aspirates)—done closed for patients with clinical states IB, IIB, IIIA, IVA, and IVB. Done open at laparotomy under general anesthesia for clinical stages IA and IIA.
8. No IVC, closed liver biopsy or GI x-rays (unless symptoms warrant).

LAPAROTOMY AND SPLENECTOMY

These procedures are performed on all patients who are not stage IVA or IVB after above studies are obtained. (Exclude patients 60 or older and those with other disease making surgery hazardous).

1. Splenectomy.
2. Open wedge biopsy of liver and needle biopsy (left and right lobes).
3. Sampling of suspicious nodes with clips placed and films taken on the table to ensure that the right node(s) has been obtained.
4. Sampling of nodes at L1 and L2 (not seen on lymphangiogram).
5. Open wedge biopsy of iliac crest.

STAGING (Simplified Form)

Stage I: Involvement of one group of nodes.
Stage II: Involvement of two groups of nodes (both on same side of
     diaphragm).

Stage III: Involvement of one or more groups of nodes on both sides of the diaphragm.

Stage IV: Involvement of nonlymphoid tissues (viscera and skin).

Footnotes

1. To the stage above the suffix A is appended to indicate absence of or B presence of constitutional symptoms consisting of fever, night sweats, or weight loss.

2. The subscript S is used to indicate spleen involvement.

3. The terms nodes and lymphoid tissues above are taken to include the tonsillar Waldeyer's ring and spleen.

THERAPY

1. Stages IA and IIA (less than 50 years old) (above the diaphragm). Mantle therapy.

2. Stages IA and IIA (over 50 years old) (above the diaphragm). Mantle therapy and/or MOPP $\times$ 6 cycles.

3. Stages IIA (below the diaphragm), IB, IIB, IIIA, IIIB—Total nodal radiation and/or MOPP $\times$ 6 cycles.

4. Stages IVA and IVB—MOPP $\times$ 6 cycles.

Footnotes

1. *Mantle Therapy* Mantle therapy refers to irradiation of 4,000 rads/4 weeks to node bearing areas above the diaphragm (cervical, supraclavicular, axillary, and mediastinal); many centers will also treat (in a separate course of 4,000 rads/4 weeks) the para-aortic nodes and splenic pedicle below the diaphragm if mediastinal disease is present.

2. *Total Nodal Irradiation* This includes mantle therapy plus a separate course to para-aortic nodes (as above) and the para-iliac nodes down to and including the inguinal nodes.

3. *Cycle of MOPP*

> (M) Nitrogen mustard: 6 mg/m^2 i.v. days 1 and 8
> (O) Vincristine: 1.4 mg/m^2 i.v. days 1 and 8
> (P) Procarbazine: 100 mg/m^2 p.o. days 1 to 14
> (P) Prednisone: 40 mg/m^2 p.o. days 1 to 14

Prednisone is given in 1st and 4th courses only. Cycles are repeated every 4 weeks. Although only 6 cycles are indicated above, some centers give MOPP cycles at 3- to 4-month intervals for an additional 2 years.

REFERENCES

Aisenberg, A. A. 1972. Hematogenous dissemination of Hodgkin's disease. Ann. Intern. Med. 77:810.

Frei, E., J. K. Luce, J. F. Gamble, C. A. Coltman, Jr., J. .J. Constanzi, R. W. Talley, R. W. Monto, H. E. Wilson, J. S. Hewlett, F. C. Delaney, and E. A. Gehan. 1973. Combination chemotherapy in advanced Hodgkin's disease. Ann. Intern. Med. 77:810.

Kaplan, H. S. 1966. Evidence for a tumoricidal dose level in the radiotherapy of Hodgkin's disease. Cancer Res. 26:1221.

Kaplan, H. S., and S. A. Rosenberg. 1966. Extended-field radical radiotherapy in advanced Hodgkin's disease: Short term results of two randomized clinical trials. Cancer Res. 26:1268.

Leavell, B. S. 1973. The significance of splenic involvement in Hodgkin's disease. Presented at the American Society of Hematology Meeting, Chicago.

Peters, M. V. 1950. A study of survivals in Hodgkin's disease treated radiologically. Amer. J. Roentgen Radium Ther. 63:299.

Rosenberg, S. A., and H. S. Kaplan. 1970. Hodgkin's disease and other malignant lymphomas. Calif. Med. 113:23.

Rosenberg, S. A., and H. S. Kaplan. 1966. Evidence for an orderly progression in the spread of Hodgkin's disease. Cancer Res. 26:1225.

Smithers, D. W. 1972. Patterns of spread. JAMA 222:1298.

Non-Hodgkin's Lymphoma

Paul F. Engstrom, M.D., F.A.C.P.

EPIDEMIOLOGY AND CLINICAL PRESENTATION

Non-Hodgkin's lymphoma (NHL) has a peak incidence period at a later age than Hodgkin's disease; namely, between 60 and 69 years of age. Males have a slight predominance over females for this disease

This work was supported in part by United States Public Health Service Grant CA-06551.

entity. The relative disease incidence of Hodgkin's disease to lympho-cytic lymphoma to histiocytic lymphoma is 2-2-1. Herpes-like viruses have been noted in cell cultures and in biopsies from patients with lymphomas, particularly Burkitt's lymphoma. Chronic immunosup-pressive therapy is related to an increased incidence of lymphoma, particularly histiocytic lymphoma.

The early signs and symptoms of NHL include glandular swell-ing, particularly in the oropharyngeal lymphoid tissue, skin rash, or gastrointestinal tract symptoms. Leukemic transformation or circula-tion of lymphosarcoma cells occurs in 13% of the cases. Patients with NHL are more susceptible to bacterial, viral, and fungus infections primarily because of the decreased circulating immunoglobulin. Auto-immune hemolytic anemia is associated with lymphocytic lymphoma.

CLASSIFICATION

These lymphomas should be anatomically staged according to the Ann Arbor Classification (Table 1) (Jones et al., 1973). Accurate differentiation of the histopathologic type has been important in fur-ther defining prognosis for this group of lymphomas. Table 2 shows the distribution of patients in NHL by the currently accepted histo-logic classification (Jones et al., 1973).

The staging work-up for patients with NHL is crucial to appro-priate management. As a rule, NHL patients, in contrast to Hodgkin's disease patients, are likely to have disseminated, extranodal disease. Therefore, the hematologic work-up is important and should include a bone marrow biopsy from both iliac crests. In a series of 218 NHL patients, Jones, Rosenberg, and Kaplan (1972) found bone marrow involvement most frequently with open bone marrow biopsy, less frequently with closed needle biopsy, and least frequently with bone marrow aspiration. The bone marrow involvement occurred most often with the mixed lymphocytic-histiocytic and with lymphocytic cell types, with splenomegaly, and with the presence of constitutional signs. The nodular or diffuse pattern did not influence the incidence of marrow involvement; however, patients with nodular lymphoma and positive marrows survived significantly longer than those marrow-positive patients with diffuse histopathology.

Bi-pedal lymphangiogram has an accuracy of 80 to 90% in NHL cases. Kim and Dorfman (1974) report that 25% of patients evaluated with staging laparotomy had asymptomatic, occult lymph-

Table 1. Non-Hodgkin's lymphomas: Ann Arbor staging classification

Clinical staging (CS)

Stage I   Involvement of a single lymph node region (I) or a single extralymphatic organ or site (I_g).

Stage II   Involvement of two or more lymph node regions on the same side of the diaphragm (II) or localized involvement of an extralymphatic organ or site and of 1 or more lymph node regions on the same side of the diaphragm (II).

Stage III   Involvement of lymph node regions on both sides of the diaphragm (III) which may also be accompanied by localized involvement of the spleen (III_s), extralymphatic site (III), or both (III_{SE}).

Stage IV   Diffuse or disseminated involvement of 1 or more extralymphatic organs or tissues with or without associated lymph node enlargement.

Pathological staging (PS)

              Involvement found at laparotomy or by any further removal of tissue for histologic examination other than that taken for the original diagnosis. Include annotations for specific sites biopsied.

              N+ or N—For other lymph node positive or negative by biopsy.

              H+ or H—For liver positive or negative by biopsy.

              S+ or S—For spleen positive or negative following splenectomy.

              L+ or L—For lung positive or negative by biopsy.

              M+ or M—For bone marrow positive or negative by biopsy or smear.

              P+ or P—For pleura or pleural fluid positive or negative by biopsy or by cytologic examination.

              D+ or D—For skin positive or negative by biopsy.

Jones et al. (1973a), p. 808.

oma in the abdomen. The mesenteric lymph nodes, splenic hilar nodes, periaortic lymph nodes, and the spleen were the most frequent sites of unsuspected disease. In another series (Bagley et al., 1973) of 46 patients evaluated for liver involvement in NHL, 11 of 44 had a positive percutaneous biopsy, 8 of 35 were positive on peritoneoscopy, and 7 of 21 were positive at laparotomy for a total of 26 of 46 with lymphomatous involvement of the liver.

Table 2. Non-Hodgkin's lymphomas: Distribution by histopathologic types (405 cases)

	Nodular	%		Diffuse	%
NH	Nodular histiocytic	7	DH	Diffuse histiocytic	29
NM	Nodular mixed histiocytic-lymphocytic	18	DM	Diffuse mixed histiocytic-lymphocytic	10
NLPD	Nodular lymphocytic poorly differentiated	17	DLPD	Diffuse lymphocytic poorly differentiated	11
NLWD	Nodular lymphocytic well differentiated	2	DLWD	Diffuse lymphocytic well differentiated	3
			DU	Diffuse undifferentiated	3
	Total nodular 178:	44		Total diffuse 227:	56

Jones et al. (1973b).

MANAGEMENT

Radiotherapy is the treatment of choice for localized stages of the disease, whether nodal or extranodal. Extended field arrangements are preferable so that all nodal and adjacent extranodal structures are included in the treatment programs, particularly for abdominal disease. Dosage levels ranging between 4,000 and 5,000 rads are indicated for the histiocytic lymphomas. The radiation-oncologist may be challenged by such complications as recurrent growth of nodes in a previously treated area, gastrointestinal involvement, mediastinal compression, spinal cord compression, osseous involvement, and recurrent pleural effusion. The results of radiotherapy in a series of 215 patients with stage I and stage II disease are seen in Table 3.

A number of important concepts have been established in the chemotherapy of non-Hodgkin's lymphoma (Table 4).

1. The lymphocytic types of lymphoma appear to respond much more readily than do the histiocytic forms of lymphoma (Luce et al., 1971).
2. Combination chemotherapy is more effective than single agent chemotherapy for all types of lymphoma except nodular lymphocytic, well differentiated subtypes (Stein et al., 1974).
3. Maintenance chemotherapy appears to be more beneficial in the lymphocytic forms of lymphoma than in the histiocytic forms (Luce et al., 1971).
4. Patients who achieve a complete remission survive significantly longer than patients who have partial remission (Luce et al., 1971).

Table 3. Non-Hodgkin's lymphoma: Radiotherapy treatment results by histopathologic class

Histology	No. of cases in Stages I-IIIE	% Probability of relapse at 1 yr	% 5-yr. survival	
			Stage I	Stage II
NLPD NM	91	19	100	63
NH	17	45	100	60
DLPD DM	45	39	52	30
DH	62	65	66	25

Jones et al. (1973b).

Table 4. Non-Hodgkin's lymphoma: Chemotherapy results by histopathologic class

Histology	Cytoxan or chlorambucil[a]			Cytoxan, oncovin, prednisone, procarbazine[b]		
	No. of cases	% C.R.	Duration (months)	No. of cases	% C.R.	Duration (months)
NH	7	28	20	0		
NM	16	31	17+	3	33	30+
NLPD	19	48	18+	14	79	9+
NLWD	0			1	100	13+
DH	19	5	5	0		
DM	13	13	6	6	16	11+
DLPD	9	22	13	4	75	16+
DLWD	0			1	100	
Favorable	42	43		19	60	
Unfavorable	41	12		10	40	

[a]Jones et al. (1972).
[b]Stein et al. (1974)

5. Patients with nodular lymphomas have a longer survival than do patients with diffuse lymphomas (Jones, Rosenberg, and Kaplan, 1972).

It is possible to define a favorable subtype of lymphoma consisting of nodular lymphocytic, well differentiated; nodular lymphocytic, poorly differentiated; nodular mixed; nodular histiocytic; and the diffuse, lymphocytic, well differentiated types. The unfavorable subtypes include diffuse, lymphocytic, poorly differentiated; diffuse, mixed; diffuse histiocytic; and diffuse undifferentiated lymphomas. Advanced mycosis fungoides and Burkitt's lymphoma are considered under the unfavorable types.

In summary, the favorable lymphomas can probably be successfully managed with an oral alkylating agent such as chlorambucil, or combinations of cyclophosphamide, vincristine, and prednisone (CVP). The latter combination (CVP) is given in 14-day courses out of each month for at least 6 months. Failures in this group should be

Table 5. Management protocols Non-Hodgkin's lymphoma

Favorable lymphoma (NLPD, NM, NLWD, DLWD)
  1. Chlorambucil, 2–4 mg/m² p.o. q day
  2. Cyclophosphamide, 70 mg/m²/day/p.o. × 14
     Vincristine, 1 mg/m²/i.v. day 1 & day 8, q 28 days × 6 mo
     Prednisone, 30 mg/m²/day p.o. × 14, then q 3 mo
  3. Cyclophosphamide, 600 mg/m²/i.v. day 1 & 8, q 28 days × 8
     Prednisone, 40 mg/m²/day p.o. × 14
  4. BCNU, 60 mg/m²/i.v. day 1
     Cyclophosphamide, 1,000 mg/m²/i.v. day 1, q 21 days × 8
     Vincristine, 1.2 mg/m²/i.v. day 1
     Prednisone, 100 mg/m²/p.o. day 1–5

Unfavorable lymphoma (DLPD, DM, DU)
  1. BCVP (See above #4)
  2. Cyclophosphamide, 600 mg/m²/i.v. day 1
     Vincristine, 1.2 mg/m²/i.v. day 1, q 21 days × 8
     Prednisone, 100 mg/m²/p.o. day 1–5
     Adriamycin, 50 mg/m²/i.v. day 1
  3. Cyclophosphamide, 1,000 mg/m²/i.v. day 1
     Prednisone, 100 mg/m²/p.o. day 1–5
     Vincristine, 1.2 mg/m²/i.v. day 15, q 21 days × 8
     Bleomycin, 10 mg/m²/i.m. day 15

Consider BCVP × 13 courses maintenance for complete responders

---

treated with more intensive combinations including 1,3-bis(2-chloro-ethyl)-1-nitrosourea (BCNU), cyclophosphamide, adriamycin, vincristine, and prednisone. Patients with unfavorable histologic subtypes should be treated with intensive chemotherapy programs utilizing vincristine, cyclophosphamide, BCNU, prednisone, adriamycin, and bleomycin. (See treatment schema, Table 5.)

REFERENCES

Bagley, C. M., V. T. DeVita, C. W. Berard, and G. P. Canellos. 1972. Advanced lymphosarcoma: Intensive cyclical combination chemotherapy with cyclophosphamide, vincristine and prednisone. Ann. Intern. Med. 76:227–234.

Bagley, C. M., L. B. Thomas, R. E. Johnson, P. B. Chretien, and V. T. DeVita, Jr. 1973. Diagnosis of liver involvement by lymphoma: Results in 96 consecutive peritoneoscopies. Cancer 31:840–847.

Jones, S. E., S. A. Rosenberg, and H. S. Kaplan. 1972. Non-Hodgkin's lymphoma. I. Bone marrow involvement. Cancer 29:954–960.

Jones, S. E., S. A. Rosenberg, and H. S. Kaplan, M. E. Kadin, and R. F. Dorfman. 1972. Non-Hodgkin's lymphoma. II. Single agent chemotherapy. Cancer 30:31–38.

Jones, S. E., Z. Fuks, M. Bull, M. E. Kadin, R. F. Dorfman, H. S. Kaplan, S. A. Rosenberg, and H. Kim. 1973a. Non-Hodgkin's lymphomas. IV. Clinicopathologic correlation in 405 cases. Cancer 31:806–823.

Jones, S. E., Fuks, H. S. Kaplan, and R. A. Rosenberg. 1973b. Non-Hodgkin's lymphomas. V. Results of radiotherapy. Cancer 32:682–690.

Kim, H., and R. F. Dorfman. 1974. Morphological Studies of 84 Untreated Patients Subjected to Laparotomy for the Staging of Non-Hodgkin's Lymphomas. Cancer 33:657–674.

Luce, J. K., J. F. Gamble, H. E. Wilson, R. W. Monto, B. L. Isaacs, R. L. Palmer, C. A. Coltman, J. S. Hewlett, E. A. Gehan, and E. Frei, III. 1971. Combined cyclophosphamide, vincristine and prednisone therapy of malignant lymphoma. Cancer 28:306–316.

Patchefsky, A. S., H. S. Brodovsky, H. Menduke, M. Southard, J. Brooks, D. Nicklas, and W. S. Hoch. 1974. Non-Hodgkin's lymphomas. A clinicopathological study of 293 cases. Cancer 34:1173–1186.

Stein, R. S., E. M. Moran, R. K. Desser, J. B. Miller, H. M. Golomb, and J. E. Ultman. 1974. Combination chemotherapy of lymphomas other than Hodgkin's disease. Ann. Intern. Med. 81:601–609.

Veronessi, U., R. Musameci, F. Pizzetti, L. Gennari, and G. Bonadonna. 1974. The value of staging laparotomy in non-Hodgkin's lymphomas. Cancer 33:446–459.

Adenocarcinoma of the Stomach

Paul F. Engstrom, M.D., F.A.C.P.

EPIDEMIOLOGY AND EARLY DETECTION

Adenocarcinoma, which accounts for 97% of the lesions, is the most common malignant tumor of the stomach. The remainder of the malignancies are sarcomas (leiomyosarcomas) and lymphomas (histiocytic type). Fifty to sixty percent of the lesions are found in the pyloric area of the stomach; 25% are in the lesser curvature; and less than 10% are located in the cardia of the stomach. Occasional tumors may involve the entire stomach area. The incidence of stomach adenocarcinoma varies throughout the world but it is most prevalent in Japan, Chile, and Iceland. In the United States, males predominate and the rate is higher in blacks than in whites (Lawrence, 1973). Even though the frequency of this neoplasm is decreasing in the United States, approximately 15,000 deaths will be attributed to stomach cancer in 1975. The etiology of the tumor has not been defined although dietary factors appear to play a major role (MacGregor, 1974). Premalignant lesions of the stomach include gastric polyps, pernicious anemia with atrophic gastritis, and recurrent chronic gastric ulcerative disease.

Techniques for the early detection of stomach cancer have been developed primarily in Japan. Mass screening may be possible by carefully following patients that are at high risk for stomach carcinoma and measuring their gastic secretions of acid and pepsin (Flood and Lattes, 1967). Cytology plus fiberoptic gastroscopy give 90% accuracy in the diagnosis of early gastric carcinoma (Schade, 1960). Upper gastrointestinal x-ray studies with barium meal are less accurate in detecting early lesions in the stomach.

This work was supported in part by United States Public Health Service Grant CA-06551.

CLASSIFICATION AND STAGING

The American Joint Committee for Cancer Staging and End Results Reporting (1971) for cancer of the stomach is based on anatomic extent of the disease. Table 1 delineates this classification program. Surgical exploration plus study of the excised surgical specimen or thorough clinical examination of the patient with advanced disease allows for staging of the patient according to the following criteria:

Stage IA: Tumor confined to mucosa (T_1) without node involvement (N-O) or distant metastases (M-O).

Stage IB: Tumor extending to but not through the serosa (T_2) without regional nodes (N-O) or remote tissue involvement (M-O).

Stage IC: Tumor extending through the serosa (T_3) without involvement of regional nodes (N-O) or remote tissues (M-O).

Stage II: Diffuse involvement of gastric wall (linitis plastica) T_4 without node (N-O) or distant spread (M-O). Also any degree of

Table 1. TNM classification of carcinoma of the stomach

T — Primary Tumor

T_1 — Confined to the mucosa.

T_2 — T_2 involves mucosa, submucosa including muscularis proprii and extends to or into serosa but does not penetrate through the serosa.

T_3 — Penetrates through serosa with or without invasion of contiguous structures.

T_4 — Diffusely involves entire thickness of the stomach wall without obvious boundaries; includes linitis plastica.

TX — Degree of penetration not determined.

N — Regional lymph nodes

NO— No metastases to nodes.

N_1 — Metastases to perigastric lymph nodes in immediate vicinity of primary tumor or on both curvatures of the stomach.

N_2 — Metastases to perigastric lymph nodes a distance from the primary tumor or on both curvatures of the stomach.

NX— Metastases of nodes not determined.

M — Distant metastases

MO— No distant metastases.

M_1 — Clinical radiographic or exploratory evidence of distant metastases including nodes beyond regional lymph nodes but excluding direct extension in continuity by a primary tumor.

gastric wall involvement (T_{1-4}) with regional node involvement (N_1) but without distant metastases (M-O).

Stage III: Any degree of involvement of gastric wall accompanied by spread to regional nodes remote from tumor (N_2) but with no distant metastases (M-O).

Stage IV: Any gastric cancer having spread to distant tissues regardless of extent of primary tumor or status of regional nodes.

It is apparent that the surgical approach is necessary in order to stage fully a stomach carcinoma patient. In addition to the laporatomy, barium studies, chest films, gastroscopy and biopsy, radioisotopic liver scan, and routine laboratory studies are indicated. If the lesion is thought to be resectable, the regional lymph nodes and hepatic wedge biopsies should be performed for staging purposes. In those situations where the patient is inoperable, bone scans should also be obtained.

PRINCIPLES OF TREATMENT

At the present time, approximately 50% of all patients with suspected gastric carcinoma are resectable. A radical subtotal gastrectomy is the treatment of choice for patients who have stage I or stage II lesions. During this procedure, the surgeon resects about 75% of the stomach, the omentum, most of the gastrohepatic ligament, the short gastric vessels, and possibly the spleen. Continuous or en-bloc dissection of suspicious lymph nodes and liver metastases are indicated. Total gastrectomy is utilized only if necessary for the removal of a large or superficially spreading tumor (linitis plastica). However, the operative morbidity and mortality are significant and the 5-year survival rate is not any better than for a radical subtotal gastrectomy (Mayo, Owens, and Weinberg, 1955).

The role of radiation therapy in the primary management of patients with gastric adenocarcinoma has not been defined. In a retrospective study (Moertel, 1975), no difference in survival was noted between a group of 24 patients with localized unresectable gastric carcinoma treated with radiation therapy and 43 patients with similar disease who received no specific treatment. Both Childs (1968) and Falkson (1969) have reported that the combination of chemotherapy with fluorouracil plus radiotherapy has an additive effect in patients with locally advanced stomach carcinoma. In both studies, the patients received 3,500 or 4,000 rads over 3 to 4 weeks to the epigastric area plus fluorouracil, 15 mg/kg daily i.v. for 3 to 5 days at the start of the radiotherapy course. The mean survival of the chemotherapy plus radiotherapy group was twice that of the radiation plus placebo group.

Comis and Carter (1974) have summarized the chemotherapy trials in gastric adenocarcinoma. Fluorouracil, the nitrosoureas, and Mitomycin C are the most active compounds and show response rates of 20 to 30% (see Table 2). The Eastern Cooperative Oncology Group (Moertel, 1975) recently completed a study using intravenous fluorouracil (325 mg/m^2, days 1 to 5) combined with methyl-1-(2-chloroethyl)-3-(4-methylcyclohexyl)-1-nitrosourea (methyl CCNU) (150 mg/m^2 on day 1); the fluorouracil is repeated on days 36 to 40 and the entire protocol is repeated at the 10th week. The response rate of 50% and median survival of 26 weeks were far superior to either fluorouracil or methyl CCNU alone. Other treatments which hold promise for adenocarcinoma of the stomach include fluorouracil

Table 2. Summary of chemotherapy studies in gastric adenocarcinoma

Drug	Dose schedule	PTS evaluable	Response No.	%
5-FU[a]	i.v. loading course	392	84	21
5-FU	i.v. weekly	46	12	26
Mitomycin C	Variable	211	63	30
BCNU[b]	50 mg/m^2/da × 5 q 6 wk	33	6	18
MeCCNU[c]	200 mg/m^2/q 7 wk	27	3	11
BCNU + 5-FU	40 mg/m^2 × 5 q 6 wk 10 mg/kg × 5 q 6 wk	37	14	38
Ara-C[d] + Mitomycin C + 5-FU	Variable 300 mg/m^2/da 1–5, 35–40 q 10 wk	27	15	55
5-FU + MeCCNU	175 mg/m^2/da 1	23	12	52

[a]5-FU, 5-fluorouracil.
[b]BCNU, 1,3-bis(2-chloroethyl)-1-nitrosourea.
[c]MeCCNU, Methyl-1-(2-chloroethyl)-3-(4-methylcyclohexyl)-1-nitrosourea.
[d]Ara-C, cytosine arabinoside.

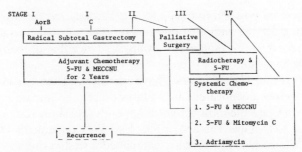

Figure 1. Suggested management schema for gastric adenocarcinoma.

plus Mitomycin C and Adriamycin alone or in combination with one of the other active medications.

Because of the availability of active combinations, postoperative adjuvant chemotherapy of stomach carcinoma should be considered. A Veterans Administrative study (1965) using thio-TEPA in the immediate postoperative period did not affect survival of patients who were resectable. A similar study (Serlin et al., 1969) utilizing 5-fluorodeoxyuridine given in two courses postoperatively was better tolerated than thio-TEPA, but again did not appear to affect survival. Because of the encouraging results noted with fluorouracil plus methyl CCNU, we use this combination as a 2-year adjuvant program for patients with stages I, II, and III gastric adenocarcinoma who have had complete resection of all known tumors. Hopefully this will improve the rather poor survival that is now reported for those patients that have locally advanced disease.

A disease-oriented approach to the management of stomach adenocarcinoma is diagrammed in Figure 1.

REFERENCES

American Joint Committee for Cancer Staging and End Results Reporting. 1971. A Staging System for Carcinoma of the Stomach, pp. 1–20. Chicago.

Comis, R. L., and S. K. Carter. 1974. A review of chemotherapy in gastric cancer. Cancer 34:1576–1586.

Flood, C. A., and R. Lattes. 1967. Premalignant lesions of the stomach. *In* Cancer of the Gastrointestinal Tract, pp. 113–125. Year Book Medical Publications Inc.

Lawrence, W. 1973. Carcinoma of the stomach. Cancer 23:286–304.

MacGregor, I. L. 1974. Carcinoma of the colon and stomach: A review with comment on epidemiologic associations. JAMA 227:911–915.

Mayo, H. W., J. K. Owens, and M. Weinberg. 1955. A critical evaluation of radical subtotal gastric resection as a definitive procedure for antral gastric carcinoma. Ann. Surg. 141:830–839.

Moertel, C. G. 1975. Clinical management of advanced gastrointestinal cancer. Cancer 36:675–682.

Schade, R. O. K. 1960. Gastric Cytology, pp. 1–81. E. Arnold & Co., London.

Serlin, O., J. S. Walkoff, J. M. Amadeo, and R. J. Keehan. 1969. Use of 5-fluorodeoxyuradine (FUDR) as an adjuvant in surgical management of carcinoma of the stomach. Cancer 24:223–238.

Veterans Administration Surgical Adjuvant Cancer Chemotherapy Group. 1965. Use of thio-TEPA as an adjuvant to surgical management of carcinoma of the stomach. Cancer 18:291–297.

Cancer of the Colon and Rectum

Richard S. Bornstein, M.D.

Cancers of the colon and rectum are the most common sites of malignancy (excluding skin cancer) in the United States. As with other gastrointestinal tumors, the incidence varies from country to country. The male to female ratio is approximately equal.

ETIOLOGY

Burkitt (1971) has stressed the fiber-deficient diet as the important factor linking the epidemiologic features of this disease. The features include the following: the increased incidence in the more industrialized countries, with low incidence in the underdeveloped countries (Doll, 1969); the associations with certain other noninfective diseases such as appendicitis, adenomatous polyps, diverticular disease, and ulcerative colitis (Burkitt, 1975). Burkitt has also commented on the epidemiologic association of other "modern" diseases such as "varicose veins, hemorrhoids, ischemic heart disease, and hiatus hernia."

DIAGNOSIS

The signs and symptoms associated with bowel cancer are dependent on the location of the tumor. Left-sided lesions are frequently associated with cramping pain and early obstruction. Right-sided lesions are frequently asymptomatic and characterized by the occult loss of blood.

Of particular importance in regard to early detection is the fact that over two-thirds of these tumors are within reach of the examining finger or the sigmoidoscope. The importance of this for mass screening cannot be overemphasized. Studies at the Cancer Detection Center of the University of Minnesota have demonstrated the prophylactic value of this simple and safe procedure (Gilbertsen, 1970). Powers (1975) has noted that 12% of tumors can be palpated, while 50% of all colon tumors are within 15 cm and 65% within 20 cm. Most studies have recommended annual sigmoidoscopy for the asymptomatic patient who is over 40 years of age.

More recently, the flexible fiberoptic colonoscope has come into use with the ability to visualize lesions up to the ileocecal valve. Further studies will define the criteria for its use.

The barium enema is the most important study for lesions beyond the sigmoidoscope. The accuracy of the procedure is very high if meticulous care is taken with the technique, including appropriate preparation. The value of air contrast studies remains controversial (Fenton and Margulis, 1975).

The most recent development in the area of cancer detection has been the carcinoembryonic antigen (CEA). The initial studies suggested that this substance might be specific for cancers of the colon. More recent large scale trials have shown less specificity, with both malignant and nonmalignant conditions giving positive results. Furthermore, it is most commonly positive in patients with transmural spread or distant metastasis, rather than the very early lesions.

It appears that the CEA assay has no value as a means of mass screening for early cancer. It does have a place in the follow-up of patients with proven colon cancer; high titers may be of value to detect early recurrence of disease in these patients.

TREATMENT

Surgery remains the only means of cure for bowel cancers. The type of resection is dictated by the lymphatic drainage in the area. Right hemicolectomy is performed for right colon lesions, whereas other lesions are treated with left hemicolectomy. A low anterior resection is used for tumors as low as 8 cm above the anorectal line, whereas abdominoperineal resections are required for lesions below this level.

One of the most interesting surgical techniques is the "no-touch" technique of Turnbull (1970). The technique involves the early ligation of the lymphovascular channels. The results have been impressive "although its value has not been substantiated by a controlled clinical trial" (Grage, 1975).

The overall 5-year survival rate remains at about 35%. The major factors correlating with prognosis are lymph node involvement and the degree of mural penetration. This correlation has been shown by Astler and Coller (1954), using a modification of Dukes' (1932) classification.

    Class A : limited to mucosa
          B-1: confined to muscularis mucosa
          B-2: extended through muscularis
          C-1: limited to wall with positive nodes
          C-2: extended through all layers with positive nodes

Radiation therapy has been used for relief of pain or bleeding. More recently, new studies have been begun to evaluate preoperative radiation therapy for the treatment of rectal carcinoma.

Chemotherapy has also been used for palliation. Fluorouracil has been recognized as the best single agent for the treatment of gastrointestinal malignancies, with a response rate of 20 to 25%. More recently the addition of a nitrosourea has been reported to yield encouraging results.

The newest area in regard to chemotherapy involves immediate postoperative chemotherapy in patients who are at a high risk for recurrence; that is, in patients who have minimal residual disease. Such a program has already yielded encouraging results in osteogenic sarcoma and breast carcinoma.

SUMMARY

Cancer of the colon remains a major cause of death. Surgery leads to cure in only a relatively small percentage of the cases and new techniques are needed for early detection and to identify high risk patients so as to make full use of the diagnostic techniques presently available. The earlier use of radiation therapy and chemotherapy may also result in an improved survival.

REFERENCES

Astler, V. B., and F. A. Coller. 1954. The prognostic significance of direct extentions of carcinoma of the colon and rectum. Ann. Surg. 139:846–851.

Burkitt, D. P. 1971. Epidemiology of cancer of the colon and rectum. Cancer 28:3–13.

Burkitt, D. P. 1975. Epidemiology and etiology. JAMA 231:517–518.

Doll, R. 1969. The geographic distribution of cancer. Brit. J. Cancer 23:1–8.

Dukes, C. E. 1932. The classification of cancer of the rectum. J. Pathol. 35:323–332.

Fenton, J. W., and A. R. Margulis. 1975. The radiologic diagnosis. JAMA 231:752–755.

Gilbertsen, V. A. 1970. Bowel cancer detections: Experience with 75,000 proctosigmoidoscopic examinations. Proc. Natl. Cancer Conf. 6:439–442.

Gold, P., and S. O. Freedman. 1965. Demonstration of tumor-specific antigens in human colonic carcinoma by immunological tolerance and absorption techniques. J. Exp. Med. 121:439–462.

Grage, T. B. 1975. Surgical management. JAMA 231:1183–1185.

Powers, J. H. 1975. Proctosigmoidoscopy in private practice. JAMA 231:750–751.

Turnbull, R. B., Jr. 1970. Ann. R. Coll. Surg. Engl. 46:243–250.

ADDITIONAL REVIEW REFERENCES

Current Concepts in Cancer. JAMA 231:(Series of articles beginning in February 1975).

Proceedings of the American Society's Second National Conference on Cancer of the Colon and Rectum. Cancer B4, September 1974 (Supplement).

Workshop in Colon Cancer. Digestive Diseases, Vol. 19, October/November 1974.

Cancer of the Kidney, Bladder, and Prostate

Richard V. Smalley, M.D., F.A.C.P.

RENAL

Renal adenocarcinoma is basically a surgical disease. If confined to the kidney or perirenal tissue the 5-year survival exceeds 60% following nephrectomy; with invasion of the vascular or lymphatic channels, it drops to 40% and to 10% with spread beyond. Irradiation to the kidney bed increases survival with involvement of the lymphatic or vascular channels. Surgery in patients with metastatic disease has received considerable attention. There appears to be some benefit in removing solitary pulmonary metastasis but there appears to be little effect on long-term survival by surgery on either the primary or metastatic lesions in other metastatic situations.

Medical treatment of metastatic disease has not been successful. Reports on the efficacy of hormone treatment (progesterone and/or testesterone) are available but prospective randomized trials indicate hormonal therapy has no benefit. Cytotoxic chemotherapeutic drugs have been universally disappointing.

BLADDER

The eventual outcome of patients with bladder carcinoma depends on the level of invasion at time of diagnosis. If deep muscle invasion can be demonstrated, the likelihood of cure becomes very small. Conservative surgery for noninvasive lesions with or without thio-TEPA instillation is used. Cystectomy with or without pelvic lymphadenectomy is advocated for invasive lesions. 5-Fluorouracil (5-FU) as an adjunct to surgery gave no better results than a placebo. Preoperative irradiation (4,500 rads/4 to 5 weeks) leads to tumor-free specimens (clinical stage B_2-C) in 35% leading to a potential 50% cure rate. The main defect in these studies has been the inability to stage accurately and clinically prior to definitive therapy.

Cytotoxic chemotherapeutic drugs (cytoxan, 5-FU, adriamycin) may give 25 to 33% response rates in advanced disease. Current prospective randomized trials are underway. Prevention (avoidance of known carcinogens) may be the most direct route for therapy. Immunotherapy would appear theoretically quite promising.

PROSTATE

Patients with a palpable nodule confined to the prostate are generally advised to have a radical prostatectomy. Impotence and rarely incontinence are sequelae. Histologic grading is important in determining outcome and well differentiated malignancies have an excellent chance at cure. There are advocates for hormone therapy exclusively in this group of patients. Orchiectomy and/or estrogen therapy are generally advocated for stage C disease (local extension). Low doses of DES (diethylstilbesterol, 1 mg p.o./day) are an effective form of treatment and do not carry the risk of cardiovascular complications that a higher dose does. Low dose DES is also effective in widespread disease. Local palliation may be achieved with irradiation and/or P_{32}. Cytotoxic chemotherapy has not been widely used and little data pro or con exist.

REFERENCES

Renal

Alberto, P., et al. 1974. Hormonal therapy of renal carcinoma alone and in association with cytostatic drugs. Cancer 33:1226.

Middleton, R. G. 1967. Surgery for metastatic renal cell ca. J. Urol. 97: 973.

Robinson, et al. 1969. Results of radical nephrectomy for renal cell ca. J. Urol. 101:297.

Skinner, et al. 1971. Renal cell ca—its diagnosis and therapy. Cancer 28: 1165.

Bladder

Barnes, et al. 1967. Control of bladder tumors by endoscopic surgery. J. Urol. 97:864.

Catalona, et al. 1974. Lymphocyte stimulation in urologic cancer patients. J. Urol. 112:373.

Marshall, V. F. 1952. Relation of preoperative estimate to the pathologic demonstration of the extent of vesical neoplasms. J. Urol. 68:714.

Prout, et al. 1970. Preoperative irradiation and 5-FU as adjuvants in the management of invasive bladder ca. J. Urol. 104:116.

Prostate

Barnes, R. W. 1969. Survival with conservative therapy. JAMA 210:331.
Byar, D. P. 1973. VA cooperative urological research group's studies of
    ca of the prostate. Cancer 32:1126.
Gleason, D. F., et al. 1974. Prediction of prognosis for prostatic adeno-
    carcinoma by combined histological grading and clinical staging. J.
    Urol. 111:58.
Jewitt, H. J. 1970. The case for radical perineal prostatectomy. J. Urol.
    103:195.

Cancer Detection by Risk Factor Analysis

Alton I. Sutnick, M.D., F.A.C.P.,
and Daniel G. Miller, M.D., F.A.C.P.

Our cancer detection program (CANSCREEN) is oriented to the detection of risk factors relevant to diseases for which a benefit from early diagnosis can be established and for which a suitable screening test is available. Selective examinations are planned on the basis of individual high risk indicators which are presumed to result in a more efficient utilization of medical resources. Screening in this program is viewed as an encounter which is part of an ongoing educational process to improve health care. Demographic historical and examination risk factors are employed in the determination of the decision logic and the design of this program. The program is also designed to afford optimal involvement of allied health personnel for examination and health counseling. A systems approach is employed with provisions for controls and evaluation.

An essential portion of the rationale in the development of this program is the utilization of risk factors to determine selective screening examinations. The utilization of selective testing, i.e., screening according to risk factor analysis, improves the efficiency of utilization of medical resources and improves the yield of positive findings. This approach is derived from the concept of prescriptive screening or evaluation of an individual for the probability of developing a disease based on historical and demographic information which in turn is used to specify the type and frequency of screening tests (McKeown, 1968; Henderson and Sherwin, 1974). An additional dimension to selectivity is provided by demographic stratification of a target population as a prescreening strategy; this allows for selection of population groups according to age, sex, race, and socioeconomic characteristics prior to screening (Henderson and Sherwin, 1974).

Another concept in this program holds that screening can do more than provide information relevant to the early diagnosis of disease. Screening can also elicit risk factors relating to primary prevention, i.e., smoking, alcoholism, and exposure to occupational pathogens. Health education relevant to primary prevention will be assessed in this program. Screening can also determine genetic or congenital disorders of structure and function or precancerous lesions such as gonadal dysplasia, undescended testes, and leukoplakia which can be prophylactically managed and carefully monitored.

A systems approach to the management of medical information has been proposed by Weed (1969), and Feinstein (1967) and these concepts are utilized in the design of this program. This approach has been successfully employed in preparing medical records and organizing the flow of information in medical facilities. Disease-specific diagnostic algorithms have been devised and are currently employed in clinic settings. The Preventive Medicine Institute—Strang Clinic and The Institute for Cancer Research, Fox Chase Cancer Center have been collaborating on the design and testing of disease-specific clinical algorithms for the early diagnosis of cancer for the CANSCREEN clinics (Sutnick, Miller, and Yarbro, 1974).

The medical questionnaire is a particularly important item in the design of a structured screening program. The questionnaire should allow for the evaluation of the effectiveness of each item, since in effect each question is a test and the information is of critical importance in decision making for selective testing. However, the questionnaire has additional purposes, i.e., the medical questionnaire may be used as an outreach tool (patients may be chosen to participate in the program based on the responses of the questionnaire); the questionnaire is also a health education tool. The use of health questionnaires relating to early detection as well as medical records used for this purpose has recently been reviewed (Eagle, 1937; Strang Clinic, 1970; Miller, 1972).

Another assumption in this program is that a large portion and perhaps all of the screening examination can be carried out by allied health professionals. The report of Sackett et al. (1974) on the randomized trial of the nurse practitioner was encouraging in this regard. The outcome of this program in terms of effectiveness and safety was judged comparable to those patients receiving conventional care. Similar and reinforcing experiences have been reported by Lewis and Resnik (1967), Collen et al. (1971), and Bates (1970).

An additional dimension in the rationale of this program relates to the role of health education as a force influencing patient behavior in matters relating to primary prevention and early detection. Experience relevant to the impact of health education on public health problems (Green, 1973) is being considered for its relevance to cancer risk factor education.

REFERENCES

Bates, B. 1970. Doctor and nurse: changing roles and relations. New Eng. J. Med. 283:129–134.

Clinical algorithms of the ambulatory care project, Beth Israel Hospital and the Lincoln Laboratory of the Massachusetts Institute of Technology, Boston, Mass.

Collen, F. B., B. Madero, K. Soghikian, et al. 1971. Kaiser-Permanente experiment in ambulant care. Amer. J. Nurs. 71:1371–1374.

Engle, R. L., Jr. 1937. History forms and self-questionnaire. In J. F. Holland and E. Frei (eds.), Cancer Medicine, pp. 309–315. Lea and Febiger, Philadelphia.

Feinstein, A. R. 1967. Clinical Judgment. The Williams & Wilkins Company, Baltimore.

Final Report of a System Concept Study for the Preventive Medicine Institute. 1970. Strang Clinic, RCA Systems Development, New York.

Green, L. W. 1973. Toward cost-benefit evaluations of health education: Some concepts, methods and examples. Presentation at Will Rogers Foundation Conference on Health Education, Saranac Lake, New York, June 22–23.

Health Education Report, March–April, Vol. 1, No. 3, 1974.

Henderson, M., and R. Sherwin. 1974. Screening—A privilege not a right. Prev. Med. 3:160–164.

Lewis, C. E., and B. A. Resnik. 1967. Nurse clinics and progressive ambulatory patient care. New Eng. J. Med. 277:1236–1241.

McKeown, T. 1968. The validation of screening. In Screening in Medical Care—Reviewing the Evidence, pp. 1–14. Oxford University Press, London.

Miller, D. G. 1972. Preventive medicine by risk factor analysis. JAMA 222:312–316.

Patient Education, Health Education Monographs, vol. 2, p. 1, Spring 1974.

Proceedings of a Conference on Cancer Public Education, July 31–August 31, 1973, Health Education Monograph, No. 36, 1973.

Sackett, D. L., W. O. Spitzer, M. Gent, et al. 1974. The Burlington randomized trial of the nurse practitioner: Health outcomes of patients. Ann. Intern. Med. 80:137–142.

Strategies for planning and evaluating cancer education, Health Education Monographs, No. 30, 1970.

Sutnick, A. I., D. G. Miller, and J. Y. Yarbro. 1974. A new approach to cancer detection. In Cancer Detection and Prevention, C. Maltoni (ed.), Excerpta Medica, Amsterdam.

Weed, L. L. 1969. Medical Records, Medical Education and Patient Care —the Problem-Oriented Record as a Basic Tool, The Press of Case Western Reserve University, Cleveland.

Investigational New Drugs

Robert E. Bellet, M.D., and Michael J. Mastrangelo, M.D., F.A.C.P.

During the early 1970's, a number of cancer chemotherapeutic agents gained conventional status. These clinically useful, commercially available, cytotoxic drugs are listed in Table 1. In 1975, BCNU and DTIC are scheduled for release from investigational status.

BCNU, the prototype nitrosourea, is a cell cycle nonspecific agent with mode of action similar to alkylating agents. This lipid-soluble drug crosses the blood-brain barrier and has manifest significant anti-tumor activity against primary brain malignancies and metastatic melanoma. BCNU is administered at a dosage of 150 mg/m² intravenously every 6 to 8 weeks. Significant toxic effects include myelosuppression and emesis.

DTIC is a cell cycle nonspecific agent with mode of action similar to alkylating agents. DTIC is the drug of choice in the treatment of metastatic melanoma and is administered intravenously at a dosage of 2 mg/kg per day for 10 consecutive days with courses repeated at 28-day intervals. Major toxic effects are myelosuppression and emesis.

This work was supported by United States Public Health Service Research Grants CA-13456 and CA-06927, National Institutes of Health Grant RR-05539, and an appropriation from the Commonwealth of Pennsylvania.

Table 1. Commercially available new drugs

Adriamycin	Sarcoma—breast—bladder
Bleomycin	Head and neck—cervix
Cytosine arabinoside	Acute myelogenous leukemia
Procarbazine	Hodgkin's disease
BCNU	Melanoma—brain
DTIC	Melanoma—sarcoma

Eleven investigational cancer chemotherapeutic agents are undergoing intensive phase II evaluation. These drugs are listed in Table 2. CCNU and Methyl-CCNU are orally administered nitrosoureas with mode of action, toxicity, and spectra of activity similar to BCNU. Of the remaining agents in Table 2, ICRF-159 and 5-azacytidine are discussed in detail in this chapter.

ICRF-159

ICRF-159, a bisdiketopiperazine structurally related to EDTA, was the 159th drug synthesized by the Imperial Cancer Research Fund facilities in London, England (Figure 1). ICRF-159 has manifest significant anti-tumor activity against both early and late murine L1210 leukemia (Woodman, 1974). In addition, this agent has significantly inhibited spontaneous metastases in mice implanted with Lewis lung carcinoma (Salsbury, Burrage, and Hellmann, 1970). This

Table 2. Investigational new drugs

5-Azacytidine
CCNU
Chromomycin A_3
cis-Platinum diamminedichloride
Hexamethylmelamine
ICRF-159
Isophosphamide
Methyl-CCNU
VM-26
VP-16-213
Yoshi-864

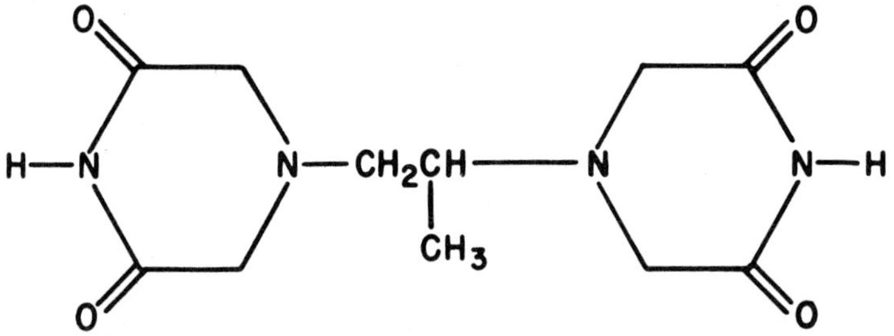

Figure 1. Structural formula of ICRF-159 (NSC-129943).

ability to inhibit metastases has been attributed to normalization of neovasculature in the primary tumor (LeServe and Hellmann, 1972).

Although its mode of action has not been well elucidated, inhibition of DNA synthesis (Sharpe, Field, and Hellmann, 1970) and alkylation (Friedman and Carter, 1970) have been described. In vitro studies reveal this drug to be most active in the G_2-M phase of the cell cycle (Sharpe et al., 1970).

A number of investigators have demonstrated synergistic activity when ICRF-159 is combined with conventional modalities of therapy. Specifically, studies in murine L1210 leukemia (Wampler, Speckhart, and Regelson, 1974) reveal anti-tumor synergism when ICRF-159 is combined with 5-fluorouracil, cyclophosphamide, hexamethylmelamine, or Adriamycin as single agents. Furthermore, synergistic anti-tumor activity is manifest when ICRF-159 is used in combination with radiation therapy in sarcoma S180 (Hellmann and Murkin, 1974). Finally, ICRF-159 has been shown to inhibit Adriamycin-induced cardiomyopathy in the isolated dog heart (Herman et al., 1972). Toxicologic studies in dogs reveal gastrointestinal and hematologic toxicity (Friedman and Carter, 1970). ICRF-159 is supplied as 500-mg scored tablets.

Phase I study of ICRF-159 in humans (Bellet et al., 1973a) revealed hematologic, gastrointestinal, and cutaneous toxicity. Leukopenia was dose limiting, resulting in a maximum tolerated oral dose of 1 g/m^2 per day for 3 successive days in divided doses every 8 hours.

A phase II study of this orally administered agent (Bellet et al., 1975) was undertaken utilizing a dose of 1 g/m^2 per day for 3 successive days in divided doses every 8 hours. Patients with a favorable response to therapy received courses of ICRF-159 at 21-day intervals. Fifty patients with a variety of advanced metastatic malignancies were treated in this manner. Toxicity experienced by 50 evaluable patients is presented in Table 3. The major toxicities were hematologic and gastrointestinal. The nadir of the white blood count occurred on day 14 (mean). With respect to response, 7 of 50 patients experienced clinically useful objective remissions. Four of 8 patients with metastatic squamous cell carcinoma of lung experienced clinically useful remissions; mean duration of remission was 4.9 months. Three of 15 patients with metastatic colorectal carcinoma experienced clinically useful objective remissions; mean duration of remission was 3.3 months. In a phase II study of ICRF-159 in colorectal carcinoma, 3 of 13 previously untreated patients experienced objective remissions (Marciniak et al., 1975).

ICRF-159 is a well tolerated oral cancer chemotherapeutic agent. Significant anti-tumor activity has been manifest in metastatic squamous cell carcinoma of lung and metastatic colorectal carcinoma. Phase III studies of ICRF-159 in squamous cell carcinoma of lung and colorectal carcinoma are therefore indicated. Since ICRF-159 has manifest significant synergistic anti-tumor activity with radiation therapy and with other cancer chemotherapeutic agents in animal tumor systems, combination chemotherapy utilizing ICRF-159 is a reasonable consideration for future studies. The ability of ICRF-159 to normalize the neo-vasculature of primary tumors in mice and rats suggests that this agent may be a useful adjuvant to surgery.

Table 3. Toxicity of ICRF-159

Type of toxicity	Incidence[a] (%)
Hematologic	62
Leukopenia (<2,000)	46
Thrombocytopenia (<100,000)	32
Anemia	22
Gastrointestinal	46
Nausea	46
Emesis	26
Diarrhea	4
Alopecia	28
Flu-like syndrome	6
No toxicity	12

[a]Fifty patients evaluable for toxicity.

5-AZACYTIDINE

5-Azacytidine is the pyrimidine analogue of cytidine with a nitrogen atom substituted for carbon in the 5-position of the ring (Figure 2). This nucleoside was synthesized in Czechoslovakia (Piskala and Sorm, 1964). 5-Azacytidine has shown significant anti-tumor activity against murine L-1210 leukemia, Walker 256 carcinosarcoma (Broder and Carter, 1970) and acute lymphoblastic leukemia in AK mice (Sorm and Vesely, 1964). This S-phase active agent (Li et al., 1970) is incorporated into RNA and DNA (Paces, Doskocil, and Sorm, 1968) with consequent inhibition of RNA, DNA, and protein synthesis. Toxicologic studies in dogs (Broder and Carter, 1970) reveal hematologic and hepatic toxicity. 5-Azacytidine is supplied in 50-mg and 100-mg vials.

Phase I studies in humans (Weiss et al., 1972) demonstrated gastrointestinal and hematologic toxicity when 5-azacytidine was administered as a bolus daily to a total dosage of 300 to 700 mg/m^2 intravenously over a 10-day period. The severe incapacitating emesis resulting from intravenous 5-azacytidine as a bolus has resulted in the drug being administered either by 24-hour infusion or by subcutaneous injection. Both routes result in a significant decrease in nausea and emesis.

The daily subcutaneous administration of 5-azacytidine for 10 days to a total dosage of 275 to 850 mg/m^2 (Bellet et al., 1974) resulted in mild gastrointestinal toxicity and dose-limiting leukopenia

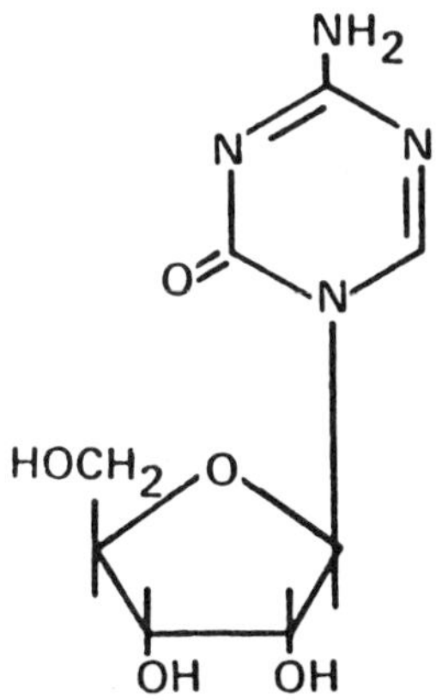

Figure 2. Structural formula of 5-azacytidine (NSC-102816).

(Table 4). Leukopenia and thrombocytopenia were dose related and delayed 21 to 35 days. In spite of severe leukopenia no patient developed life-threatening sepsis. However, the appearance of thrombocytopenia signaled a serious hemorrhagic diathesis. Liver function abnormalities were demonstrated in 5 of 20 evaluable patients; 3 of these individuals (all with significant hepatic metastatic disease) died of rapidly progressive hepatic failure. Hepatic toxicity was not dose related. A retrospective evaluation of patients dying in hepatic coma and matched patients with hepatic metastatic disease revealed the serum albumin value to be predictive of hepatocellular toxicity (Bellet et al., 1973b). Specifically patients with hepatic metastatic disease and serum albumin values less than 2.8 g % are at high risk for the development of 5-azacytidine-induced hepatotoxicity.

Phase II studies of intravenously administered 5-azacytidine have demonstrated marginal therapeutic efficacy in colorectal carcinoma (Moertel et al., 1972). Four of 8 patients with metastatic adenocarcinoma of ovary responded to 5-azacytidine administered subcutaneously at a dosage of 35 mg/m² per day for 10 successive days with courses repeated at 5-week intervals (Bellet, unpublished data).

Table 4. Toxicity of subcutaneous 5-azacytidine

Type of toxicity	Incidence[a] (%)	
Hematologic	60	
Leukopenia (<2,000)		60
Thrombocytopenia (<100,000)		15
Anemia		10
Gastrointestinal	40	
Nausea		40
Emesis		20
Diarrhea		15
Hepatic	25	
Liver function abnormalities		25
Hepatic coma		15
Stomatitis	5	
No toxicity	40	

[a]Twenty patients evaluable for toxicity.

The most significant anti-tumor activity resulting from 5-azacytidine systemic chemotherapy has been noted in acute myelogenous leukemia of childhood (Karon et al., 1973). Five of 14 patients refractory to standard therapy experienced complete remissions when 5-azacytidine was administered in a dosage of 150 to 200 mg/m^2 per day for 5 successive days. Patients with a favorable response were retreated at 14- to 21-day intervals. Phase II studies of intravenous 5-azacytidine presently utilize 24-hour infusions at a dosage of 150 mg/m^2 per day for 5 successive days (Lomen, Vaitkevicius, and Samson, 1975).

5-Azacytidine, a new anti-metabolite, has manifest significant anti-tumor activity against refractory acute myelogenous leukemia in children. Phase II studies in adults with acute myelogenous leukemia are indicated. In addition this agent is potentially useful in the treatment of metastatic adenocarcinoma of ovary refractory to standard therapy.

CONCLUSION

At least 50% of all cancer patients ultimately manifest metastatic disease and therefore require systemic therapy. The recent trend toward combination chemotherapy has been productive of increased response rates, prolonged remissions, and increased survival; multi-drug combinations for the treatment of metastatic solid tumors will further favorably influence survival as new agents are added to our therapeutic armamentarium. In addition, the discovery of effective cancer chemotherapeutic agents for signal solid tumor groups will result in effective postoperative adjuvant therapy and consequent increased survival. Perhaps ICRF-159 and 5-azacytidine will be useful additions to cancer chemotherapy.

APPENDIX—LIST OF COMPOUNDS

Adriamycin: NSC-123127.

5-Azacytidine: NSC-102816; s-triazin-2(1H)-one, 4-amino-1-α-D-ribofuranosyl-.

BCNU: NSC-409962; urea, 1,3-bis(2-chloroethyl)-1-nitroso-.

Bleomycin: NSC-125066.

CCNU: NSC-79037; urea, 1-(2-chloroethyl)-3-cyclohexyl-1-nitroso-.

Chromomycin A$_3$: NSC-58514; Toyomycin.

244   Bellet and Mastrangelo

cis-Platinum diamminedichloride: NSC-119875; *cis*-diamminedichloroplatinum.

Cytosine arabinoside: NSC-63878; cytosine, 1-β-D-arabinofuranosyl-, monohydrochloride; ara-C.

DTIC: NSC-45388; imidazole-4-carboxamide, 5-(3,3-dimethyl-1-triazeno)-; DIC.

Hexamethylmelamine: NSC-13875.

ICRF-159: NSC-129943; 2,6-piperazinedione, 4,4'-propylenedi-, (±)-.

Isophosphamide: NSC-109724; CAS reg. No. 3778-73-2; 1,3,2-oxazaphosphorine, 3-(2-chloroethyl)-2-[(2-chloroethyl)amino]tetrahydro-, 2-oxide; Z-4942.

Methyl-CCNU: NSC-95441; urea, 1-(2-chloroethyl)-3-(4-methylcyclohexyl)-1-nitroso-.

Procarbazine: NSC-77213; *p*-toluamide, *N*-isopropyl-α-(2-methylhydrazino)-, monohydrochloride.

VM-26: NSC-122819; 4'-demethyl-9-(4,6-*O*-2-thenylidene-β-D-glucopyranoside).

VP-16-213: NSC-141540; 4'-demethyl-epipodophyllotoxin-β-D-ethylidene glucoside.

Yoshi-864: NSC-102627; 1-propanol,3,3'-iminodi-dimethanesulfonate (ester) hydrochloride.

REFERENCES

Bellet, R. E., M. J. Mastrangelo, L. M. Dixon, and J. W. Yarbro. 1973a. Phase I study of ICRF-159 (NSC-129943) in human solid tumors. Cancer Chemother. Rep. 57:185–189.

Bellet, R. E., M. J. Mastrangelo, P. F. Engstrom, and R. P. Custer. 1973b. Hepatotoxicity of 5-azacytidine (NSC-102816) (A clinical and pathologic study). Neoplasma 20:303–309.

Bellet, R. E., M. J. Mastrangelo, P. F. Engstrom, J. G. Strawitz, A. J. Weiss, and J. W. Yarbro. 1974. Clinical trial with subcutaneously administered 5-azacytidine (NSC-102816). Cancer Chemother. Rep. 58:217–222.

Bellet, R. E., M. J. Mastrangelo, R. H. Creech, and P. F. Engstrom. 1975. Phase II study of ICRF-159 (NSC-129943) in human solid tumors. Proc. Amer. Soc. Clin. Oncol. 16:224.

Broder, L. E., and S. K. Carter. 1970. Clinical Brochure: 5-Azacytidine. National Cancer Institute, Bethesda. 25 pp.

Friedman, M. D., and S. K. Carter. 1970. Clinical Brochure: ICRF-159. National Cancer Institute, Bethesda, 35 pp.

Hellmann, K., and G. E. Murkin. 1974. Synergism of ICRF-159 and radiotherapy in treatment of experimental tumors. Cancer 34:1033–1039.

Herman, E. H., R. M. Mhatre, I. P. Lee, and V. S. Waravdekar. 1972. Prevention of the cardiotoxic effects of Adriamycin and Daunomycin in the isolated dog heart. Proc. Soc. Exp. Biol. Med. 140:234–239.

Karon, M., L. Sieger, S. Leimbrock, J. Z. Finklestein, M. E. Nesbit, and J. J. Swaney. 1973. 5-Azacytidine: A new active agent for the treatment of acute leukemia. Blood 42:359–365.

LeServe, A. W., and K. Hellmann. 1972. Metastases and the normalization of tumour blood vessels by ICRF-159: A new type of drug action. Brit. Med. J. 1:597–601.

Li, L. H., E. J. Olin, T. J. Fraser, and B. K. Bhuyan. 1970. Phase specificity of 5-Azacytidine against mammalian cells in tissue culture. Cancer Res. 30:2770–2775.

Lomen, P. L., V. K. Vaitkevicius, and M. K. Samson. 1975. Phase I study of 5-azacytidine using 24 hrs continuous infusion for 5 days. Proc. Amer. Assoc. Cancer Res. 16:52.

Marciniak, T. A., C. G. Moertel, A. J. Schutt, R. G. Hahn, and R. J. Reitemeier. 1975. A phase II study of ICRF-159 (NSC-129943) in advanced colorectal carcinoma. Cancer Chemother. Rep. In press.

Moertel, C. G., A. J. Schutt, R. J. Reitemeier, and R. G. Hahn. 1972. Phase II study of 5-Azacytidine (NSC-102816) in the treatment of advanced gastrointestinal cancer. Cancer Chemother. Rep. 56:649–652.

Paces, V., J. Doskocil, and F. Sorm. 1968. Incorporation of 5-Azacytidine into nucleic acids of "Escherichia coli." Biochim. Biophys. Acta 161:352–360.

Piskala, A., and F. Sorm. 1964. Nucleic acids components and their analogues. LI. Synthesis of 1-glycosyl derivatives of 5-azauracil and 5-azacytosine. Coll. Czech. Chem. Commun. 29:2060–2076.

Salsbury, A. J., K. Burrage, and K. Hellmann. 1970. Inhibition of metastatic spread by ICRF-159: Selective deletion of a malignant characteristic. Brit. Med. J. 4:344–346.

Sharpe, H. B. A., E. O. Field, and K. Hellmann. 1970. Mode of action of the cytostatic agent "ICRF-159." Nature 226:524–526.

Sorm, F., and J. Vesely. 1964. The activity of a new antimetabolite, 5-Azacytidine, against lymphoid leukemia in AK mice. Neoplasma 11:123–130.

Wampler, G. L., V. J. Speckhart, and W. Regelson. 1974. Phase I clinical study of Adriamycin-ICRF-159 combination and other ICRF-159 drug combinations. Proc. Amer. Soc. Clin. Oncol. 15:189.

Weiss, A. J., J. E. Stambaugh, M. J. Mastrangelo, J. F. Laucius, and R. E. Bellet. 1972. Phase I study of 5-azacytidine (NSC-102816). Cancer Chemother. Rep. 56:413–419.

Woodman, R. J. 1974. Enhancement of antitumor effectiveness of ICRF-159 (NSC-129943) against early L-1210 leukemia by combination with cis-diamminedichloroplatinum (NSC-119875) or Daunomycin (NSC-82151). Cancer Chemother. Rep. 4(2):45–52.

Hemostasis and Cancer

Isadore Brodsky, M.D., F.A.C.P.,
Anthony A. Fuscaldo, Ph.D.,
and Kathryn E. Fuscaldo, Ph.D.

BLOOD COAGULATION AND FIBRINOLYSIS IN NEOPLASTIC DISEASE

Recently, renewed interest has developed in the role of the blood coagulation and fibrinolysin systems in neoplastic disease. In an attempt to bring the field into sharper focus a symposium entitled "Anticoagulation in the Treatment of Cancer" was organized at Hahnemann in December 1972. The proceedings of this symposium were recently published (Brodsky, 1974a). It was emphasized that alterations in the blood coagulation and fibrinolysin system could influence neoplasia by a variety of mechanisms. A resumé of the current thinking concerning the influence of blood coagulation on oncology was presented at a workshop on "Anticoagulation in the Control of Cancer" held at the National Cancer Institute in November 1973. The key factors considered were: 1) hemorrhagic and thromboembolic complications in cancer patients, 2) metastases, 3) fibrinolysis, 4) the megakaryocyte and leukemia, and 5) therapy. Each of these factors is discussed briefly in this review.

INFLUENCE OF COAGULATION ON ONCOLOGY

Hemorrhagic and Thromboembolic Complications in Cancer Patients

After infection, hemorrhage and/or thromboembolism was the second leading cause of death in patients with cancer. In a study performed

at Roswell Park (RPMI) of 506 deaths in cancer patients, hemorrhage and/or thromboembolism was the main direct cause in 18%
and a contributing cause in 43%. Neoplastic disease is a well recognized cause of secondary thrombocytosis and the hypercoagulable
state (Brodsky, 1974b; Brugarolas et al., 1973; Davis, Theologides,
and Kennedy, 1969; Levin and Conley, 1964). Brugarolas et al.
(1973) found that of 100 patients with lung cancer, 93 exhibited
hyperfibrinogenemia and increased levels of fibrin degradation products. The results suggested local defibrination in the tumor. An exacerbation of such a hypercoagulable state may be responsible for the
increasing documentation of disseminated intravascular coagulation
(DIC) in clinical oncology. Presumably this hypercoagulable state
is caused by the release of thromboplastic material by the tumor.
Certainly effective chemotherapy may result in release of thromboplastic factors from injured cancer or leukemic cells, further potentiating an existing hypercoagulability and thereby precipitating DIC
(Brodsky, 1974b).

Metastases
Studies indicate that fibrin deposition is important for the growth of
primary tumors and their metastatic spread. Fibrin is deposited, particularly at the periphery; and this provides an important latticework
for tumor growth (Laki, 1974). The intravascular events associated
with metastasis formation have been demonstrated by cinemicrog-
raphy using the rabbit ear chamber (Wood, 1958). Once circulating
tumor cells adhere to the capillary endothelium, a coagulum consisting of fibrin and platelets rapidly forms around the cells. Vascular
permeability increases and the tumor penetrates into the perivascular
tissues with the ultimate development of a metastatic focus. Agostino,
Clifton, and Girolami (1966) demonstrated that damage to the
endothelium by either trauma or radiation potentiated the tendency
for tumor cell adherence. However, anticoagulation and antiplatelet
drugs in the experimental animal decrease tumor cell adherence and
the formation of metastases (Wood, 1958; Gasic, Gasic, and Stewart,
1968). Fibrin deposition may also be essential for the development of
the tumor's blood supply, i.e., neovascularization (Laki, 1974; Folkman, 1975). Folkman (1975) has emphasized the importance of
tumor angiogenesis factor (TAF) in this phenomenon. It is conceivable that TAF is a coagulative protein (factor XIII) that leads to

fibrin deposition and increased platelet consumption (Laki, 1974; Yancey and Laki, 1972).

Fibrinolysis

Reich and associates (Unkeless et al., 1973) reported that neoplastic transformation by oncogenic viruses or carcinogens in culture or in vivo greatly increases fibrinolytic activity (plasminogen activation content) of cultured cells. Thornes et al. (1972) observed that treatment of some patients with cancer and leukemia with brinase (a proteolytic enzyme from *Aspergillus oryzae*) resulted in sharp decrease in antiplasmin levels, resulting in destruction of leukemic cells in vivo. He postulated that brinase aided in the return of immunologic competence (Thornes, 1969). The presumption is that the hypercoagulable state blocks the fibrinolytic mechanism which is necessary for the proper function of the immune mechanism. In this regard the "tangled web" of hemostasis and the immune system must be considered. Factor XII (Hageman factor) not only plays a role in initiating the coagulation cascade, but also has a central role in activating fibrinolysis, the Kallikrein-Kinin system, and in the activation of the first component of complement.

The Megakaryocyte and Leukemia

The megakaryocyte and platelet in experimental animals are undoubtedly major reservoirs and perhaps sites of replication of the C-type oncornaviruses (Brodsky, 1973; Brodsky and Dimitrov, 1967). Electron microscopy studies have demonstrated that the oncornaviruses are characteristically present in the megakaryocytes and platelets of both spontaneous and experimentally induced murine and feline leukemias (Dalton et al., 1961; Laird et al., 1968). Altered megakaryocytopoiesis and thrombopoiesis may be the earliest manifestations of leukemia. Many analogies exist clinically between the leukemic process in the experimental animals and in human beings (Brodsky, 1973). Preliminary electron microscopic studies suggest that viruslike particles with some of the characteristics of oncornaviruses may be present in the platelets of patients with myeloproliferative disorders (Figure 1). Biochemical studies aimed at characterizing an enzyme, presumably of viral origin (reverse transcriptase), have also been productive. An RNA-dependent DNA polymerase has been detected in platelets from patients with either thrombocythemia or polycythemia vera. Normal controls were negative in both the exogenous and

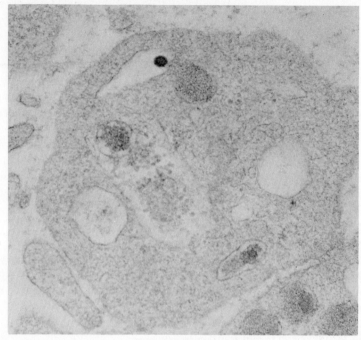

Figure 1. Virus-like particle budding into vacuolar space of human platelet. × 67,000.

endogenous reactions for reverse transcriptase. The electron microscopic and biochemical studies, although at this stage preliminary, are highly suggestive of the presence of viral particles in preneoplastic human platelets (Brodsky et al., 1975).

Therapy

Millar and Ketcham (1974), following a review of their own experiments and the literature, suggested that such anticoagulants as heparin and warfarin affected metastasis formation by interfering with the lodgement of tumor cell emboli in capillary beds. This point has been clearly demonstrated in mice with both transplanted and spontaneous tumors (Ryan, Ketcham, and Wexler, 1968a, 1968b). Anticoagulation prolonged the time that circulating tumor cells were found in the blood. This increased exposure to destructive processes, i.e., the immune and macrophage systems, results in a decrease in metastases formation. Anticoagulation by interfering with neovascularization of already established tumors may potentiate the action of chemotherapeutic drugs.

The metabolism of tumors can be divided into a gycolytic phase (anaerobic and aerobic) and oxidative phosphorylation (Laki, 1974). The former is generally avascular, whereas the latter is highly vascular and is the phase of rapid tumor growth (Folkman, 1975). It has been postulated that prevention of the vascular phase, i.e., neovascularization, will force a tumor to depend entirely on the gycolytic pathways of metabolism. Such a therapeutic maneuver might serve to limit tumor growth, increase the tumor's susceptibility to radiation therapy and chemotherapy, and raise the threshold between therapeutic effectiveness and toxicity to the normal tissues. Fibrinolytic therapy, as already indicated, may activate the immune system and thereby further enhance the action of chemotherapeutic agents and radiation therapy modalities.

In man experimental protocols have already been established to evaluate the role of anticoagulation plus chemotherapy in the treatment of lung and colon cancer, brain tumors, and osteogenic sarcomas (Elias, 1974; Kirsch et al., 1974). The results to date are too limited to draw any definitive conclusions as to the possible effectiveness of anticoagulation in these neoplastic disorders. Such protocols should study the role of anticoagulation as adjuncts to chemotherapy in the prevention of metastases following "curative" surgery or radiation therapy as well as in the advanced neoplastic state.

Although many of the issues raised above are speculative and theoretical, it is important to emphasize that a knowledge of thrombopoiesis and blood coagulation is essential in understanding the pathogenesis and present therapy of cancer and, in particular, the leukemic disorders.

Recently Gralnick, Marchasi, and Gwelber (1972), by means of fibrinogen kinetic studies, divided the hypercoagulable state in the acute leukemias into three categories: 1) patients with increased fibrinogen catabolism without laboratory or clinical evidence of DIC; 2) patients with increased fibrinogen catabolism and laboratory evidence of DIC but with no clinical evidence of hemorrhage or thrombosis; and 3) the syndrome of DIC with severe hemorrhage and thrombosis.

In our laboratory we have been investigating platelet and fibrinogen kinetics in the chronic myeloproliferative disorders. Simultaneous platelet and fibrinogen kinetics utilizing [^{75}Se] selenomethionine have been performed in patients with polycythemia vera (PV), patients with myelofibrosis and myeloid metaplasia (MF), and patients with chronic myelogenous leukemia (CML) (Brodsky et al., 1972).

The data are presented in Table 1. Untreated PV and MF are characterized clinically by an increased incidence of thrombosis and hemorrhage, which are the major factors in the morbidity and mortality in these diseases. However, to date we have not encountered laboratory or clinical evidence of disseminated intravascular coagulation in polycythemia vera and myelofibrosis and myeloid metaplasia. However, it is possible that antiplatelet drugs may be important in preventing some of the thrombotic complications in these disorders. In the acute leukemias the hypercoagulable state is probably initiated by the release of coagulative or thromboplastic substances from the leukemic cells. As a rule, hypercoagulability is more common in the acute leukemias associated with very high white blood cell (WBC) counts.

In PV and MF the hypercoagulable state is probably initiated by marked increase in megakaryocytopoiesis with an associated thrombocytosis, decreased platelet survival, and increased platelet turnover. Therefore, either the coagulation mechanism through the excessive intravascular conversion of fibrinogen to fibrin or increased numbers and consumption of functionally active platelets can induce hypercoagulability. Of course, it is conceivable that under certain conditions both mechanisms will be operative.

In this regard it is important to indicate that in early CML hypocoagulability develops. These patients, from a hemostatic standpoint, are usually characterized by a mild bleeding diathesis, even with an associated thrombocytosis. Platelet and fibrinogen survivals are distinctly prolonged as compared to PV and MF as well as control subjects (Table 1). The prolonged platelet survival in CML is due to the underutilization of functionally abnormal platelets. The studies in the chronic myeloproliferative disorders suggest definite interrelationship between platelet and fibrinogen turnover. In vitro platelet function, as measured by platelet adhesiveness and platelet aggregation, is frequently abnormal in the chronic myeloproliferative disorders; but in our studies only platelet and fibrinogen turnover correlated with a history of a thrombotic or bleeding diathesis (Brodsky et al., 1972).

Table 1. Platelet and fibrinogen kinetics in chronic myeloproliferative disorders

Disorder	Platelets			Fibrinogen		
	Count (platelets/μl)	Survival (days)	Turnover (platelets/μl/day)	Concentration	Survival (days)	Turnover (mg/ml/day)
CML (7) + [a]						
Mean	402,000	13.2	31,700	271	12.8	0.24
Range	218,000–715,000	10.5–16.0	15,600–51,100	206–350	6.5–190	0.11–0.39
PV (9) [a]						
Mean	536,000	7.2	75,700	219	5.6	0.44
Range	354,000–747,000	5.5–8.5	41,700–122,000	162–340	3.5–7.0	0.25–0.97
MF (8) [a]						
Mean	1,094,000	6.6	176,800	318	6.8	0.52
Range	56,000–3,353,000	4.0–11.5	9,600–609,600	233–373	4.0–9.0	0.30–0.85
Controls (10) [a]						
Mean	378,000	10.6	38,000	218	7.8	0.42
Range	168,000–475,000	7.0–11.0	22,000–52,000	225–400	6.5–9.5	0.33–0.49

[a]ELT, euglobulin lysis time.

Although the hypercoagulable state leading to DIC can develop spontaneously (Polliack, 1971), it is becoming apparent that chemotherapy in leukemia can initiate DIC. We have reported one of two cases in which chemotherapy precipitated DIC in patients with acute leukemia (Leavey, Kahn, and Brodsky, 1970). One patient had acute myelomonocytic and the other acute lymphoblastic leukemia. Each case was treated with the VAMP program (vincristine, methotrexate, 6-mercaptopurine, and prednisone), which produced a precipitous drop in the WBC count along with clinical and laboratory evidence of DIC. It was postulated that destruction of WBC resulted in the release of thromboplastic material which then triggered the coagulopathy. Both cases were successfully treated with heparin, and a summary of events is presented in Tables 2 and 3. Gralnick et al. (1972) also indicated the importance of this consideration in the treatment of acute leukemia.

In conclusion, the hypercoagulable state is of major significance in the pathogenesis of neoplastic disease. In this paper particular emphasis was placed on the acute and chronic leukemic disorders. Various stages and degrees of hypercoagulability have been described in the acute leukemias and the chronic myeloproliferative disorders. Simultaneous platelet and fibrinogen kinetic studies are essential in such investigations. The development of DIC following chemotherapy is a serious complication and should be considered in all patients with acute leukemia and particularly in those presenting with high WBC counts. However, many questions remain unresolved. At what point and under what conditions should anticoagulation be instituted in the acute leukemias? With the onset of DIC the answer is obvious, but should anticoagulation be combined with chemotherapy in the less severe stages of hypercoagulability? What are the anticoagulants of choice? One must consider the relative merits of the coumarin congeners, heparin, fibrinolytic agents (urokinase, streptokinase), Malayan pit viper (Arvin), and finally drugs that will intrinsically alter the fibrinogen molecule, i.e., L-asparaginase.

The latter drug is of particular interest, since it is therapeutically effective in acute lymphatic leukemia and the lymphomas. L-asparaginase routinely causes hypofibrinogenemia and an abnormal third stage of coagulation as monitored by the thrombin time. Our studies suggest that L-asparaginase can interfere with asparagine metabolism, leading to the synthesis of an abnormal fibrinogen (dysfibrinogenemia) with a decreased fibrinogen survival (Brodsky et al., 1971). Is

Table 2. Effect of chemotherapy and heparin therapy on coagulation profile in a patient with acute myelomonocytic leukemia

Days of chemotherapy	WBC × (10³/mm³)	Thrombin time at incubation of 10 min (sec)	Platelet count × (10³/mm³)	Fibrinogen (mg/100 ml)	ELT[a] (hr)
0 (chemotherapy begun)	192	3.2	277		5–6
3 (heparin begun)	128	16.5	122	45	5–6
4	8.4	10.0	106	45	5–6
6	3.7	4.8	191	165	5–6
9 (heparin discontinued)	3.8	3.2	164		5–6
Normal range		3.9–6.0	150–450	150–300	4.5–6.0

[a]ELT, euglobulin lysis time.

Table 3. Effect of chemotherapy and heparin therapy on coagulation profile in a patient with acute lymphoblastic leukemia

Days of chemotherapy	WBC × (10^3/mm^3)	Thrombin time at incubation of 10 min (sec)	Platelet count × (10^3/mm^3)	Fibrinogen (mg/100 ml)	ELT^a (hr)	Fi-test	Protamine test
0 (chemotherapy begun)	137	6.2	134	260	4–6		
3	73		110				
4	4.6	7.7	28	100	4–6		
5 (heparin begun)	4.2	12.4	37	80	4–6	1:32	+3
6 (platelets given)	17.2	10.6	28	80	4–6	1:32	+2
7	21.3	6.5	154	95	4–6	1:16	
8 (heparin discontinued)		5.1	230	240	4–6	neg.	
Normal range		3.9–6	150–450	150–300	4.5–6.0		

^{a}ELT, euglobulin lysis time.

this merely an undesirable side effect or do the resulting hypo-fibrinogenemia and dysfibrinogenemia have therapeutic implications?

A major question is whether anticoagulation, either alone or combined with chemotherapy, should be used in the acute leukemias when the patients are in complete remission. The chronic myeloproliferative disorders, i.e., PV and MF, pose even different problems. Here, adequate control of abnormal megakaryocytopoiesis may be all that is required to control hypercoagulability. Given the present state of the art, it is quite apparent that we are faced with more questions than answers.

However, even now it is apparent that the role of thrombopoiesis, blood coagulation, and the fibrinolytic systems deserves intensive study vis-à-vis the pathogenesis and treatment of neoplasia. This author suspects that such studies will rapidly stimulate the development of new interdisciplinary fields in cancer research with a level of interest that now already exists in the closely allied field of immunology and immunotherapy.

REFERENCES

Agostino, D., E. Clifton, and A. Girolami. 1966. Effect of prolonged coumadin treatment on production of pulmonary metastases in the rat. Cancer 19:284–288.

Brodsky, I. 1973. Role of the megakaryocyte and platelet in the leukemic process in mice and men: A review and hypothesis. J. Natl. Cancer Inst. 51:329–335.

Brodsky, I. 1974a. Anticoagulation in the Treatment of Cancer. Journal of Medicine. Vol. 5, No. 1-3. S. Karger, Basel, Switzerland. 148 pp.

Brodsky, I. 1974b. Leukemia and the hypercoagulable state. In I. Brodsky (ed.), Anticoagulation in the Treatment of Cancer. Journal of Medicine, pp. 38–49. S. Karger, Basel, Switzerland.

Brodsky, I., and N. V. Dimitrov. 1967. Platelet metabolism in Rauscher virus leukemia. J. Natl. Cancer Inst. 43:385–390.

Brodsky, I., Fuscaldo, A., Fuscaldo, K., Erlick, B., Kingsbury, E., and Schultz, G. 1975. Analysis of human platelets in thrombocythemia for reverse transcriptase and virus-like particles. J. Natl. Ca. Inst. 55: 1069–1074.

Brodsky, I., S. B. Kahn, E. M. Ross, and G. Petkov. 1972. Platelet and fibrinogen kinetics in the chronic myeloproliferative disorders. Cancer 30:1444–1450.

Brodsky, I., S. B. Kahn, G. Vash, E. M. Ross, and G. Petkov. 1971. Fibrinogen survival with (^{75}Se) selenomethionine during L-asparaginase therapy. Brit. J. Haematol. 20:477–487.

Brugarolas, A., E. G. Elias, H. Takita, I. B. Mink, A. Mittleman, and S. L. Ambrus. 1973. Hyperfibrinogenemia and lung cancer. J. Med. (Basel) 4:96.

Dalton, A. J., L. W. Law, J. Maloney, and R. A. Manaker. 1961. An electron microscopic study of a series of murine lymphoid neoplasms. J. Natl. Cancer Inst. 27:747–791.

Davis, R. P., A. Theologides, and B. J. Kennedy. 1969. Comparative studies of blood coagulation and platelet aggregation in patients with cancer and non-malignant disease. Ann. Intern. Med. 71:67–80.

Elias, G. E. 1974. Heparin anticoagulation as adjuvant to chemotherapy in carcinoma of the lung. J. Med. (Basel) 5:114–132.

Folkman, J. 1975. Tumor angiogenesis: A possible control point in tumor growth. Ann. Intern. Med. 82:96–100.

Gasic, J., B. Gasic, and C. C. Stewart. 1968. Antimetastatic effects associated with platelet reduction. Proc. Natl. Acad. Sci. USA 61:46–52.

Gralnick, H. R., S. Marchasi, and H. Gwelber. 1972. Intravascular coagulation in acute leukemia. Blood 40:709–718.

Kirsch, W. M., D. Schultz, J. J. Van Buskirk, and H. E. Young. 1974. Effects of sodium warfarin and other carcinostatic agents on malignant cells: A study of drug synergy. J. Med. (Basel) 5:69–82.

Laird, H. M., O. Jarrett, G. W. Grighton, and W. F. H. Jarrett. 1968. An electron microscopic study of virus particles in spontaneous leukemia in the cat. J. Natl. Cancer Inst. 41:867–878.

Laki, K. 1974. Fibrinogen and metastases. J. Med. (Basel) 5:32–37.

Leavey, R. A., S. B. Kahn, and I. Brodsky. 1970. Disseminated intravascular coagulation. A complication of chemotherapy in acute myelomonocytic leukemia. Cancer 26:142–145.

Levin, J., and C. L. Conley. 1964. Thrombocytosis associated with malignant disease. Arch. Intern. Med. 114:497–500.

Millar, R. C., and S. Ketcham. 1974. The effect of heparin and warfarin on primary and metastatic tumors. J. Med. (Basel) 5:23–31.

Polliack, A. 1971. Acute promyelocytic leukemia with DIC. Amer. J. Clin. Pathol. 56:155–161.

Ryan, J. J., A. S. Ketcham, and H. Wexler. 1968a. Warfarin treatment of mice bearing autochthonous tumors: Effect on spontaneous metastases. Science 162:1493–1494.

Ryan, J. J., A. S. Ketcham, and H. Wexler. 1968b. Reduced incidence of spontaneous metastases with long-term coumadin therapy. Ann. Surg. 168:163.

Thornes, R. D. 1969. Inhibition of antiplasmin and effect of protease 1 in patients with leukemia. Lancet ii:1220–1223.

Thornes, R. D., P. F. Deasy, R. Carroll, D. J. Reen, and J. D. MacDonell. 1972. The use of the proteolytic enzyme brinase to produce autocytotoxicity in patients with acute leukemia and its possible role in immunotherapy. Cancer Res. 32:280–284.

Unkeless, J. C., A. Tobia, L. Ossowski, J. P. Quigley, D. B. Rifkin, and E. Reich. 1973. An enzymatic function associated with transformation of fibroblasts by oncogenic viruses. J. Exp. Med. 137:85–111.

Wood, S., Jr. 1958. Pathogenesis of metastasis formation observed in vivo in the rabbit ear chamber. Pathology 66:550–568.

Yancey, S. T., and K. Laki. 1972. Tranaglutaminase and tumor growth. Ann. N.Y. Acad. Sci. 202:344–348.

Anemia in Cancer

Stanley Zucker, M.D., F.A.C.P.,
and Rita M. Lysik, B.A.

Anemia develops at some point in the clinical course of most patients with cancer (Ley, 1956; Price and Greenfield, 1958; Holland and Frei, 1973). The degree of anemia varies depending on the type of malignancy and the duration of disease. In general, because of the insidious onset of anemia in cancer, the symptoms are usually mild. Weakness, fatigue, pallor, and weight loss commonly occur in malignancy with or without anemia and it is, therefore, difficult to determine whether these symptoms are due to anemia, per se, or to the malignancy. Other explanations for the lack of symptoms related to anemia in cancer are the voluntary limitation of physical activity and the increased red cell 2,3-diphosphoglycerate (DPG) (Douglas and Adamson, 1975) and increased tissue oxygen delivery that accompanies the anemia of cancer. On occasion, however, symptoms due to severe anemia may be the presenting complaints of the patient with cancer. Each patient with anemia associated with cancer, therefore, should be approached as a fresh hematologic problem, and the same care in precise diagnosis should be observed, since appropriate therapeutic measures may produce substantial symptomatic relief (Ley, 1956).

This work was supported by Veterans Administration General Research funds and by Public Health Service Research Grant CA-15629-01 from the National Cancer Institute.

The observation that the anemia of malignancy shares many clinical similarities with the anemias occurring in chronic infection and inflammation has led several authors to use the term "Anemia of Chronic Disorders" (ACD) (Cartwright and Lee, 1971; Ward, Kurnick, and Pisarczyk, 1971). The term ACD is useful to physicians since the clinical and laboratory features of anemia in these diseases are quite similar; but from a research point of view, this grouping of disorders has tended to obscure differences in pathophysiology.

LABORATORY FEATURES

The anemia of cancer has traditionally been described as normocytic and normochromic; however, more recent observations suggest the frequent occurrence of hypochromic or microcytic red cells (Cartwright and Lee, 1971). The hemoglobin concentration usually stabilizes between 8 and 12 g/100 ml and the packed cell volume varies between 26 and 38% (Ley, 1956; Price and Greenfield, 1958; Ward et al., 1971; Cartwright and Lee, 1971; Holland and Frei, 1973; Zucker, Friedman, and Lysik, 1974; Douglas and Adamson, 1975). The use of the hemoglobin concentration as a criterion of anemia has been criticized on the basis that a concentration value cannot distinguish between an actual change in hemoglobin mass and an apparent change resulting from an alteration in blood volume. Most investigators have also found, however, a significantly lower red cell mass and an increased plasma volume in patients with cancer. In ACD the absolute reticulocyte count is within the normal range or slightly elevated. The white cell count and platelet counts are normal or elevated. The pattern of alteration of iron metabolism is important in confirming the diagnosis of anemia of cancer. Characteristically there is a significant reduction in serum iron (hypoferremia) and a moderate decrease in serum iron binding capacity (transferrin), resulting in a mild decrease in saturation of transferrin with iron. In the anemia of cancer, Prussian blue stains of bone marrow particles reveal normal or increased iron stores (hemosiderin), but decreased numbers of bone marrow sideroblasts. This phenomenon of decreased plasma iron in the face of increased storage iron in the reticuloendothelial system (RES) is a major factor in the pathophysiology of ACD (Cartwright and Lee, 1971). The marrow is normocellular and the erythroid to myeloid ratio is generally normal or somewhat reduced in malignancy, indicating a failure of compensatory erythroid hyperplasia (Zucker et al., 1974). Other findings of lesser importance are a decreased concentration of serum albumin, and an increased concentration of free red cell protoporphrin (Cartwright and Lee, 1971). Evidence for significant hemolysis is usually lacking in routine testing. However, using red cells labeled with radioactive chromium (^{51}Cr), a mildly shortened red cell life span can usually be demonstrated in the anemia of cancer.

DIFFERENTIAL DIAGNOSIS

The diagnosis of the anemia of cancer is made primarily by exclusion of other causes. Iron deficiency anemia frequently occurs in patients with cancer especially with ulcerative lesions of the gastrointestinal tract, head and neck, urinary bladder, and after extensive surgery. Iron deficiency can be differentiated from the anemia of cancer by the absence of stainable iron in the marrow in the former condition. In patients with advanced cancer and iron deficiency the serum iron binding capacity is often decreased rather than increased as anticipated. Occasionally a therapeutic trial of iron is required to determine the etiology of anemia in a patient with cancer and decreased iron stores. When the test becomes more readily available, the measurement of serum ferritin should simplify this diagnostic dilemma since serum ferritin levels are increased in the anemias of chronic disorders and decreased in iron deficiency anemia (Douglas and Adamson, 1975). Also, dilutional anemia, infection, inflammation, liver disease, renal impairment, folate deficiency, hemolysis, and metastatic replacement of the bone marrow must be ruled out as contributing causes for anemia in patients with cancer. In patients with gastric carcinoma the development of vitamin B_{12} deficiency following extensive gastric resections must also be considered.

Anemia commonly develops after extensive chemotherapy or radiotherapy and is related to an impairment of erythropoiesis. The pancytopenia and marrow hypoplasia that follows vigorous myelosuppressive therapy is usually reversible after discontinuing the offending drug.

MYELOPHTHISIC ANEMIA

In certain types of malignancies, metastases commonly localize and proliferate in the bone marrow. Carcinomas of the prostate, breast, lung (small cell type), adrenal, thyroid and kidney, as well as neuroblastoma, malignant melanoma, and lymphomas frequently metastasize to bone marrow (Shen and Homburger, 1951; West, Ley, and Pearson, 1955). The bone marrow is invariably extensively involved in acute and chronic leukemias and multiple myeloma.

Tumor invasion of the marrow frequently results in definite signs, such as bone pain and tenderness and/or radiologic evidence of bone involvement. Splenomegaly may be present.

Myelophthisic or leukoerythroblastic anemia is the term used to describe the anemia associated with infiltrative lesions of the bone marrow, usually of a malignant nature (Shen and Homburger, 1951; West, Ley, and Pearson, 1955; Zucker, Lysik, and Friedman, in press). The peripheral blood findings include anemia of variable degree and increased or decreased numbers of leukocytes and platelets. The hallmark of this type of anemia is the appearance in peripheral blood of immature red cells (nucleated red cells and reticulocytes) and immature granulocytes (myelocytes and metamyelocytes). Marked anisocytosis and poikilocytosis, with bizarre-shaped red cells, are frequently present. The finding of nucleated erythrocytes in the peripheral blood in a patient with cancer should alert the physician to the probability of marrow invasion. Bone marrow metastases are also frequently accompanied by marrow fibrosis, which further decreases the quantity of functioning myeloid tissue (Shen and Homburger, 1951; West, Ley, and Pearson, 1955; Myers et al., 1974; Zucker et al., in press). For appropriate diagnosis of myelophthisic anemia, it is essential to examine a marrow biopsy specimen, as well as a marrow aspiration specimen, since the latter technique alone has a high incidence of false negative results, especially in the presence of myelofibrosis.

Ineffective erythropoiesis with intramedullary destruction of developing normoblasts and reticulocytes is another component of anemia due to malignant invasion of the marrow and is observed most prominently in erythroleukemia. Ineffective erythropoiesis and a fall in the number of stem cells available for erythroblastic differentiation appear to be the principal mechanisms responsible for anemia in acute myelogenous leukemia (Gavosto et al., 1970).

PATHOGENESIS OF ANEMIA IN CANCER

At least three factors are implicated in the pathogenesis of anemia in cancer (without marrow invasion): 1) shortened red cell survival; 2) impaired flow of iron from the reticuloendothelial system to erythropoietic marrow; and 3) relative failure of bone marrow to increase red cell production (end organ failure) (Cartwright and Lee, 1971; Zucker et al., 1974).

A shortened red cell survival has been demonstrated in most patients with the anemia of cancer. In the majority of patients with cancer, the red cell survival is between 60 and 90 days as compared to 120 days in normal subjects (Ley, 1956; Price and Greenfield, 1958). In leukemias and other types of cancer in advanced stages an even greater degree of red cell destruction has been noted. The nature of the extracorporeal factor in red cell destruction in cancer has not been defined, but it has been suggested that the RES of the host may be overactive in destroying red cells (Ley, 1956; Price and Greenfield, 1958; Holland and Frei, 1973). Splenic sequestration and destruction of red cells by the splenic RES are often an important clinical phenomenon especially in leukemias and lymphomas. The concept that neoplastic tissue elaborates substances that have a destructive action against red cells was popular before 1960. The clinical importance of "tumor hemolysins" has not been substantiated in recent years (Ley, 1956; Price and Greenfield, 1958; Holland and Frei, 1973).

Since normal bone marrow can increase the red cell production rate by a factor of 5 times the basal rate, a 50% decrease in red cell survival theoretically should not lead to anemia (Cartwright and Lee, 1971; Ward et al., 1971; Zucker et al., 1974). Therefore, the major factor in the anemia of cancer is a relative failure of the bone marrow to increase red cell production sufficiently to compensate for the mildly shortened red cell survival.

FAILURE OF ERYTHROPOIESIS IN CANCER

Three mechanisms have been suggested to explain the relative failure of erythropoiesis in cancer: 1) inadequate iron supply for erythropoiesis; 2) inadequate production of erythropoietin, and 3) impaired bone marrow response to erythropoietin stimulation.

Haurani, Young, and Tocantins (1963) have demonstrated the sequestration of iron in the RES and a decreased reutilization of iron in patients with cancer. A decreased plasma iron concentration in patients with cancer has been correlated with a failure of erythropoiesis to increase to more than twice normal (Douglas and Adamson, 1975). Thus, the bone marrow is "starved of iron in the face of plenty" in the RES (Cartwright and Lee, 1971).

The effect of malignancy on erythropoietin production remains disputed. In most other forms of anemia, as the hemoglobin level is depressed below 10 g/100 ml, the level of plasma erythropoietin is elevated in roughly a linear fashion. Ward et al. (1971) noted significantly lower serum erythropoietin levels in malignancy. Zucker et al. (Zucker, Friedman, and Lysik, 1974; Zucker, Lysik, and Distefano, 1975), however, reported that erythropoietin levels in malignancy (human and animal studies) were appropriately elevated for the degree of anemia.

The possibility of impaired bone marrow response to erythropoietin in malignancy has recently been evaluated in patients with advanced malignancy and anemia. In these studies, assessment of bone marrow response to erythropoietin was made by measuring ^{59}Fe-heme synthesis in bone marrow suspensions cultured for 3 days with and without the addition of erythropoietin (Zucker et al., 1974). The results showed that the erythropoietin-induced increase in marrow heme synthesis in malignancy ($31 \pm 5\%$ increase) was significantly less than observed in normal patients ($66 \pm 8\%$) or patients with anemia of infection or inflammation ($101 \pm 10\%$). Additional studies in patients with extensive neoplastic bone marrow invasion (chronic lymphocytic leukemia, lymphoma, myeloma, prostate, and lung cancer) revealed an even greater decrease in marrow responsiveness to erythropoietin (Zucker et al., in press). As a result of these studies we propose the following hypothesis to explain the development and progression of anemia in malignancy: 1) some malignant cells produce factor(s) that lead to diminished erythropoiesis as a result of bone marrow hyporesponsiveness to erythropoietin (Figure 1B); dissemination of malignant cells to the bone marrow further depresses the responsiveness of erythroid precursor cells (ERC) to erythropoietin (Figure 1C); malignant cells, then, continue to populate the marrow at the expense of normal myeloid (erythroid) elements, eventuating in almost total marrow replacement with tumor (myelophthisic anemia). A second hypothesis that remains to be evaluated is that advanced cancer might alter the marrow microenvironment to the extent that erythroid proliferation would no longer be adequately supported.

A. NORMAL ERYTHROPOIESIS

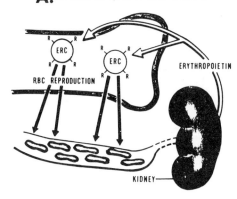

B. ERYTHROPOIESIS IN MALIGNANCY
WITHOUT MARROW METASTASIS

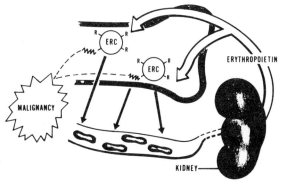

Figure 1. A postulated mechanism for the development of diminished erythropoiesis in myelophthisic anemia. *A* represents normal red cell production. Erythropoietin acts on erythropoietin responsive cells (*ERC*) presumably through a receptor mechanism (*R*) to enhance hemoglobin synthesis. *B* displays decreased erythropoietin responsiveness in malignancy, possibly by interference with the ERC receptor mechanism. *C* depicts the markedly diminished erythropoiesis with extensive marrow invasion. The number of ERC is diminished and the receptor mechanism for erythropoietin is "blocked" by the metastatic cells (*M*). As noted in *B* and *C* the production of erythropoietin increases as the anemia progresses, but end-organ hyporesponsiveness to hormone prevents augmented erythropoiesis.

INFREQUENT CAUSES OF ANEMIA IN CANCER

Autoimmune Hemolytic Anemia

Immune hemolytic anemia due to the production of red cell auto-antibodies may be seen in association with neoplastic diseases, especially those involving the lymphatic and reticuloendothelial systems (Ley, 1956; Price and Greenfield, 1958; Holland and Frei, 1973). In these cases, overt hemolysis, characterized by moderate to severe anemia, polychromasia and spherocytosis of red cells, increased plasma indirect bilirubin, increased urine and fecal urobilinogen excretion, decreased serum haptoglobin, and splenomegaly can be demonstrated. The absolute reticulocyte count is usually elevated and the bone marrow may exhibit erythroid hyperplasia depending on the extent of malignant cell infiltration. The red blood cell survival is markedly shortened and a positive direct Coomb's test (direct antiglobulin test) is usually present. Coomb's positive hemolytic anemia occurs most commonly in patients with chronic lymphocytic leukemia (possibly 10 to 20%) and non-Hodgkin's lymphoma. Adrenocorticosteroids in association with primary treatment for the underlying neoplasm are the primary form of treatment for this complication. In some instances, irradiation of the spleen or splenectomy are required to control the hemolytic anemia.

Microangiopathic Hemolytic Anemia

Microangiopathic hemolytic anemia is an unusual form of intravascular hemolysis that has been described in patients with metastatic adenocarcinoma, usually of the mucin-producing type (Brain et al., 1970). This anemia is characterized by overt hemolysis, red cell distortion and fragmentation, hemoglobinemia, hemoglobinuria or hemosiderinuria, and increased excretion of bile metabolites in the urine. Often these patients also have evidence of disseminated intravascular coagulation, as characterized by thrombocytopenia, decreased levels of coagulation factors, and elevated levels of fibrin degradation products.

Red Cell Aplasia

Anemia due to "pure" red cell aplasia is another rare type of anemia described in patients with cancer, especially thymomas (Safdar, Krantz, and Brown, 1970). This anemia is characterized by a marked diminution of erythroid precursors in the bone marrow which presumably is the result of auto-antibodies directed against host erythroblasts. Remissions have been obtained after thymectomy alone, or combined with corticosteroids, androgens, or splenectomy.

TREATMENT OF ANEMIA IN CANCER

Anemia occurring in a patient with cancer should be investigated to rule out specific deficiencies or complications. Patients with concomitant iron or folate deficiency should be treated with oral ferrous salts or folic acid, respectively. Most patients with cancer appear to tolerate a stable hemoglobin level above 8 g/100 ml without physiologic decompensation. Transfusion of packed red cells, however, will be required in patients in whom the anemia becomes symptomatic.

Effective therapy of the underlying malignancy generally results in simultaneous improvement in the anemia. In a recently reported series of patients with Hodgkin's disease involving the bone marrow, chemotherapy with "MOPP" resulted in complete remission, including a normal bone marrow free of tumor, for 25+ months in 13 of 19 patients (Myers et al., 1974).

Testosterone and related steroids have been shown to ameliorate the anemia in several malignant hematologic disorders (chronic lymphocytic leukemia, lymphoma, multiple myeloma, acute and subacute leukemia) and in patients with bone marrow depression secondary to radiotherapy and chemotherapy (Sanchez-Medal, 1971). Responses are achieved only with large doses of androgens given for a minimum period of 2 to 3 months. Androgens appear to act by increasing the production of erythropoietin and by a direct stimulatory effect on red cell precursors (stem cells). The side effects of androgen therapy and the minimal disability resulting from anemia in most patients with cancer have, however, limited the usefulness of androgens in cancer.

SUMMARY

Anemia commonly develops in the advanced stages of malignancy. In most patients with cancer the anemia does not become symptomatic and requires no specific therapy. Secondary factors such as blood loss, infection, and extensive hemolysis need to be identified and treated.

Anemia in cancer is due to a relative failure to increase red cell production in response to mild shortening of red cell survival. The major factors in the defective erythropoiesis in cancer are: 1) RES blockade in the reutilization of iron; and 2) decreased bone marrow responsiveness to erythropoietin (end-organ failure).

REFERENCES

Brain, M. C., J. G. Azzapardi, L. R. I. Baker, et al. 1970. Microangiopathic hemolytic anemia and mucin-forming adenocarcinoma. Brit. J. Haematol. 18:183.

Cartwright, G. E., and G. R. Lee. 1971. The anemia of chronic disorders. Brit. J. Haematol. 21:147–152.

Douglas, S. W., and J. W. Adamson. 1975. The anemia of chronic disorders: Studies of marrow regulation and iron metabolism. Blood 45: 55–65.

Gavosto, F., V. Gabutti, P. Masera, and A. Pilari. 1970. The problem of anemia in acute leukemia. Kinetic study. Eur. J. Cancer 6:33–38.

Haurani, F. I., K. Young, and L. M. Tocantins. 1963. Reutilization of iron in anemia complicating malignant neoplasms. Blood 22:73–81.

Holland, J. F., and E. Frei. 1973. Cancer Medicine, p. 1086. Lea & Febiger, Philadelphia.

Ley, A. B. 1956. Mechanism of anemia in cancer. Med. Clin. North Amer. 857–870.

Myers, C. E., B. A. Chabner, V. T. Devita, and H. R. Gralnick. 1974. Bone marrow involvement in Hodgkin's disease: Pathology and response to MOPP chemotherapy. Blood 44:197–204.

Price, V. E., and R. E. Greenfield. 1958. Anemia in cancer. Adv. Cancer Res. 5:199–290.

Safdar, S. H., S. B. Krantz, and E. B. Brown. 1970. Successful immunosuppressive treatment of erythroid aplasia appearing after thymectomy. Brit. J. Haematol. 19:435–443.

Sanchez-Medal, L. 1971. The hemopoietic action of androstanes. Prog. Hematol. 7:111–136.

Shen, S. C., and F. Homburger. 1951. Anemia of cancer patients and its relation to metastasis to bone marrow. J. Lab. Clin. Med. 37:182–198.

Ward, H. P., J. E. Kurnick, and M. J. Pisarczyk. 1971. Serum level of erythropoietin in anemias associated with chronic infection, malignancy, and primary hematopoietic disease. J. Clin. Invest. 50:332–335.

West, C. D., A. B. Ley, and O. H. Pearson. 1955. Myelophthisic anemia in cancer of breast. Amer. J. Med. 18:923–931.

Zucker, S., S. Friedman, and R. M. Lysik. 1974. Bone marrow erythropoiesis in anemia of infection, inflammation and malignancy. J. Clin. Invest. 53:1132–1138.

Zucker, S., R. M. Lysik, and J. F. DiStefano. 1975. Pathogenesis of anemia of malignancy. Clin. Res. 33:286.

Zucker, S., R. M. Lysik, and S. Friedman. Diminished bone marrow responsiveness to erythropoietin in myelophthisic anemia. Cancer. In press.

Bacterial and Fungal Infections

Kristen Ries, M.D.,
and Donald Kaye, M.D., F.A.C.P.

Infections are common and are the leading cause of death in patients with malignant diseases (Inagani, Rodriguez, and Bodey, 1974; Levine et al., 1974). With the advent of modern cancer therapy, which can produce prolonged remissions or cure, it becomes imperative that infectious complications be diagnosed and treated early. Common bacterial pathogens account for the majority of infections in patients with cancer. During recent years, antibiotics that are active against most of these organisms have become available. With improved therapy for these infectious complications, an increasing incidence of serious infections caused by the more unusual bacteria and fungi has been noted. This review considers both the common and unusual bacterial and fungal infections that pose a threat to the lives of patients with neoplastic disease.

PREDISPOSING FACTORS

The pattern of infections in patients with malignancies varies depending upon the nature and stage of the malignancy, because the type of infection is directly related to the type and degree of loss of host defenses (e.g., obstruction to drainage, damage to skin or mucosal surfaces, loss of antibody production, decrease in phagocytes, loss of cellular immunity). Hospitalization for therapy of the malignancy also introduces the dangers of urethral catheterization, intravascular catheters, and respiratory equipment which act as portals of entry for infecting microorganisms.

Local Factors (Obstruction to Drainage and Damage to Skin or Mucosal Surfaces)

Infection is prone to occur behind obstructing lesions blocking drainage of an area with an indigenous or introduced microbial flora. Examples are: pneumonia behind a bronchial lesion, pyelonephritis and bacteremia behind urinary tract obstruction, and purulent sinusitis behind a lesion obstructing drainage of a sinus. The usual microorganisms involved are those most likely normally to be present at the site involved (e.g., anaerobic bacteria in infections resulting from obstruction to the bronchi or sinuses and gram-negative enteric bacilli in urinary tract obstruction). Initial antimicrobial therapy should be directed against these presumptive infecting microorganisms. The results of therapy will depend not only on giving appropriate antimicrobial therapy but also on removing the obstruction and promoting drainage.

Loss of skin such as occurs in patients with leukemia and lymphoma who bleed easily and extensively may predispose to serious infections caused by group A streptococci, *Staphylococcus aureus* and gram-negative bacilli (most importantly *Pseudomonas aeruginosa*). Damage to mucosal surfaces as occurs in malignancies of the gastrointestinal and female genital tracts may permit the local normal flora (predominantly anaerobic) to invade tissues; necrosis related to the malignancy lowers the oxidation-reduction potential and may allow multiplication of the anaerobes.

Decrease in Antibody Production

Patients with multiple myeloma, chronic lymphatic leukemia, lymphosarcoma, and to a lesser extent other leukemias and lymphomas have a high incidence of bacterial infections which is in large part due to the failure to produce and maintain normal levels of immunoglobulins (Silver, 1963). This defect is also important in some patients with other malignancies who have received antineoplastic therapy. These patients have frequent infections with encapsulated bacteria (e.g., pneumococci, group A streptococci, and even *Hemophilus influenzae*) which are usually well controlled by antibiotics (Chernik,

Armstrong, and Posner, 1973; Levin et al., 1974). However, infection may also occur with less virulent but more antibiotic-resistant gram-negative enteric bacilli as well as with the more unusual bacteria and fungi.

Decrease in Phagocytes

Polymorphonuclear leukocytic mediated defenses are important. Patients with acute leukemia or patients receiving cancer chemotherapy frequently suffer from lack of adequate numbers of granulocytes and perhaps granulocytes that are defective. These patients are especially predisposed to staphylococcal infections and infections caused by gram-negative aerobic bacilli (e.g., *Escherichia coli, Klebsiella-Enterobacter-Serratia* sp., *Proteus* sp., and *Pseudomonas*) (DeVita and Young, 1973).

Bacteremia is sometimes caused by several different gram-negative bacilli simultaneously, especially in granulocytopenic patients. When the polymorphonuclear leukocyte count is less than $500/mm^3$, *Pseudomonas* bacteremia is likely.

Decrease in Cellular Immunity

Alteration in cellular immunity (i.e., diminished T cell function as measured by decreased delayed hypersensitivity) is seen in patients with Hodgkin's disease and other lymphomas, and after antineoplastic chemotherapy. These patients are especially predisposed to developing infection caused by *Mycobacterium tuberculosis, Nocardia asteroides, Listeria monocytogenes, Salmonella* sp., *Brucella* sp., *Cryptococcus neoformans, Candida* sp., and *Pneumocystis carinii* as well as other intracellular viruses and parasites (Armstrong et al., 1974).

Iatrogenic Factors

In addition to the effect of antineoplastic chemotherapy in interfering with host defense mechanisms, certain procedures which are commonly used in hospitalized patients markedly increase the risk of infection. Hospitalized patients tend to acquire *Staphylococcus aureus* and gram-negative bacilli including *Pseudomonas aeruginosa* as part of their skin and mucosal flora. With antimicrobial therapy the rate and frequency of acquisition are enhanced. The common use of indwelling urethral catheters increases the risk of urinary tract infection and subsequent gram-negative bacillary bacteremia. Intravascular catheters increase the risk of bacteremia caused by staphylococci,

gram-negative bacilli, and fungi (especially *Candida*). Use of respiratory equipment with nebulizers (which tend to become contaminated) increases the risk of pneumonia caused by gram-negative
bacilli. Contaminated blood platelet transfusions and intravenous
fluids may also result in serious infection.

INFECTIONS CAUSED BY GRAM-POSITIVE BACTERIA

Gram-positive bacteria still cause serious infections in patients with
malignancies, and *Staphylococcus aureus* is the leading cause of
infections due to gram-positive organisms. However, its importance
has greatly diminished over the past 20 years. Most of the serious
infections caused by *S. aureus* are either pneumonia or bacteremia.
Soft tissue infection (e.g., related to intravenous catheters or surgical
procedures) may also occur (Armstrong et al., 1974). Fortunately,
most of these infections, if recognized early, can be successfully
treated with one of the semisynthetic penicillins or cephalosporins.

Streptococci cause a small percentage of serious infections in
cancer patients. Although group A streptococci are the most frequent
causes, groups B, C, D (enterococci), and G streptococci have been
isolated as definite causes of infections in such patients (Armstrong et
al., 1970; Henkel et al., 1970). Although these organisms usually
cause skin or wound infections, they have been isolated as the primary
infectious agent in patients with pneumonia, meningitis, and urinary
tract infections. Streptococcal infections have been most commonly
associated with surgery and with patients with solid tumors.

Pneumococcal infections occur frequently and are usually pneumonia, meningitis, or bacteremia without apparent localization. Infections due to this organism have been noted to occur especially in
the patient with hypogammaglobulinemia or with abnormal serum
proteins (e.g., multiple myeloma or chronic lymphatic leukemia)
(Silver, 1963). However, in a recent review of 48 cases of pneumococcal bacteremia in patients with neoplastic diseases, the most frequently associated condition was leukopenia (Armstrong et al.,
1974). Treatment with penicillin is still highly effective.

Listeria monocytogenes, a short gram-positive bacillus, has been
isolated as the causative agent of septic arthritis and meningitis in
patients with lymphatic malignancies (Louria et al., 1967b; Louria
and Armstrong, 1970). The most common presentation is that of an
indolent meningitis. Since the organism is frequently misidentified as a
diphtheroid by the laboratory, special tests must be requested on

specimens reported as contaminated by diphtheroids. The best therapy is probably penicillin, although ampicillin, erythromycin, or tetracycline have been used.

INFECTIONS CAUSED BY GRAM-NEGATIVE BACILLI

Unlike the normal host, the patient with a neoplasm frequently becomes colonized with gram-negative aerobic bacilli in areas such as the skin and respiratory tract. This change in body flora is most frequently related to antineoplastic chemotherapy, antimicrobial therapy, and debilitation and is most likely to occur in the hospital. Therefore, the etiology of infection in these patients must be considered in light of their abnormal flora. For example, serious head and neck infections in these patients (e.g., purulent sinusitis) should be treated for presence of gram-negative organisms (including *P. aeruginosa*) as well as the usual gram-positive organisms until results of cultures are known. In fact over the past 20 years gram-negative bacilli have replaced the staphylococcus as the most important causes of infections in patients with neoplastic diseases.

Organisms

Escherichia coli is still the most frequently encountered gram-negative aerobic bacillus causing either localized infection or bacteremia in cancer patients, but *Klebsiella-Enterobacter-Serratia* sp., *Proteus* sp., and *Pseudomonas* sp. are also important causes of gram-negative bacillary infections. Unusual organisms such as *Mimae* or *Herellea* are also more frequently found as causative organisms in patients with cancer. *Pseudomonas* accounts for only about 15 to 20% of all gram-negative bacillary bacteremias in this group; however, bacteremia due to *P. aeruginosa* accounts for 50% of the fatal gram-negative bacteremias in patients with neoplastic diseases. This is especially true in patients with hematologic malignancies; in patients with leukemia *P. aeruginosa* has been reported to cause about 80% of all fatal bacteremias (Fishman and Armstrong, 1972; Schimpff et al., 1974; Tapper and Armstrong, 1974). Although all bacteremias caused by gram-negative bacilli are more common in patients with defects in granulocyte function or numbers, *P. aeruginosa* bacteremia is especially likely to occur in this setting.

Wolfe et al. (1971) found a striking association of *Salmonella typhimurium* bacteremia with patients with leukemia and lymphoma.

They suggested that the hemolytic component in those diseases may predispose to *S. typhimurium* bacteremia similar to the predisposition in sickle cell disease and malaria. *Salmonella* infection was also associated with recent surgery in this study.

Site of Infection

Gram-negative bacilli can cause many varieties of infections in patients with cancer. As in the normal host the urinary and gastrointestinal tracts are the most common sites of infection due to gram-negative bacilli. However, gram-negative bacilli more frequently cause bacteremia, soft tissue infection, pneumonia, and meningitis in patients with malignant diseases (Twomey, 1973). This is especially true if the patient has been receiving intensive cancer chemotherapy or has a granulocyte defect.

A recent study of pneumonia in patients with leukemia revealed that over half of all pneumonias were caused by gram-negative bacilli and that the majority of these infections originated in the respiratory tract (Sickles et al., 1973). There was an especially high incidence of bacteremia in those patients with pneumonia due to *Pseudomonas* or *E. coli*. Mortality was significantly related to granulocytopenia.

One of the common sites of infection in patients with neoplastic diseases with or without granulocytopenia is the anorectal area (Schimpff, Wernik, and Block, 1972; Schimpff et al., 1972; Steinberg, Gold, and Brodin, 1973). Although these infections are frequently caused by anaerobic bacteria, gram-negative bacilli (including *P. aeruginosa* in the granulocytopenic patient) are common causative microorganisms. Thus, the rectal examination becomes most important when searching for the localization of infection in patients with malignancy.

In many patients with neoplastic disease and bacteremia, it is impossible to find the primary site of infection. This is especially true in granulocytopenic patients (i.e., <500 polymorphonuclear leukocytes/mm^3) who acquire *Pseudomonas bacteremia*. The likely source of these infections is the ulcerated gastrointestinal tract which has been previously colonized by *Pseudomonas*.

Therapy of Gram-negative Bacterial Infections

Gram-negative bacillary infections, especially bacteremia, may very rapidly be fatal. Thus, whenever an episode of fever occurs and bacteremia is suspected, appropriate gram stains and cultures should

be performed and therapy immediately initiated. In the nongranulo-
cytopenic patient, therapy should be aimed at *E. coli, Klebsiella-
Enterobacter* sp., and *Proteus* sp. as well as the more common
gram-positive coccal causes. Appropriate therapy should include
gentamicin; it is our policy to add a cephalosporin. Appropriate doses
for serious infections would be: gentamicin, 1.7 mg/kg intramuscularly or intravenously every 8 hr for patients with normal renal function, plus cephalothin, 2 g intravenously every 4 hr, or cefazolin, 1 g,
intramuscularly or intravenously every 6 to 8 hr. In the granulocytopenic patient with a high likelihood of *Pseudomonas* infection,
carbenicillin should be given with the gentamicin and cephalosporin.
The dose of carbenicillin is 500 mg/kg/day intravenously in divided
doses every 4 hr. When results of cultures become available, appropriate changes in therapy can be made. In a recent study it is stated
that despite widespread uses of carbenicillin and gentamicin the majority of *Pseudomonas* organisms remain sensitive (Fishman et al., 1972).

Pseudomonas Vaccine

Recently, a polyvalent vaccine against *P. aeruginosa* has been developed primarily for use in burn patients. It has been shown that this
vaccine may be useful in patients with solid tumors who develop
P. aeruginosa infection at a time when they have normal quantities of
granulocytes (Fisher, 1974; Young, Meyer, and Armstrong, 1973).
However, it is not protective in the granulocytopenic patient and can
cause significant fever and local pain. At present, it appears that *P.
aeruginosa* vaccine will have limited use in the patient with cancer.

Leukocyte Transfusions

Leukocyte transfusions from HLA matched donors have been used
with some success along with antibiotic therapy in granulocytopenic
patients who had bacteremia caused by gram-negative bacilli. This
modality of therapy may be particularly helpful in patients with
Pseudomonas bacteremia.

INFECTIONS CAUSED BY ANAEROBIC BACTERIA

Infections caused by anaerobic bacteria occur most frequently in
association with tumors which obstruct the bronchi and with tumors
which interrupt the integrity of the oral, gastrointestinal, or genito-
urinary mucosa. Anaerobic streptococci and *Bacteroides* sp. (usually

B. fragilis) are the organisms most commonly isolated (Kagnoff, Armstrong, and Blevins, 1972). *B. fragilis* is found in only 15% of pulmonary infections, but is almost always present in intra-abdominal and pelvic infections.

Most intra-abdominal, pararectal, and pelvic infections (excluding gonorrhea) in patients with or without neoplasms are caused by anaerobic bacteria; these infections often follow surgery. *Bacteroides fragilis* is the anaerobic organism that most frequently produces bacteremia and the frequency is increased in patients with malignancies. Although the primary site of infection in the patient with *B. fragilis* bacteremia is usually in the abdomen or pelvis, no localized infection may be apparent. The key to diagnosis of all anaerobic infections is use of proper anaerobic culture techniques.

Therapy of anaerobic infection involves drainage of pus, removal of necrotic tissue, and appropriate antimicrobial therapy. Clindamycin and chloramphenicol both have an excellent spectrum against anaerobes and have been shown to be effective in these infections. The doses are: 50 mg/kg/day of chloramphenicol in divided doses every 6 hr orally or intravenously; and 300 to 600 mg of clindamycin orally, intramuscularly, or intravenously every 8 hr (the higher dose and parenteral route are used in more serious infections). Chloramphenicol must be used in intracranial lesions as clindamycin does not penetrate the blood-brain barrier well.

Recently, bacteremia caused by *Clostridia* (usually *C. perfrigens*) has been recognized more frequently in the cancer patient (Wynne and Armstrong, 1972). This complication does not appear to be related to a specific type of malignancy, but rather to far advanced malignancy, intensive chemotherapy, and lesions of the bowel (either due to the malignancy itself or chemotherapy). The diagnosis should be suspected if bowel obstruction or cholecystitis is present or if there is cellulitis of the flanks or trunk (Armstrong et al., 1974). Therapy includes drainage and high dose penicillin therapy.

INFECTIONS CAUSED BY HIGHER BACTERIA

Nocardia

Among the higher bacteria, infections caused by *Nocardia asteroides* but not *Actinomyces* are more common in cancer patients. Nocardia infections are particularly likely to occur in patients with leukemia or lymphoma who are receiving adrenocorticosteroid therapy (Young et al., 1971). The respiratory tract is the usual portal of entry for infection, and pneumonia is the most common infection. The chest x-ray shows infiltrates with or without cavities (Grossman, Bragg, and Armstrong, 1970). If dissemination occurs, the kidneys, subcutaneous tissues, and brain may become involved.

The organism is a gram-positive, partially acid-fast, branching rod. Since the organism grows slowly and is easily overgrown by other flora of the upper respiratory tract, the microbiology laboratory should be specifically notified to search for this organism if it is to be isolated from sputum.

Therapy includes drainage and antimicrobial agents. Sulfonamides given in doses that produce peak serum concentrations of 12 to 15 mg/100 ml are often successful (e.g., 75 mg/kg/day in divided doses every 6 hr). In a few patients who did not respond to sulfonamides, minocycline or the combination of erythromycin plus ampicillin has been used (Bach, Monaco, and Finland, 1973). We would recommend beginning therapy with a sulfonamide and then tailoring therapy depending upon in vitro testing and patient response.

INFECTIONS CAUSED BY MYCOBACTERIUM TUBERCULOSIS

Tuberculosis can be fulminant in patients who are receiving adrenocorticosteroids or other immunosuppressive therapy for cancer. Thus all patients with malignancies, especially those with leukemias and lymphomas, should be PPD (purified protein derivative) skin tested at the time of diagnosis of the malignancy. If the skin test is negative, it is important to perform a battery of skin tests (e.g., *Trichophyton, Candida*, and mumps) to be sure the patient is not anergic. If the PPD is positive, the patient should be followed with chest x-rays every 6 to 12 months. If steroids or other immunosuppressive therapy is used to treat the patient with a positive skin test, isoniazide or rifampin should be given to prevent activation of the tuberculosis. In past years isoniazide therapy was recommended for all patients with leukemias or lymphomas who had positive skin tests. With recent knowledge of the high incidence of serious hepatotoxicity from isoniazide (especially in patients over the age of 35 or with underlying liver disease), such blanket recommendations are no longer justifiable. However, 12 to 18 months of isoniazide therapy can still be justified in leukemia or lymphoma patients below the age of 35 who have a positive PPD skin test.

Tuberculosis appears to be found with increased frequency in patients with carcinoma of the lung. Thus it is important to be suspicious of tuberculosis in these patients and to do proper smears and cultures.

In the patient with cancer who is receiving immunosuppressive therapy, tuberculosis may disseminate and may be fulminant. Pulmonary findings may be completely absent. Therefore a high index of suspicion for tuberculosis must be present, and bone marrow or liver biopsy must be performed for histology and culture in such patients. The disease is treated as in the normal host.

FUNGAL INFECTIONS

Invasive fungal infections have become increasingly important as causes of morbidity and mortality in patients who have altered host defenses due to malignancy, cancer chemotherapy, antibiotic therapy, or intravenous catheters. Although any fungus may be the cause of the infection, *Candida* sp., *Aspergillus* sp., and *Mucor* sp. are the most frequent invaders with *Candida* being the most important and *Mucor* the least frequent of the three. There appears to be an actual increase in incidence of these infections rather than a simple increase in identification of the infections (Levine et al., 1974). The increase in incidence is most strongly correlated with cancer chemotherapy. Cryptococcosis and disseminated histoplasmosis occur more frequently in patients with chronic lymphatic leukemia and lymphomas than in the general hospital population; however, the incidence of these infections does not appear to be increasing. Other fungal infections (including blastomycosis, sporotrichosis, coccidioidomycosis, chromoblastomycosis, and maduromycosis) are not found more frequently in patients with cancer, but may present in an atypical manner in these patients.

Candidiasis

Candidiasis is the most frequent of the fungal diseases seen in the patient with neoplasia. Most infections have been due to *C. albicans,* but infections caused by other *Candida* species have also been reported (Louria et al., 1967a). Localized forms of candidiasis (e.g., thrush, vaginitis, esophagitis) are frequent and usually indicate superficial colonization; dissemination can develop from any superficial area (i.e., mouth, gastrointestinal tract, or urinary tract).

Candida fungemia with subsequent dissemination of infection usually occurs in patients with indwelling intravascular catheters. Once infection disseminates, the organs primarily involved are the kidneys, lungs, meninges, heart, and eyes; however, any organ may be involved secondary to fungemia (Louria, Stiff, and Bennett, 1962). Serologic studies (e.g., agglutinating antibodies) may suggest invasion if there is a rising titer; however, these studies may be falsely negative or positive (Preisler et al., 1969). Recently, *Candida* endophthalmitis has been recognized more frequently and has been very useful in suggesting the presence of disseminated disease. Thus, visual complaints in the compromised host should lead to prompt ophthalmoscopic examination; these examinations should be performed repeatedly in the patient suspected of having disseminated *Candida* infection (Meyers, Lieberman, and Ferry, 1973; Edwards et al., 1974). Although candidemia has frequently been reported to be benign and transient in a general hospital population (almost always in association with intravascular catheters), candidemia in a compromised host such as one with leukemia or lymphoma usually means disseminated disease (Levine et al., 1974).

Every effort must be made to prevent disseminated candidiasis by avoiding the use of intravascular catheters and treating localized candidiasis. Once the disseminated disease is suspected, a vigorous diagnostic search including blood and urine cultures and tissue biopsies, if indicated, must be performed. The treatment is intravenous amphotericin B therapy (Bennett, 1974).

Aspergillosis

Aspergillosis is the second most common fungal infection in patients with leukemia and lymphoma. Patients with solid tumors also develop disseminated aspergillosis in the setting of corticosteroid therapy, cytotoxic therapy, and/or leukopenia (Meyer et al., 1973). The most frequent species isolated are *Aspergillus fumigatus* and *Aspergillus flavus;* however, *Aspergillus glaucus* and other species have been involved. Invasive aspergillosis most frequently causes pulmonary disease. Although there is no pathognomonic x-ray finding, multiple nodular infiltrates, crossing fissures, which rapidly progress is suggestive. Aspergillosis of the lung may mimic pulmonary emboli because the fungus has the propensity to involve blood vessels and cause thrombosis and infarction. Other sites of invasive aspergillosis have included the gastrointestinal tract, brain, liver, and kidney.

Antemortem diagnosis is difficult because positive cultures of sputum, for example, do not necessarily mean disease and cultures are often negative in the presence of disease; blood cultures rarely are positive. Serologic studies have not proven very useful. Thus, in order to diagnose the disease antemortem, a vigorous diagnostic work-up such as transtracheal aspiration, bronchial brushing, closed needle biopsy, and/or open lung biopsy is necessary; tissue biopsy is most rewarding.

The antimicrobial therapy of choice for disseminated aspergillosis is intravenous amphotericin B, but the results of therapy are poor.

Mucormycosis

Mucormycosis includes a group of infections caused by the non-septate fungi of the order *Mucorales. Rhizopus, Absidia,* and *Mucor* species are most frequently involved. These infections have been classically reported in patients with diabetes with sinusitis and orbital cellulitis. Although patients with leukemia and lymphoma may occasionally present with this classic syndrome, disseminated pulmonary and central nervous system mucormycosis is more common. In fact, the most common presentation in one report on the disease in the compromised host was fever and progressive pulmonary infiltration despite antibiotics (Meyer, Rosen, and Armstrong, 1972). Other organs involved included the spleen, kidney, heart, liver, and stomach. In mucormycosis like aspergillosis, the blood vessels are invaded and the presentation may be similar to that of pulmonary emboli or cerebral infarction. Blood cultures and cultures of sputum and urine, and even cultures of the involved tissues, tend to be negative. Thus, diagnosis is made premortem only with vigorous work-up including tissue biopsies for histology (which is most apt to be rewarding) and culture. Treatment is intravenous amphotericin B therapy.

Cryptococcosis

Cryptococcus neofomans causes acute or chronic meningeal, pulmonary, or disseminated disease which is seen with increased frequency in patients with lymphoma and chronic lymphatic leukemia. The portal of entry appears to be the respiratory tract. Any suspicion of central nervous system disease should lead to lumbar puncture with appropriate studies including India ink preparation and search for cryptococcal polysaccharide in the cerebrospinal fluid (Goodman,

Kaufman, and Koenig, 1971); large amounts of CSF must be cultured. Culture of sputum and urine for cryptococcus should be performed in all patients suspected of having cryptococcosis. The therapy is intravenous amphotericin B (Newberry, 1972).

Histoplasmosis

Histoplasma capsulatum is a dimorphic fungus which usually causes pulmonary disease in the normal host. Patients with leukemia or lymphoma may develop disseminated disease involving the reticuloendothelial system, lungs, brain, and/or mucosa. Although the incidence of disseminated histoplasmosis is not greatly increased in patients with malignancies, it should be considered in the appropriate setting. Although the diagnosis can sometimes be made by isolation of *Histoplasma capsulatum* from blood or sputum, histologic examination and culture of biopsy specimens (e.g., liver, marrow, mucosal ulcerations) are usually more rewarding. The therapy is amphotericin B (Bennett, 1974).

Therapy of Fungal Diseases

Amphotericin B is the recommended therapy for all of these deep fungal diseases. Although newer agents such as 5-fluorocytosine have been reported to give favorable results in some patients with candidiasis and cryptococcosis, these drugs should not be used as primary therapy in the compromised host at present (Newberry, 1972). After initial doses of 1 mg and 5 mg, amphotericin B is given in doses of 0.5 mg/kg/day or 1.0 mg/kg every other day in an intravenous drip over a period of 6 hr. Intrathecal administration may be necessary in meningitis.

Transfer factor, a dialyzable substance isolated from peripheral blood leukocytes, is being investigated to determine its efficacy in the restoration of cutaneous delayed hypersensitivity and cellular immunity in patients with cancer (Lawrence, 1972). Its mechanism of action has not been established at present. It has been used in patients with mucocutaneous candidiasis, disseminated coccidioidomycosis, and tuberculosis. Although there have been no serious trials of this agent in cancer patients, it may prove to be of benefit in the future for the treatment of refractory fungal and mycobacterial infection in these patients.

MANAGEMENT OF PATIENT WITH
NEOPLASTIC DISEASE WHO DEVELOPS FEVER

The sudden onset of fever in a patient with a neoplasm, especially with leukemia or lymphoma, is strongly suggestive of bacterial infection, either bacteremia or pneumonia (Levine et al., 1974). About two-thirds of febrile episodes in patients with leukemia and lymphoma are caused by infections, over 90% of which are bacterial or fungal (Levine et al., 1974). Of life-threatening infections in patients with leukemia and lymphoma, bacteremia caused by gram-negative aerobic bacilli accounts for about 40%, fungemia for about 10%, bacterial pneumonia for about 20%, and fungal pneumonia for about 10%.

The therapeutic approach will depend upon the absolute numbers of polymorphonuclear leukocytes present.

Patient with Adequate Numbers of Polymorphonuclear Leukocytes

Any patient with neoplastic disease who suddenly develops fever should have a complete history and physical examination with emphasis on probable portals of entry (e.g., urethral catheters, intravascular catheters) and sites with a high probability of infection (e.g., pneumonia). Gram stains and cultures of pus should be obtained as well as at least two to three sets of blood cultures. Chest x-ray should always be performed because pneumonia is common and physical signs may be absent. In the patient with adequate polymorphonuclear leukocytes in whom the above examination does not point to a specific organism causing infection, antimicrobial therapy should be begun to cover the common gram-positive and gram-negative bacteria. A reasonable regimen would be a cephalosporin plus gentamicin as described in the section on gram-negative bacilli. If intra-abdominal or pelvic infection is suspected, clindamycin or chloramphenicol may be added. If cultures are positive, therapy can be altered as indicated. If fever continues for days and cultures are negative, infection caused by fungi, higher bacteria, mycobacteria, and other microorganisms becomes more likely. At this time, antibiotics should be discontinued and further work-up including tissue biopsies of areas of suspected infection should be performed.

Patient with Inadequate Numbers of Polymorphonuclear Leukocytes ($<500/mm^3$)

In a patient with granulocytopenia, the evaluation including a history, physical examination, and cultures should also be performed. Gram stains should be performed of all suspicious areas even in the absence of pus as these patients may not be able to produce pus. Once cultures are taken, antimicrobial therapy should be begun including therapy against the *Pseudomonas*. A reasonable combination would be a cephalosporin plus carbenicillin and gentamicin as described in the section on gram-negative bacilli. If subsequent evidence does not support bacterial infection (i.e., negative cultures) and fever continues, the possibility of tuberculosis or fungal infection must be evaluated.

PREVENTION OF INFECTION IN PATIENTS WITH NEOPLASTIC DISEASE

The prevention of infection in patients with neoplasia is of utmost importance. Hospitalization with exposure to antibiotic-resistant organisms should be avoided whenever possible. Once hospitalization becomes necessary, prolonged venous or urinary catheterization should be avoided. If venous catheters are necessary, they should be cared for by scrupulously clean techniques. Closed sterile drainage systems should be used when indwelling urinary catheters are necessary. Any respiratory equipment must be handled with careful asepsis.

The granulocytopenic patient (polymorphonuclear leukocytes, $<500/mm^3$) is at particular risk in the hospital environment. This patient should be in reverse isolation, served food and water that are preferably sterile or have a low bacterial content, and given sterilized clothes and sheets. The use of laminar flow rooms in combination with oral nonabsorbable antibiotics has been shown to decrease the numbers of serious infections and infectious deaths in leukopenic patients with leukemia and lymphoma. However, these techniques are very expensive and require special expertise and thus are still research tools for prevention of infection.

SUMMARY

Patients with malignant diseases are highly susceptible to infections because of altered host defenses and an altered indigenous bacterial flora. The majority of infections are caused by common pathogens; however, unusual infecting microorganisms may cause infection in these patients. Many of the organisms producing infection are resistant to many antimicrobial agents; therefore, it is of great importance to use a vigorous diagnostic approach and to look for the more unusual pathogens. Of utmost importance is the prevention of infections whenever possible by avoiding use of intravascular catheters and other equipment and procedures that predispose to infection. Therapy must be vigorous and specific.

REFERENCES

Armstrong, D., A. Blevins, D. B. Louria, J. S. Henkel, M. D. Moody, and M. Sukany. 1970. Groups B, C, and G streptococcal infections in a cancer hospital. Ann. N.Y. Acad. Sci. 174:511–522.

Armstrong, D. L., L. S. Young, R. D. Meyer, and A. H. Blevins. 1974. Infectious complications of neoplastic disease. Med. Clin. North Amer. 55:729–745.

Bach, M. C., A. P. Monaco, and M. Finland. 1973. Pulmonary Nocardiosis: Therapy with minocycline and with erythromycin plus ampicillin. JAMA 224:1378–1381.

Bennett, J. E. 1974. Chemotherapy of systemic mycoses. New Eng. J. Med. 290:30–32.

Chernik, N. L., D. Armstrong, and J. B. Posner. 1973. Central nervous system infections in patients with cancer. Medicine 52:563–581.

DeVita, V. T., and R. C. Young. 1973. Infection and cancer: Old friends. Ann. Intern. Med. 79:597–599.

Edwards, J. E., Jr., R. Y. Foos, J. Z. Montgomerie, and L. B. Guze. 1974. Occular manifestations of candida septicemia: Review of seventy-six cases of hematogenous candida endophthalmitis. Medicine 53:47–75.

Fisher, M. W. 1974. Development of immunotherapy for infections due to *Pseudomonas aeruginosa*. J. Infect. Dis. 130 (Suppl.):S149–S151.

Fishman, L. S., and D. Armstrong. 1972. *Pseudomonas aeruginosa* bacteremia in patients with neoplastic disease. Cancer 30:764–773.

Goodman, J. S., L. Kaufman, and M. G. Koenig. 1971. Diagnosis of cryptococcal meningitis: Value of immunologic detection of cryptococcal antigen. New Eng. J. Med. 285:434–436.

Grossman, C. B., D. G. Bragg, and D. Armstrong. 1970. Roentgen manifestations of pulmonary Nocardiosis. Radiology 96:325–330.

Henkel, J. S., D. Armstrong, A. Blevins, and M. D. Moody. 1970. Group A, B-hemolytic Streptococcus bacteremia in a cancer hospital. JAMA 211:983–986.

Inagani, J., V. Rodriguez, and G. P. Bodey. 1974. Causes of death in cancer patients. Cancer 33:568–573.

Kagnoff, M. F., D. Armstrong, and A. Blevins. 1972. Bacteroides bacteremia: Experience in a hospital for neoplastic diseases. Cancer 29:245–251.

Lawrence, H. S. 1972. Immunotherapy with transfer factor. New Eng. J. Med. 287:1092–1094.

Levine, A. S., S. C. Schimpff, R. G. Graw, Jr., and R. C. Young. 1974. Hematologic malignancies and other marrow failure states: Progress in the management of complicating infections. Semin. Hematol. 11:141–202.

Louria, D. B., and D. Armstrong. 1970. Listeria infections. Ann. N.Y. Acad. Sci. 174:545–551.

Louria, D. B., A. Blevins, D. Armstrong, R. Burdick, and P. Lieberman. 1967a. Fungemia caused by "non-pathogenic" yeasts. Arch. Intern. Med. 119:247–256.

Louria, D. B., T. Hensle, D. Armstrong, H. S. Collins, A. Blevins, D. Krugman, and M. Buse. 1967b. Listerosis complicating malignant disease: A new association. Ann. Intern. Med. 67:261–281.

Louria, D. B., D. P. Stiff, and B. Bennett. 1962. Disseminated moniliasis in the adult. Medicine 41:303–337.

Meyer, R. D., P. Rosen, and D. Armstrong. 1972. Phycomycosis complicating leukemia and lymphoma. Ann. Intern. Med. 77:871–879.

Meyer, R. D., L. S. Young, D. Armstrong, and B. Yu. 1973. Aspergillosis complicating neoplastic disease. Amer. J. Med. 54:6–15.

Meyers, B. R., T. W. Lieberman, and A. P. Ferry. 1973. Candida endophthalmitis complicating candidemia. Ann. Intern. Med. 79:647–653.

Newberry, W. M. 1972. Drug treatment of the systemic mycoses. Semin. Hematol. 2:313–329.

Preisler, H. D., H. F. Hasenclever, A. A. Levitan, and E. S. Henderson. 1969. Serologic diagnosis of disseminated candidiasis in patients with acute leukemia. Ann. Intern. Med. 70:19–30.

Schimpff, S. C., W. H. Greene, V. M. Young, and P. H. Wiernik. 1974. Significance of *Pseudomonas aeruginosa* in the patient with leukemia or lymphoma. J. Infect. Dis. 130 (Suppl.):S24–S31.

Schimpff, S. C., P. H. Wiernik, and J. B. Block. 1972. Rectal abscesses in cancer patients. Lancet 2:844–847.

Schimpff, S. C., V. M. Young, W. H. Greene, G. D. Vermeulen, M. R. Moody, and P. H. Wiernik. 1972. Origin of infection in acute non-lymphocytic leukemia. Ann. Intern. Med. 77:707–714.

Sickles, E. A., V. M. Young, W. H. Greene, and P. H. Wiernik. 1973. Pneumonia in acute leukemia. Ann. Intern. Med. 79:528–534.

Silver, R. T. 1963. Infections, fever and host resistance in neoplastic diseases. J. Chronic Dis. 16:677–701.

Steinberg, D., J. Gold, and A. Brodin. 1973. Necrotizing enterocolitis in leukemia. Arch. Intern. Med. 131:538–544.

Tapper, M. L., and D. Armstrong. 1974. Bacteremia due to *Pseudomonas aeruginosa* complicating neoplastic disease: A progress report. J. Infect. Dis. 130 (Suppl.):S14–S23.

Twomey, J. J. 1973. Infections complicating multiple myeloma and chronic lymphocytic leukemia. Arch. Intern. Med. 132:562–565.

Wolfe, M. S., D. Armstrong, D. B. Louria, and A. Blevins. 1971. Salmonellosis in patients with neoplastic disease. Arch. Intern. Med. 128:546–554.

Wynne, J. W., and D. Armstrong. 1972. Clostridial septicemia. Cancer 29:215–221.

Young, L. S., D. Armstrong, A. Blevins, and P. Lieberman. 1971. *Nocardia asteroides* infection complicating neoplastic disease. Amer. J. Med. 50:356–367.

Young, L. S., R. D. Meyer, and D. L. Armstrong. 1973. *Pseudomonas aeruginosa* vaccine in cancer patients. Ann. Intern. Med. 79:518–527.

Viral and Protozoan Infections in Cancer Patients

Richard K. Root, M.D.

Systemic infections with bacteria and fungi account for most of the infection-related mortality in patients with advanced malignancies, particularly those involving the hematopoietic system or in patients on high dose cytotoxic and steroid therapy (Levine, Graw, and Young, 1972; Levine et al., 1974). On the other hand, a great deal of morbidity and some fatalities in such patients can be ascribed to infections by certain viruses and protozoans. Table 1 indicates which viral and protozoan infections are seen with increased frequency and severity in cancer patients (Levine, Graw, and Young, 1972; Levine et al., 1974). It is the purpose of this chapter to discuss the mechanisms responsible for infection by those agents, to indicate the mode of their presentation and their particular complications, and finally to develop rational approaches to diagnosis and therapy in clinical situations in which infection by these agents is suspected or proven.

HOST AND EPIDEMIOLOGIC FACTORS LEADING TO VIRAL OR PROTOZOAN INFECTION IN PATIENTS WITH CANCER

The integrity of local mucocutaneous barriers, the patency of normal drainage tracts, and an adequate acute inflammatory response all

Table 1. Protozoan and viral infections occurring with increased frequency or severity in cancer patients

Protozoan
Pneumocystis carinii
Toxoplasma gondii
Viral
Herpes group viruses
Cytomegalovirus
Varicella-Zoster virus
Herpes simplex virus
Vaccinia
Rubeola
Hepatitis B

play a critical role in the initial host defenses against systemic invasion by bacteria and fungi, whereas antibody formation and cellular immunity become significant only in the event of prolonged infection. The increased incidence and severity of bacterial and fungal infections in patients with malignancy who are receiving cytotoxic therapy can largely be ascribed to alterations in the acute inflammatory response with neutropenia being the major factor along with disruption of the local defense barriers (Bodey et al., 1966, 1972; Green et al., 1973).

In contrast, relatively little is known about the initial defense mechanisms against viral and protozoan infections and how they might be altered by malignancy or its therapy. Certain viruses such as herpes simplex may gain entry into the body through local inoculation at skin break sites (Stern et al., 1959; Foley et al., 1970). Local irradiation may precipitate symptomatic herpes zoster infection in the exposed site (Stern et al., 1959; Rifkind, 1966). Interferon production occurs early in the course of most viral infections and may aid in shortening their course. Patients with advanced lymphomas on steroid therapy exhibit reduced cutaneous interferon production when infected with varicella-zoster virus (Armstrong et al., 1970).

The role that phagocytosis plays in protection against viral infection is unknown; however, it may be significant in providing protection against infection by protozoans. *Toxoplasma gondii* organisms are known to be capable of surviving inside granulocytes and macrophages for an extended period of time due to an inhibition of the fusion of lysosomes with the phagocytic vacuole (Jones and Hirsch, 1972). Whether or not another parasitic protozoan, *Pneumocystis carinii,* exerts the same effect on these cells is unknown. Neutropenia produced by hematopoietic malignancies, marrow replacement, or cytotoxic therapy may therefore play a role in predisposing patients to protozoan infections as might the anti-inflammatory effects of corticosteroids by depressing the phagocytic defenses.

Given the capability of viruses and protozoans to survive for prolonged periods within the host, it is not surprising that an accumulating body of evidence supports a major role for humoral and cellular immunity in controlling infection by these agents (Merigan, 1974). Neutralizing antibody against viruses may prevent infection by blocking attachment of the virus to the host target cell or rendering it nonviable. It seems likely that antibody may also play a role in opsonizing protozoans for ingestion by granulocytes and macrophages. The role of antibodies, then, can be seen to limit spread of organisms in the extracellular location from one site to another. Certain patients with lymphomas or lymphatic leukemias may have depressed antibody formation as do patients with myeloma (Fahey and Boggs, 1969; Hersh, 1971). Corticosteroid and cytotoxic therapy will impair humoral immune responses to new antigens while leaving established antibody levels relatively intact (Kass, Kendrick, and Finland, 1955; Santos, Owens, and Sensenbrenner, 1964; Makindan, Santos, and Quinn, 1970; Hersh et al., 1971; Leventhal, Cohen, and Triem, in press).

Macrophages that have been "activated" by contact with extracellular materials (lymphokines) formed and released by T-lymphocytes under specific antigenic stimulation will increase in size, become more avidly phagocytic, and develop an increased metabolic and microbicidal capacity (Steinman and Cohn, 1974). Such cells are capable of killing intracellular organisms such as protozoans, which may have survived in the initial postphagocytic period. It is possible that they might also kill viruses by a similar mechanism, although proof for this is lacking. Advanced Hodgkin's disease is characteristically accompanied by cutaneous anergy (Hersh and Oppenheim, 1965; Aisenberg, 1966; Young et al., 1972) and recent evidence indicates that this is also true of other malignant states when the tumor burden is high (Eilber and Morton, 1970). Malnutrition and corticosteroid therapy also suppress cellular immune mechanisms broadly (MacGregor et al., 1969; Smythe et al., 1971; Yu, Clements, and Paulus, 1974; Fauci and Dale, 1975), whereas cytotoxic drugs exert their primary effects on newly developing cellular immunity (Makindan, Santos, and Quinn, 1970).

Table 2 summarizes diseases and therapies that are associated with depressions in host defenses in the different areas discussed above. The infectious complications of such impairments are as follows.

When granulocytopenia is present, particularly when coupled with corticosteroid treatment, the major infections are produced by pyogenic bacteria and fungi such as *Aspergillus* and *Candida*. Depressions of antibody formation have as their consequence an increased incidence of infection with bacteria that require opsonization for irradication as well as infection by *Pneumocystis carinii* and vaccinia. In the face of impaired cellular immunity infection by intracellular bacteria, such as tuberculosis and listeria, is observed. In addition, disseminated infections with protozoans, the DNA viruses belonging to the herpes group, and measles and vaccina viruses may develop (Levine, Graw, and Young, 1972; Levine et al., 1974). Given the fact that multiple defects in host defense may exist in the same patient, simultaneous or sequential infection with a variety of different organisms is a common event and must be considered in the diagnostic and therapeutic approaches to the patient.

Besides alterations in host defenses, epidemiologic factors play a significant role in the pathogenesis of viral and protozoan infections in this patient group. Transfusion of blood products has been re-

Table 2. Host impairments in malignancy responsible for protozoan and viral infections

System	Impairment
Local	Irradiation Mucosal or skin ulceration
Phagocytic	Neutropenia, steroids
Interferon production	Lymphoma, steroids
Antibody production	Lymphoma, myeloma cytotoxic agents steroids
Cell-mediated immunity	Lymphoma, carcinomatosis cytotoxic agents steroids

sponsible for the subsequent development of hepatitis (Cherubin and Prince, 1971), cytomegalovirus (CMV) (Stevens et al., 1970), and Ebstein-Barr virus (EBV) (Turner, MacDonald, and Cooper, 1972) infections and toxoplasmosis (Siegel et al., 1971). Hospital epidemics of *Pneumocystis carinii* (Johnson and Johnson, 1970; Perera et al., 1970), zoster-varicella viruses (Schimpff et al., 1972), and vaccinia (Lane et al., 1969) have been well documented resulting from the exposure of susceptible individuals to other patients with these infections. Epidemiologic factors also play the primary role in the development of type B hepatitis virus infection in this patient population, whereas altered immunity appears to make its major impact by modifying the form the disease takes as is discussed below.

CHARACTERISTICS OF SPECIFIC VIRAL AND PROTOZOAL INFECTIONS IN CANCER PATIENTS

Pneumocystis carinii

Infection by this protozoan is almost exclusively limited to the lungs (Rifkind, Faris, and Hill, 1966; Walzer et al., 1974), although at least one case of extrapulmonary infection has been described (Jarnum et al., 1968). The patient population that develops this disease as reported to the Center for Disease Control (Walzer et al., 1974; Western, Perera, and Schultz, 1970) almost exclusively falls into three categories: 1) neonates, particularly premature infants, 2) individuals with hypogammaglobulinemia, and 3) patients receiving steroid therapy for a variety of underlying diseases, including malignancy. The precise source of the organism is not known although animal vectors are possible, person to person transmission has been documented (Johnson and Johnson, 1970; Perera et al., 1970), and some asymptomatic patients dying of other causes have been found to have *Pneumocystis* in pulmonary sections, suggesting that some infections are of the reactivation type (Esterly, 1968). The typical clinical picture is that of an interstitial pneumonia developing over several days to several weeks with associated fever, dry cough, and progressive dyspnea and hypoxia (Rifkind, Faris, and Hill, 1966; Western, Perera, and Schultz, 1970; Walzer et al., 1974). Clinical manifestations often develop during the period of tapering of steroid therapy (Western, Perera, and Schultz, 1970). While the incidence of this agent as a cause for interstitial pneumonia shows considerable variation among institutions, in at least one major center involved extensively in the treatment of cancer patients *Pneumocystis carinii* has been found to be responsible for 50% of interstitial pneumonias (Goodell et al., 1970). Variant clinical pictures have been described in which patients have had localized nodular infiltrates rather than diffuse disease or dyspnea, hypoxia, and fever without roentgenographic manifestations until late in the caurse (Sheldon, 1959; Cross and Steigbeigel, 1974; Friedman et al., 1975).

Since the disease is invariably fatal if untreated (Rifkind, Faris, and Hill, 1966; Western, Perera, and Schultz, 1970) and effective treatment involves the use of a highly toxic drug (pentamidine isethionate), every effort should be made to establish the diagnosis in clinically suspect patients before committing them to therapy. Examination of expectorated or aspirated sputum for the characteristic cup-shaped cysts, which are best revealed when stained with materials that deposit silver in the cyst walls (e.g., methenamine silver), should be performed. However, these studies are usually unrevealing. The use of fibroptic bronchoscopy, coupled with bronchial washing (Drew et al., 1974), or brush biopsy (Repshir, Schroter, and Hammond, 1972), has been much more useful with yields approaching 50% in active cases. Failing diagnosis by these maneuvers, lung biopsy is indicated, under cover of platelet transfusions if necessary (Western, Perera, and Schultz, 1970).

Therapy with pentamidine isethionate (4 mg/kg/day, i.m.) for 10 to 14 days results in a 60 to 65% cure rate with a small percentage of survivors exhibiting pulmonary fibrosis of varying degrees (Rifkind, Faris, and Hill, 1966; Western, Perera, and Schultz, 1970). This treatment is complicated by azotemia, hypoglycemia, and local muscle necrosis in an appreciable number of patients. Anaphylactoid reactions have been described in patients receiving intravenous therapy so that the intramuscular route of administration is preferred. Some therapeutic successes with combined use of pyramethamine and sulfadiazine have been described (Kirby, Kenamore, and Guckian, 1971); however, this author has had one striking failure with these drugs (as have others) and at present there seem to be no compelling reasons for their use.

Toxoplasmosis

The high incidence of seropositivity to toxoplasmosis in normal adults indicates that infection by this obligate intracellular protozoan is a common and often unrecognized event (Feldman, 1968). Most symptomatic infections in normal hosts are mild and may produce an illness that mimics infectious mononucleosis (Felman, 1968) or, on rare occasion, localized central nervous system disease (Sexton, Eyles, and Dillman, 1963), myositis (Greenlee et al., 1975) or persistent localized lymph node enlargement that superficially resembles lymphoma (Barlotta et al., 1969). In patients with hematologic malignancies or those receiving immunosuppressive therapy post-organ transplantation, a severe, highly lethal disseminated infection may develop with diffuse involvement of the central nervous system, heart, liver, kidneys, and lungs (Reynolds, Walls, and Pfeiffer, 1966; Carey et al., 1973; Gleason and Hamlin, 1974). An encephalitis-like picture is characteristic, often with cranial nerve palsies, together with interstitial pulmonary infiltrates, hepatosplenomegaly, lymphadenopathy, congestive heart failure, and fever.

The definitive host of this organism is the cat which sheds oocysts in the stool which are infectious by the oral route (Krogstad, Juranek, and Walls, 1972). A more common way of developing infection is by the ingestion of raw or partially cooked meat which contains the encysted form of the protozoan. This danger is avoided when meat is frozen since the cysts are destroyed by this process (Jacobs, Remington, and Melton, 1960). On rare occasion infection has been transmitted by the infusion of blood products (Siegel et al., 1971). The diagnosis is made by documentation of the organism in infected tissue or characteristic changes in infected lymph nodes (a unique reticulum cell hyperplasia) (Dorfman ánd Remington, 1973) together with high or rising titers of antibody. Characteristically IgM antibodies can be documented by indirect fluorescence assay (Remington, Miller, and Brownlee, 1968) during active infection. Specific therapy is available with the combined use of pyramethamine (25 mg daily) and sulfadiazine (1 g 4 times daily). Folinic acid (10 mg daily p.o. or i.m.) should be given to avoid marrow suppression. Treatment is given for at least 4 weeks (Feldman, 1968).

Viruses: Herpes Group

Varicella-Zoster Localized zoster is a common occurrence in adults receiving irradiation therapy for malignancy, with the characteristic vesicular lesions appearing in the dermatomes involved in the irradiation portal (Sokal and Firat, 1965; Rifkind, 1966). The disease is particularly prevalent in subjects with Hodgkin's disease, appearing with a frequency of 25% in one series (Schimpff et al.,

1972). In the same series, 8% of patients with lymphoma, 1% of patients with leukemia, and 2% of patients with solid tumors developed zoster at some point in their course. In the majority of patients clinical disease represents reactivation of endogenous infection (Chang, 1971), although rare examples of epidemic exogenous reinfection have been documented (Schimpff et al., 1972; Goffinet, Glastkin, and Merigan, 1972). Approximately one-third of actively infected patients will develop a disseminated form of the infection with widespread skin lesions and, in the most severe cases, pulmonary, hepatic, and central nervous system involvement. Dissemination is favored by advanced disease and cutaneous anergy, indicative of the important role that cell-mediated immunity plays in localizing infection (Merigan, 1974).

Along the same lines high dose corticosteroid therapy may be associated with dissemination. Mortality may result when dissemination occurs and may approach 2 to 3%. Similar to adults, children with malignancies and on high dose corticosteroid treatment are more prone to a potentially lethal dissemination of primary varicella infections (Pinkel, 1961; Prager, Bruder, and Jawitsky, 1971).

If given early after exposure, passive humoral immunity administered in the form of zoster immune globulin (ZIG) may prevent or blunt clinical disease in susceptible patients. It has no value in the treatment of actively infected patients (Brunell, Gershon, and Hughes, 1972; Brunell and Gershon, 1973; Gershon, Steinberg, and Brunell, 1974). Supplies are limited and must be obtained through the Center for Disease Control, Atlanta, Georgia. Although initial case reports using cytosine arabinoside (ARA-C) or iodoxyuridine (IUDR) appeared promising as effective chemotherapy against this DNA virus, recent controlled studies have demonstrated no value for these agents, and in fact treated patients frequently develop major myelosuppression from these drugs which increases both morbidity and mortality (Stevens et al., 1973; Zaky et al., 1974). It is too early to say if treatment with adenosine arabinoside (ARA-A) will offer more therapeutic benefit with less toxicity (Johnson et al., 1975). IUDR dissolved in dimethylsulfoxide has been partially successful in treating localized zoster (Juel-Jensen et al., 1970). The primary management of active infection in these patients involves reduction of dosages of cytotoxic and steroid therapies. Most importantly, infection prevention is key to controlling the disease in this patient population. Therefore, all patients with zoster or varicella should be placed on isolation until the lesions crust over. Virus shedding in the respiratory tract during active zoster infection has not been clearly documented in patients with disseminated infection, unless they have pneumonia (Schimpff et al., 1972), so that contact isolation should be sufficient to prevent infection spread.

Herpes Simplex Viruses (HSV)   Most patients with infection by these viruses develop localized vesicles in the oral (herpes virus type I) or genital (herpes virus type II) regions. In adults the appearance of oral lesions usually represents reactivation of latent infection and is promoted by concurrent febrile illnesses, or, on occasion, exposure to ultraviolet rays in sunlight (Nahmias and Roizman, 1973). Children and adolescents with primary herpes virus type I infections can have oral ulcers, exudative tonsilitis, cervical adenopathy, and high fever (Nahmias and Roizman, 1973).

In patients with leukemia or lymphoma or other malignancies in which cytotoxic and steroid therapy is employed an extensive necrotizing cellulitis may develop at the infection site (Montgomerie et al., 1969; Arora et al., 1974). Fatalities may occur because of secondary bacterial infection.

Disseminated herpes virus infections may also develop in this population with widespread skin lesions and pulmonary and central nervous system involvement (Lynfield, Farhangi, and Runnels, 1969; Muller, Herrmann, and Winkelmann, 1972). In some patients only pulmonary or CNS infection may be seen. In the former, rather than presenting as diffuse interstitial disease, characteristic of other viral pneumonias, a severe necrotizing tracheobronchitis and confluent bronchopneumonia may be seen (Case Records, 1973). CNS infection by herpes type I or II may take the form of a mild aseptic meningitis, or a severe necrotizing focal cerebritis often localized to the temporal region of the cerebrum. This latter form of infection is more typical of type I HSV (Juel-Jensen and MacCallum, 1972; Nahmias and Roizman, 1973; Morrison et al., 1974). Headache, seizures, and a hemorrhagic CSF may mimic localized bleeding into the cerebrum or a space-occupying lesion. While this picture is characteristic of HSV encephalitis in normal subjects, in immunosuppressed patients a more indolent and diffuse process may develop which mimics progressive multifocal leukoencephalopathy (Price et al., 1973).

Since antibody formation develops with primary illness, a common occurrence in the pediatric and adolescent population, serologic assays for antibodies are not reliable as a diagnostic aid in the adult unless they are done serially and a conversion from negative to positive or a 4-fold rise in titer occurs (Nahmias and Roizman, 1973). Definitive diagnosis is made by demonstrating typical intranuclear inclusions of the Cowdry type A ("owls eye") in infected tissue and the virus can be positively identified by fluorescent antibody tagging or growth in tissue culture (Juel-Jensen and MacCallum, 1972; Nahmias and Roizman, 1973).

Effective topical therapy is provided by photoinactivation techniques, employing neutral red dye or proflavine (Felber et al., 1973) or the topical application of IUDR (Weinstein and Chang, 1973). Systemic IUDR has been tried with variable success for life-threatening disease involving the CNS or other organs. A well controlled recent study indicates that this form of therapy probably does not alter the natural history of the disease and in fact may add to myelosuppression caused by chemotherapy (Boston Interhospital Virus Study Group, 1975).

Like varicella-zoster infections disseminated HSV infection may be very difficult to eradicate. The best treatment is prevention. Interferon inducers may also offer some potential usefulness; however, no controlled studies of their effectiveness exist (Bellanti, Catalana, and Chambers, 1971).

Cytomegalovirus (CMV)   Infections by CMV are ubiquitous and protean in their clinical manifestations (Weller, 1971). Serologic surveys detect specific antibodies in 60 to 80% of normal adults indicative of previous infection. Man to man transfer may occur by oral or venereal routes (Jordan et al., 1973) and disease has been induced by the transfusion of infected blood products (Stevens et al., 1970). Clinical illness may be undetectable, or it may present an infectious mononucleosis-like picture with fever, atypical lymphocytosis, a maculopapular skin rash, and hepatic involvement (Jordan et al., 1973). Localized or extensive ulceration of the oral and GI tract may occur as may cryptogenic fever, nodular interstitial pneumonia, hepatitis, or encephalitis (Weller, 1971). CMV has also been implicated in the pathogenesis of the Guillain-Barre syndrome (Klemola et al., 1967). Cytotoxic or steroid therapy may activate latent infection in cancer patients or promote viral shedding without obvious evidence of infection (Henson et al., 1972). Some patients dying with malignancy have evidence of widespread organ invasion with the virus, although the agent appears rarely to be a cause of fatal infection by itself (Bodey, Westlake, and Douglas, 1965; Rifkind, Goodman, and Hill, 1967; Dyment et al., 1968; Fine et al., 1970; Myers et al., 1975).

Definitive diagnosis of active infection by CMV depends upon the occurrence of a compatible clinical picture together with demonstration of the virus in infected tissue or its shedding into the urine or saliva and 4-fold or greater rises in complement-fixing antibodies against the organism. The latter will detect all three serologic subtypes of the virus (Weller, 1971). Some patients with hematologic malignancies may have positive antibody titers during infection without specific antibody rises, whereas other patients may shed virus in the urine for months without evidence of active disease (Henson et al., 1972). Thus, specific documentation of active infection may be difficult, and requires satisfaction of the criteria stated above.

ARA-C, IUDR, and 2-deoxy-5-fluorouridine all have specific antiviral activity against this DNA virus (Weller, 1971; Levine, Graw, and Young, 1972; Weinstein and Chang, 1973; Levine et al., 1974), however, controlled clinical trials of their efficacy in treating active infection are lacking.

Vaccinia

Infections with this agent occur through accidental or purposeful inoculation and illustrate the point that live virus vaccines should not be used in patients with malignancies, particularly those involving the hematopoietic system or requiring steroid and cytotoxic therapy as treatment. Extensive infection by this virus may take the form of progressive localized disease (*Vaccinia gangrenosa* or *exczema vaccinatum*) or generalized vaccinia (Kempe, 1960; Lane et al., 1969). Fatalities may occur from secondary bacterial infection or through primary involvement of the lungs or central nervous system.

The diagnosis is made by a history of contact with the virus and its recovery from the typical umbilicated vesiculo-pustules. Vaccinia immune globulin (VIG) is an effective prophylactic agent when given early after contact and may aid in active treatment of infections where viremia is a component (Kempe, 1960; Kempe et al., 1961; Lane et al., 1969). After viremia occurs the virus remains intracellular where it is protected from circulating antibody; however, VIG may still serve a role in limiting further viremic episodes and should be administered. The dose is 0.6 ml/kg i.m. (maximum 5 ml) and the globulin can be obtained from the American Red Cross. A thiosemicarbazone, Marboran, has antiviral activity against vaccinia and has been used to treat inoculation complications in some patients with apparent success (Bauer, 1965). The dose is 200 mg/kg orally as initial therapy, followed by 50 mg/kg p.o. q 6 hr for 3 days. Rifampin may also have activity against this agent (Levine et al., 1974).

Prevention of contact of susceptible patients with recently vaccinated individuals is crucial to prevention of infection.

Measles

Rubeola virus is highly contagious among nonimmune subjects, and therefore infection with this virus presents a problem predominantly in unvaccinated children or those without a history of infection. In children with hematologic malignancies or susceptible patients on steroid therapy fatal giant cell pneumonia may develop during the course of infection, sometimes without an exanthem (Mitus et al., 1959). Vaccination against measles of nonimmune individuals with malignancy is contraindicated since it is necessary to use a live virus vaccine. Passive immunization with pooled immune serum globulin (0.25 ml/kg i.m.) is effective in preventing disease if given within 48 hr after exposure and disease may be modified even if given within 5 days of exposure (Stokes et al., 1944). There is no evidence that immune serum globulin can modify active measles or prevent the development of potentially fatal pulmonary infection. Thus, once measles has developed in the immunosuppressed patient with malignancy the only therapy available is supportive. As a rule, viral shedding is prolonged in infected individuals with hematologic malignancies in contrast to normals in which it disappears rapidly from the respiratory tract after infection becomes clinically apparent (Mitus et al., 1959).

Hepatitis

Because transfusion of blood products is often required as supportive therapy in patients with malignancy, and the opportunity for exposure to type B hepatitis is enhanced by the need for frequent hospitalization, some oncology units are reporting an increase in infection rates with this agent in their patients (Wands et al., 1974). Furthermore, as in patients with advanced renal failure or those on immunosuppressive therapy after organ transplantation, a prolonged carrier state of the hepatitis B–associated antigen (HbAg) may develop in up to 50% of patients with leukemia or lymphoma or other subjects on cytotoxic therapy (London et al., 1969; Sutnick et al., 1970, 1971;

Wands et al., 1974). When antibody against HbAg is looked for in addition to the antigen, documentation of previous infection in leukemia and lymphoma patients may reach 80% (Wands et al., 1974). Clinical manifestations of the disease are usually mild in contrast to those in nonimmune normal subjects who develop overt type B hepatitis. For these reasons patients with malignancy should undergo periodic surveillance for the presence of the antigen whether symptomatic or not, since they may represent a significant health hazard to the staff responsible for their care or their intimate contacts (Wands et al., 1974). Recent evidence indicates that HbAg-positive patients may be infectious not only by the parenteral route but by nonparenteral means also (Villarejos et al., 1974). The viral particle has been identified in the tears, saliva, stool, urine, and semen of infected individuals. Fortunately, the virus is much more infectious when inoculated by the parenteral route than by other means (Barker et al., 1970); however, a small but finite risk of infection remains after prolonged contact with infected subjects, even without overt evidence of contamination by blood.

Pooled immune serum globulin is of no value in preventing or modifying disease (Krugman and Giles, 1973). Initial trials with type B hepatitis hyperimmune serum have indicated that this material provides a significant protective effect to exposed subjects when administered within 1 to 2 weeks after parenteral inoculation of serum containing the virus (Krugman and Giles, 1973; Szmuness et al., 1974). Unfortunately this serum can be obtained only through laboratories engaged in its investigative use. Upon completion of clinical trials, commercial preparations should become available for general use.

All patients with leukemia or lymphoma and others with a transfusion or hepatitis contact history should have their serum evaluated for HbAg when first seen and at monthly intervals thereafter during cytotoxic therapy. Such therapy has been documented to be associated with marked rises in titers (Wands et al., 1974), and it is reasonable to assume that a corresponding rise in infectiousness of the patient may occur also. Patients who are found to be positive should have single rooms or share rooms with other HbAg-positive patients and be placed on stool, urine, and syringe precautions. In addition educational programs which point out the risk and mechanisms of transfer of the virus should be directed at the staff responsible for the care of these patients. It is also reasonable to screen these personnel for HbAg and antibody to HbAg at periodic (e.g., monthly) intervals. Since the presence of antibody is protective, it is reasonable to have antibody-positive staff assume primary care responsibility for HbAg-positive patients.

Table 4 summarizes available specific prophylactic and therapeutic agents to be used in the management of the viral and protozoan infections discussed above.

SUMMARY: DIFFERENTIAL DIAGNOSTIC APPROACH TO INFECTIOUS SYNDROMES IN WHICH VIRAL OR PROTOZOAN INFECTION IS POSSIBLE

Fever

Previous information- indicates that the granulocytopenic patient (<500 PMN/mm^3) with fever is likely to have an infectious cause for fever approximately 80% of the time (Raab et al., 1960; Silver, 1963; Bodey et al., 1966; Bodey et al., 1972; Levine, Graw, and Young, 1972; Tattersal, Spiers, and Darrell, 1972; Levine et al., 1974). The incidence of infection as a cause for fever is less in patients with normal granulocyte counts; however, it is still appreciable and a thorough evaluation of every febrile patient for infection is indicated. Whereas bacterial and deep fungal infections are more likely to be lethal causes of infection responsible for fever and require rapid diagnostic and therapeutic measures, a careful search for viral and/or protozoan infection should be undertaken in patients in whom a bacterial or fungal etiology cannot be proven and when the patient is not responding to antimicrobial treatment. Table 3 summarizes diagnostic measures that are available to document infection by the agents discussed above and Table 4 indicates treatment regimens that might be employed.

Interstitial or Nodular Pneumonia

Since many of the agents discussed above may produce a pulmonary infection as part of their clinical picture, and effective therapy is available for systemic protozoan and helminthic (e.g., *Stronglyoides stercoralis*) infections, these should be looked for carefully when the chest x-ray discloses interstitial or nodular infiltrates. An important point to keep in mind is that these infections are often mixed with bacterial and fungal agents. Table 5 divides pulmonary infiltrative diseases producing an interstitial pattern on x-ray into noninfectious

Table 3. Diagnostic measures in protozoan and viral infections

	Culture	Histology	Serology
Toxoplasmosis	No	Yes	CF, dye titer, FA
Pneumocystis carinii	No	Yes	Not generally available
Herpes group viruses			
Cytomegalovirus	Yes	Inclusions not specific	CF
Ebstein-Barr virus	Yes	No	CF, precipitating, heterophile
Varicella-Zoster	Yes	Inclusions not specific	Available but not necessary
Herpes simplex	Yes	Inclusions not specific	FA
Vaccinia	Yes	Yes	Not generally available
Rubeola	Yes	Giant cells	Neutralizing, CF
Hepatitis A	No	No	Not generally available
Hepatitis B	No	No	HbAg, Antibody to HbAg

ªAbbreviations: CF, complement fixation; FA, fluorescent antibody; HbAg, hepatitis B–associated antigen.

and infectious etiologies and subdivides the latter into the causes for which specific treatment is available and those for which there is no specific therapy. Vigorous diagnostic approaches must be taken to document the nature of the infecting agent. If expectorated or aspirated sputum does not reveal a specific cause for the pneumonia, the next diagnostic step to take is to conduct a fiberoptic bronchoscopic exam of the tracheal bronchial tree. This should be coupled with localized lavage with saline of the affected segments and a bronchial brush biopsy. If the patient is severely thrombocytopenic, platelet transfusions should be given before this procedure is undertaken, since hemorrhage may occur after biopsy. Recent evidence suggests that these relatively innocuous techniques may yield a diagnosis in over 50% of patients (Walzer et al., 1974). If they are not diagnostic, then the physician should resort to open or closed lung biopsy, again under appropriate platelet "coverage," if necessary. "Touch preps" and methenamine silver and periodic acid-Schiff (PAS) stains of the material obtained at biopsy or bronchoscopy

Table 4. Therapy and prophylaxis of protozoan and viral infections

	Prophylaxis[a]	Therapy
Toxoplasmosis	None	Pyramethamine, 25 mg q.d. Sulfadiazine, 1 g 4 i.d. p.o. Folinic acid, 10 mg q.d. p.o.
Pneumocystis carinii	None	Pentamidine isethionate, 4 mg/kg/day i.m.
Rubeola	ISG, 0.25 ml/kg <5 days	None
Varicella-Zoster	ZIG, 0.2 ml/kg ZIP, 2–4 ml/kg <3 days	None effective
Vaccinia	VIG, 0.6 ml/kg <5 days	Marboran 200 mg/kg p.o. then 50 mg/kg p.o. q 6 hr × 3 days
Cytomegalovirus	None	None effective
Herpes simplex virus	None	None effective, except topical IUDR
Hepatitis A	ISG, 0.2 ml/kg <15 days	None
Hepatitis B	HIG <7 days	None

[a]The periods of time in the prophylaxis section refer to the upper limit of days after which therapy is no longer effective. Abbreviations: ISG, immune serum globulin; ZIG, zoster immune globulin; ZIP, zoster immune plasma; VIG, vaccinia immune globulin; HIG, hepatitis immune globulin.

should be made and a careful search made for fungi, protozoan forms, and the inclusion bodies of CMV, in addition to obtaining routine fungal and AFB cultures. Since the agents required to treat pneumocystis pneumonia are nephrotoxic, particularly when combined with aminoglycoside antibiotics or amphotericin, every effort should be made to make a specific diagnosis before resorting to blind "shotgun" therapy to treat this syndrome.

Finally, as pointed out earlier, agents such as *Pneumocystis carinii* may produce pulmonary infection and fever without observable x-ray abnormalities until late in their course (Sheldon, 1959; Cross and Steigbeigel, 1974; Friedman et al., 1975). Obtaining arterial blood gases should therefore be a routine part of the work-up of fever in which no immediately obvious etiology can be determined, and

Table 5. Interstitial pneumonia in patients with malignancy

I. Noninfectious
   Lymphangitic spread of tumor
   Irradiation pneumonitis
   Miscellaneous toxic exposures
   Pulmonary edema

II. Infectious
   A. Treatable
      Pyogenic bacteria: *Staphylococcus aureus*—β-streptococcus,
         Klebsiella, Pseudomonas
      Mycobacteria
      Fungi: histoplasmosis, candidiasis, aspergillosis
      Mycoplasma
      Protozoans: pneumocystis, toxoplasma
      Strongyloides stercoralis
   B. No effective treatment available
      Cytomegalovirus
      Herpes simplex
      Varicella-zoster
      Measles
      Adenovirus
      Other viruses

---

the same diagnostic measures pursued as outlined for overt interstitial pneumonias.

Hepatocellular Dysfunction

Chemotherapeutic agents, particularly the purine derivatives, may produce hepatic necrosis and fever as may other drugs such as α-methyldopa, isoniazid, or dilantin when used in an older patient population who have diseases other than their malignancies (Martin and Arthand, 1970; Noble, 1971; Brodsky and Kahn, 1972). On the other hand, toxoplasmosis and all of the viral agents described in detail above (except for measles) may infect the liver. Appropriate diagnostic measures to document the specific nature of viral or protozoan agents producing a hepatitis-like syndrome are indicated in Table 3.

Finally, this review has concentrated upon infection by unusual pathogens which rarely produce clinically significant illness in normal subjects or unique manifestations of infection by ubiquitous pathogens in an immunosuppressed patient population with malignancy. It should not be forgotten, however, that cancer patients have the same risk and incidence of infection with viruses and mycoplasma species which cause fever and upper respiratory tract symptoms as do the normal patient population. Present evidence indicates that the manifestations and complications of infection by these agents in cancer patients are no different from those in the population at large (Levine, 1973). Therefore, before esoteric infectious syndromes are considered in the cancer patient, the more "routine" pathogens should be sought for carefully and dealt with appropriately.

REFERENCES

Aisenberg, A. L. 1966. Manifestations of immunologic unresponsiveness in Hodgkin's Disease. Cancer Res. 26:1152.

Armstrong, R. W., M. J. Gurwith, D. Waddell, and T. C. Merigan. 1970. Cutaneous interferon during varicella and vaccinia infections in patients with malignancies. New Eng. J. Med. 283:1182.

Arora, K. K., R. Karalakulasingam, M. J. Roff, and D. G. Martin. 1974. Cutaneous herpes virus Hominis (type 2) infection after renal transplantation. JAMA 230:1174.

Barker, L. F., N. R. Shulman, R. Murray, R. J. Hirschman, F. Ratner, W. C. L. Diefenbach, and H. M. Geller. 1970. Transmission of serum hepatitis. JAMA 211:1509.

Barlotta, F. M., M. Ochoa, Jr., H. C. Neu, and J. E. Ultmann. 1969. Toxoplasmosis, lymphoma, or both? Ann. Intern. Med. 70:517.

Bauer, D. J. 1965. Clinical experience with the antiviral drug marboran (1-methyl isatin-3-thio semicarbazone). Ann. N.Y. Acad. Sci. 130:110.

Bellanti, J. A., L. W. Catalana, Jr., and R. W. Chambers. 1971. Herpes simplex encephalitis: virologic and serologic study of a patient treated with an interferon inducer. J. Pediatr. 78:136.

Bodey, G. P., M. Buckley, Y. S. Sathe, and E. J. Freireich. 1966. Quantitative relationships between circulating leukocytes and infection in patients with acute leukemia. Ann. Intern. Med. 64:328.

Bodey, G. P., E. Middleman, T. Umsawadi, and V. Rodriguez. 1972. Infections in cancer patients: Results with gentamicin sulfate therapy. Cancer 29:1697.

Bodey, G. P., P. T. Westlake, and G. Douglas. 1965. Cytomegalic inclusion disease in patients with acute leukemia. Ann. Intern. Med. 62:899.

Boston Interhospital Virus Study Group and the NIAID-sponsored antiviral clinical study. Failure of high-dose 5-Iodo-2-deoxyuridine for herpes simplex encephalitis. 1975. New Eng. J. Med. 292:599.

Brodsky, I., and J. B. Kahn (eds). 1972. Cancer Chemotherapy, Vol. II. 2nd Ed. Grune and Stratton, New York.

Brunell, P. A., and A. A. Gershon. 1973. Passive immunization against varicella-zoster infections and other modes of therapy. J. Infect. Dis. 127:415.

Brunell, P. A., A. A. Gershon, and W. T. Hughes. 1972. Prevention of varicella in high risk children. Pediatrics 50:718.

Carey, R. M., A. C. Kimball, D. Armstrong, and P. H. Lieberman. 1973. Toxoplasmosis: Clinical experiences in a cancer hospital. Amer. J. Med. 54:30.

Case Records of the Massachusetts General Hospital. 1973. New Eng. J. Med. 289:91.

Chang, T. W. 1971. Recurrent viral infection (reinfection). New Eng. J. Med. 284:765.

Cherubin, C. E., and A. M. Prince. 1971. Serum hepatitis specific antigen in commercial and volunteer sources of blood. Tranfusion 11:25.

Cross, A. S., and R. T. Steigbeigel. 1974. Pneumocystis carinii pneumonia presenting as local nodular densities. New Eng. J. Med. 291:831.

Dorfman, R. F., and J. S. Remington. 1973. Value of lymph node biopsy in the diagnosis of acute acquired toxoplasmosis. New Eng. J. Med. 289:878.

Drew, W. L., T. N. Finley, L. Mintz, and H. Z. Klein. 1974. Diagnosis of Pneumocystis carinii pneumonia by bronchopulmonary lavage. JAMA 230:713.

Dyment, P. G., S. J. Orlando, H. Isaacs Jr., and H. T. Wright. 1968. The incidence of cytomegaloviruria and postmortem cytomegalic inclusions in children with acute leukemia. J. Pediatr. 72:533.

Eilber, F. R., and D. L. Morton. 1970. Impaired immunologic reactivity and recurrence following cancer surgery. Cancer 25:362.

Esterly, J. A. 1968. Pneumocystis carinii in lungs of adults at autopsy. Amer. Rev. Respir. Dis. 97:935.

Fahey, J. L., and D. R. Boggs. 1969. Serum protein changes in malignant diseases. Blood 16:1479.

Fauci, A. S., and D. C. Dale. 1975. The effect of in vivo hydrocortisone on subpopulations of human lymphocytes. J. Clin. Invest. 53:240.

Felber, T. D., E. E. Smith, J. M. Knox, C. Wallis, and J. L. Melnick. 1973. Photodynamic inactivation of Herpes simplex: report of a clinical trial. JAMA 223:289.

Feldman, H. A. 1968. Toxoplasmosis. New Eng. J. Med. 279:1370.

Fine, R. N., C. M. Grishkin, S. Anand, E. Lieberman, and H. T. Wright. 1970. Cytomegalovirus in children. Amer. J. Dis. Child. 120:197.

Foley, F. D., K. A. Greenwald, G. Nash, and B. A. Pruitt, Jr. 1970. Herpes virus infection in burned patients. New Eng. J. Med. 282:652.

Friedman, B. A., B. D. Wenglin, R. N. Hyland, and D. Rifkind. 1975. Roentgenographically atypical Pneumocystis carinii pneumonia. Amer. Rev. Respir. Dis. 111:89.

Gershon, A. A., S. Steinberg, and P. A. Brunell. 1974. Zoster immune globulin: A further assessment. New Eng. J. Med. 290:243.

Gleason, T. H., and W. B. Hamlin. 1974. Disseminated toxoplasmosis in the compromised host. Arch. Intern. Med. 134:1059.

Goffinet, D. R., E. J. Glatskin, and T. C. Merigan. 1972. Herpes Zoster-varicella infection and lymphoma. Ann. Intern. Med. 76:235.

Goodell, B., J. B. Jacobs, R. D. Powell, and V. T. DeVita. 1970. *Pneumocystis carinii:* the spectrum of diffuse interstitial pneumonia in patients with neoplastic disease. Ann. Intern. Med. 72:337.

Green, W. H., S. C. Schimpff, V. M. Young, and P. H. Wiernik. 1973. Empiric carbenicillin, gentamicin, and cephalothin therapy for presumed infection. Ann. Intern. Med. 78:825.

Greenlee, J. E., W. D. Johnson, Jr., J. F. Campa, L. S. Adelman, and M. A. Sande. 1975. Adult toxoplasmosis presenting as polymyositis and cerebellar ataxia. Ann. Intern. Med. 82:367.

Henson, D., S. E. Siegel, D. A. Fucillo, E. Matthew, and A. S. Levine. 1972. Cytomegalovirus infections during acute childhood leukemia. J. Infect. Dis. 126:469.

Hersh, E. M. 1971. Immunological defects in Hodgkin's disease. Proceedings Symposium on Hodgkin's Disease. St. Louis, Mo., October 7–9, 1971.

Hersh, E. M., and J. J. Oppenheim. 1965. Impaired *in vitro* lymphocyte transformation in Hodgkin's disease. New Eng. J. Med. 273:1006.

Hersh, E. W., J. P. Whitecar, K. B. McCredie, G. P. Bodey, and E. J. Freireich. 1971. Chemotherapy, immunocompetence immunosuppression and prognosis in acute leukemia. New Eng. J. Med. 285:1211.

Jacobs, L., J. S. Remington, and M. L. Melton. 1960. The resistance of the encysted form of *Toxoplasma gondii.* J. Parisitol. 46:11.

Jarnum, A., E. F. Rasmussen, A. S. Ohlsen, and A. S. Sorenson. 1968. Generalized *Pneumocystis carinii* infection with severe idiopathic hypoproteinemia. Ann. Intern. Med. 68:138.

Johnson, H. D., and W. W. Johnson. 1970. *Pneumocystis carinii* pneumonia in children with cancer. JAMA 214:1067.

Johnson, M. T., J. P. Luby, R. A. Buchanan, and D. Mikulec. 1975. Treatment of varicella-zoster virus infections with adenosine arabinoside. J. Infect. Dis. 131:225.

Jones, T., and J. G. Hirsch. 1972. The interactions between Toxoplasma gondii and mammalian cells. II. The absence of lysosomal fusion with phagocytic vacuoles containing living parasites. J. Exp. Med. 136:1173.

Jordan, M. C. C., W. E. Rousseau, G. R. Noble, J. A. Stewart, and T. D. Y. Chin. 1973. Association of cervical cytomegaloviruses with venereal disease. New Eng. J. Med. 288:932.

Jordan, M. C. C., W. E. Rousseau, J. A. Stewart, G. R. Noble, and T. D. Y. Chin. 1973. Spontaneous cytomegalovirus mononucleosis. Ann. Intern. Med. 79:153.

Juel-Jensen, B. E., and F. O. MacCallum. 1972. Herpes simplex, varicella and zoster: Clinical manifestations and treatment. Lippincott, Philadelphia.

Juel-Jensen, B. E., F. O. MacCallum, A. M. Mackenzie, and M. C. Pike. 1970. Treatment of zoster with idoxuridine in dimethylsulfoxide. Brit. Med. J. 4:776.

Kass, E. H., M. I. Kendrick, and M. Finland. 1955. Effects of corticosterone, hydrocortisone and corticotropin on production of antibodies in the rabbit. J. Exp. Med. 102:767.

Kempe, C. H. 1960. Studies on smallpox and complications of smallpox vaccination. Pediatrics 26:176.

Kempe, C. H., et al. 1961. The use of vaccinia immune globulin in the prophylaxis of smallpox. Bull. WHO 25:41.

Kirby, H. I. S., B. Kenamore, and J. C. Guckian. 1971. *Pneumocystis carinii* pneumonia treated with pyramethamine and sulfadiazine. Ann. Intern. Med. 75:505.

Klemola, E., N. Weckman, K. Haltia, and L. Kaariainen. 1967. The Guillian-Barre syndrome associated with acquired cytomegalovirus infection. Acta Med. Scand. 181:603.

Krogstad, D. J., D. D. Juranek, and K. W. Walls. 1972. Toxoplasmosis with comments on risk of infection from cats. Ann. Intern. Med. 77: 773.

Krugman, S., and J. P. Giles. 1973. Viral hepatitis Type B (MS-2 strain): Further observation on natural history, and prevention. New Eng. J. Med. 288:755.

Lane, T., F. L. Ruben, J. M. Neff, and J. D. Millar. 1969. Complications of smallpox vaccination. New Eng. J. Med. 281:1201.

Leventhal, B. G., P. Cohen, and S. C. Triem. The effect of chemotherapy on the immune response in acute leukemia: A review. Israel J. Med. Sci. In press.

Levine, A. S. 1973. Germ-free biology and the patient with malignant disease: Clinical and preclinical studies. Cancer Chemother. Rep. Part 3, 4(3).

Levine, A. S., R. G. Graw, Jr., and R. C. Young. 1972. Management of infections in patients with leukemia and lymphoma: Current concepts and experimental approaches. Semin. Hematol. 9:141.

Levine, A. S., S. C. Schimpff, R. G. Graw, Jr., and R. C. Young. 1974. Hematologic malignancies and other marrow failure states: Progress in the management of complicating infections. Semin. Hematol. 11:141.

London, W. T., M. DiFiglia, A. I. Sutnick, and B. S. Blumberg. 1969. An epidemic of hepatitis in a chronic dialysis unit. Australia antigen and differences in host response. New Eng. J. Med. 281:571.

Lynfield, Y. L., M. Farhangi, and J. L. Runnels. 1969. Generalized herpes simplex complicating lymphoma. JAMA 207:944.

MacGregor, R. R., J. N. Sheagren, M. L. Lipsett, and S. M. Wolff. 1969. Alternate day prednisone therapy. New Eng. J. Med. 26:1427.

Makindan, T., G. W. Santos, and R. P. Quinn. 1970. Immunosuppressive drugs. Pharmacol. Rev. 22:189.

Martin, C. E., and J. B. Arthand. 1970. Hepatitis after isoniazid administration. New Eng. J. Med. 282:433.

Merigan, T. C. 1974. Host defenses against viral disease. New Eng. J. Med. 290:323.

Mitus, A., J. F. Enders, J. M. Craig, and A. Holloway. 1959. Persistence of measles virus and depression of antibody formation in patients with giant cell pneumonia after measles. New Eng. J. Med. 261:882.

Montgomerie, J. Z., D. M. O. Becroft, M. C. Croxson, P. B. Doak, and J. D. K. North. 1969. Herpes simplex viral infection after renal transplantation. Lancet ii:867.

Morrison, R. E., M. H. Miller, L. W. Lyon, J. M. Griffiss, and M. S. Artenstein. 1974. Adult meningoencephalitis caused by Herpes-virus Hominis type 2. Amer. J. Med. 56:540.

Muller, S. A., E. C. Herrmann, and R. K. Winkelmann. 1972. Herpes simplex infections in hematologic malignancies. Amer. J. Med. 52:102.

Myers, J. D., H. C. Spencer, Jr., J. C. Watts, M. B. Gregg, J. A. Stewart, R. H. Troupin, and E. D. Thomas. 1975. Cytomegalovirus pneumonia after human marrow transplantation. Ann. Intern. Med. 82:181.

Nahmias, A. J., and B. Roizman. 1973. Infection with Herpes Simplex viruses 1 and 2 (3 parts). New Eng. J. Med. 289:667, 719, 781.

Noble, J. 1971. Isoniazid prophylaxis reexamined. New Eng. J. Med. 285:687.

Perera, D. R., K. A. Western, H. D. Johnson, W. W. Johnson, M. G. Schultz, and P. V. Akers. 1970. *Pneumocystis carinii* pneumonia in a hospital for children. JAMA 214:1074.

Pinkel, D. 1961. Chickenpox and leukemia. J. Pediatr. 58:729.

Prager, D., M. Bruder, and A. Jawitsky. 1971. Disseminated varicella in a patient with acute myelogenous leukemia: Treatment with cytosine arabinoside, J. Pediatr. 78:321.

Price, R., N. L. Chernik, L. Horta-Barbosa, and J. B. Posner. 1973. Herpes simplex encephalitis in an anergic patient. Amer. J. Med. 54:22.

Raab, S. O., P. D. Hoeprich, M. M. Wintrobe, and G. E. Cartwright. 1960. The clinical significance of fever in acute leukemia. Blood 16:1609.

Remington, J. S., M. J. Miller, and I. Brownlee. 1968: IgM antibodies in acute toxoplasmosis. I. Diagnostic significance in congenital cases and a method for their rapid identification. Pediatrics 41:1082.

Repshir, L. H., G. Schroter, and W. S. Hammond. 1972. Diagnosis of *Pneumocystis carinii* pneumonia by means of endobronchial brush biopsy. New Eng. J. Med. 287:340.

Reynolds, E. J., K. W. Walls, and R. I. Pfeiffer. 1966. Generalized toxoplasmosis following renal transplantation. Arch. Intern. Med. 118:401.

Rifkind, D. 1966. The activation of varicella-zoster virus infections by immunosuppressive therapy. J. Lab. Clin. Med. 68:463.

Rifkind, D., T. D. Faris, and R. B. Hill, Jr. 1966. *Pneumocystis carinii* pneumonia. Studies on the diagnosis and treatment. Ann. Intern. Med. 65:943.

Rifkind, D., N. Goodman, and R. B. Hill, Jr. 1967. The clinical significance of cytomegalovirus infections in renal transplant recipients. Ann. Intern. Med. 66:1116.

Santos, G. W., A. H. Owens, and L. C. Sensenbrenner. 1964. Effects of selected cytotoxic agents on antibody formation in man. Ann. N.Y. Acad. Sci. 114:404.

Schimpff, S. C., A. Serpick, B. Stoler, B. Rumack, H. Mellin, J. M. Joseph, and J. Block. 1972. Varicella-Zoster infection in patients with cancer. Ann. Intern. Med. 76:241.

Sexton, R. C., D. E. Eyles, and R. E. Dillman. 1963. Adult Toxoplasmosis. Amer. J. Med. 14:366.

Sheldon, W. H. 1959. Subclinical neumocystis pneumonitis. Amer. J. Dis. Child. 97:287.

Siegel, S., M. N. Lunde, A. H. Gelderman, R. H. Holterman, J. A. Brown, A. S. Levine, and R. G. Graw, Jr. 1971. Transmission of toxoplasmosis by leukocyte transfusion. Blood 37:388.

Silver, R. T. 1963. Infection, fever, and host resistance in neoplastic disease. J. Chronic. Dis. 16:677.

Smythe, P. M., M. Schonland, G. J. Brereton-Stiles, H. M. Coovida, H. J. Grace, et al. 1971. Thymo-lymphatic deficiency and depression of cell-mediated immunity in protein calorie malnutrition. Lancet ii:939.

Sokal, J. E., and J. E. Firat. 1965. Varicella-Zoster infection in Hodgkin's Disease. Amer. J. Med. 39:452.

Steinman, R. M., and Z. A. Cohn. 1974. Mononuclear Phagocytes. In B. W. Zwiebach, L. Grant, and R. T. McCluskey (eds.), The Inflammatory Process, 2nd Ed., Vol. 1. Academic Press, New York.

Stern, H., S. D. Elek, D. M. Millar, et al. 1959. Herpetic whitlow: a form of cross-infection in hospitals. Lancet 2:871.

Stevens, D. A., G. W. Jordan, T. F. Waddell, and T. C. Merigan. 1973. Adverse effect of cytosine arabinoside in disseminated zoster in a controlled trial. New Eng. J. Med. 289:873.

Stevens, D. P., L. F. Barker, A. S. Ketcham, and H. M. Meyer, Jr. 1970. Asymptomatic cytomegalovirus infection following blood transfusions in tumor surgery. JAMA 211:1341.

Stokes, J., Jr., E. P. Maris, and S. S. Gellis. 1944. The use of concentrated normal human serum globulin in the prophylaxis and treatment of measles. J. Clin. Invest. 23:531.

Sutnick, A. I., P. H. Levine, W. T. London, and B. S. Blumberg. 1971. Frequency of Australia antigen in patients with leukemia in different countries. Lancet i:1200.

Sutnick, A. I., W. T. London, B. S. Blumberg, L. A. Yankee, B. J. Gerstley, and I. Millman. 1970. Australia antigen (a hepatitis associated antigen) in leukemia. J. Natl. Cancer Inst. 44:1241.

Szmuness, W., A. M. Prince, M. Goodman, C. Ehrich, R. Pick, and M. Ansari. 1974. Hepatitis B immune serum globulin in prevention of non-parenterally transmitted hepatitis B. New Eng. J. Med. 290:701.

Tattersal, N. M. H., A. S. D. Spiers, and J. H. Darrell. 1972. Initial therapy with a combination of five antibiotics in febrile patients with leukemia and neutropenia. Lancet i:162.

Turner, A. R., R. N. MacDonald, and B. A. Cooper. 1972. Transmission of infectious mononucleosis by transfusion of pre-illness plasma. Ann. Intern. Med. 77:751.

Villarejos, V. M., K. A. Visona, A. Gutierrez, and A. Rodriguez. 1974. Role of saliva, urine and feces in the transmission of Type B hepatitis. New Eng. J. Med. 291:1375.

Walzer, P. P., D. P. Perl, D. J. Krogstad, D. J. Krogstead, P. G. Rawson, and M. G. Schultz. 1974. *Pneumocystis carinii* pneumonia in the United States. Ann. Intern. Med. 80:83.

Wands, J. R., J. A. Walker, T. T. Davis, L. A. Waterbury, A. H. Owens, and C. C. J. Carpenter. 1974. Hepatitis B in an oncology unit. New Eng. J. Med. 291:1371.

Weinstein, L., and T. W. Chang. 1973. The chemotherapy of viral infections. New Eng. J. Med. 289:725.

Weller, T. H. 1971. The cytomegaloviruses: ubiquitous agents with protean clinical manifestations. New Eng. J. Med. 285:203, 267.

Western, K. A., D. R. Perera, and M. G. Schultz. 1970. Pentamidine isethionate in the treatment of *Pneumocystis carinii* pneumonia. Ann. Intern. Med. 73:695.

Young, R. C., M. P. Corden, H. A. Haynes, and V. T. DeVita. 1972. Delayed hypersensitivity in Hodgkin's Disease. Amer. J. Med. 52:63.

Yu, D. T. Y., P. J. Clements, and H. E. Paulus. 1974. Human lymphocyte subpopulations: Effect of corticosteroids. J. Clin. Invest. 53:536.

Zaky, D. A., R. F. Belts, R. G. Douglas, and G. L. Moyer. 1974. Double blind study of cytarabine (CA) in localized Herpes Zoster (HZ). Clin. Res. 22:458A.

Paraneoplastic and Cancer-Associated Syndromes

Richard H. Creech, M.D., F.A.C.P.

Although cancer causes most of its clinical problems by local extension of the primary tumor or its metastases into adjacent normal tissues, many clinically important syndromes are caused by the systemic effects of cancer. These indirect effects on distant end organs comprise the paraneoplastic syndromes. This discussion concentrates on these paraneoplastic syndromes as well as on the symptom complexes associated with, but not caused by, cancer. These cancer-associated syndromes, if recognized by the physician, may result in the early diagnosis and treatment of otherwise unsuspected malignancy.

In this overview many of the rarer syndromes are discussed briefly, but most attention is paid to the more common clinical problems. These syndromes are subdivided by clinical presentation as seen by medical subspecialists in the fields of hematology, endocrinology, gastroenterology, rheumatology, and dermatology.

HEMATOLOGIC PRESENTATION

Patients may be referred for hematologic consultation because of elevated or depressed hemoglobin, white blood cell counts, or platelet counts. They also may have coagulation problems.

Leukocytosis may be seen in patients with lung cancer (Fahey, 1951) or with extensive hepatic carcinoma. The leukocytosis in the latter group of patients may be caused by the elaboration of by-products of tumor necrosis. Thrombocytosis secondary to marrow hyperactivity is often seen in patients with the myeloproliferative disorders, but the mechanism of elevated platelet counts in most solid tumor patients is poorly understood (Levin and Conley, 1964).

Leukopenia and thrombocytopenia in the untreated patient with malignancy may be caused by splenic sequestration without cellular destruction in splenomegalic patients (Rosenbaum, Murphy, and Swisher, 1966) or by immune destruction. The patients with hyper-cellular bone marrows and splenic nonimmune cytopenias may be benefited by splenectomy. Immune thrombocytopenia is seen in patients with lymphoproliferative disorders, particularly chronic lymphocytic leukemia. Reversal of immune thrombocytopenia may occur after therapy with corticosteroids, after chemotherapy, or, in refractory cases, after splenectomy (Ebbe, Wittels, and Dameshek, 1962).

Erythrocytosis

The patient presenting with an elevated hemoglobin is always a diagnostic challenge to the clinician, who must decide whether the patient has polycythemia vera, spurious polycythemia, or polycythemia secondary to pulmonary disease, cyanotic heart disease, defective oxygen transport, benign renal disease, or malignancy. The polycythemia vera patients have generalized marrow hyperactivity (elevated hemoglobin, white count, and platelet count), splenomegaly, normal arterial oxygen saturation, and elevations of red cell mass, serum vitamin B_{12}, unsaturated B_{12} binding capacity, and leukocyte alkaline phosphatase. Patients with spurious polycythemia have an elevated hematocrit due to a normal red cell mass with low plasma volume.

The secondary polycythemia patients are most often found to have a decreased arterial oxygen saturation due to pulmonary disease. Occasionally, patients may have erythrocytosis secondary to methemoglobinemia or familial amino acid substitutions in areas of the α or β chains of the hemoglobin molecule critical for the proper molecular changes during deoxygenation.

Polycythemia secondary to erythropoietin stimulation or ectopic production occurs in both benign and malignant conditions. Thirty percent of renal diseases causing polycythemia are benign and include cystic kidneys (20%), hydronephrosis (8%), hemangiomas (1%), and adenomas (1%). The other 70% of renal diseases associated with erythrocytosis are malignant, including hypernephroma (67%), Wilms' tumor (2%), and sarcoma (1%) (Hammond and Winnick, 1974). Renal tumors are the most common polycythemia-associated malignancies (55%); hepatomas (20%) (McFadzean, Todd, and Tso, 1967), cerebellar hemangioblastomas (15%) (Cramer and Kimsey, 1952), uterine fibroids (7%) (Hertko, 1968), pheochromocytomas, adrenal adenomas, virilizing ovarian tumors, and lung cancers (Waldmann, Rosse, and Swarm, 1968) also may induce erythrocytosis.

Erythropoietin activity is found in greater than 75% of tissue extracts of the affected organs in patients with cystic kidneys, hypernephromas, and the cerebellar hemangioblastomas. Extracts of uterine fibroids and hepatomas have a 25% incidence of erythropoietin activity (Hammond and Winnick, 1974). Since not all polycythemia-associated tumors secrete erythropoietin, it has been hypothesized that the large intra-abdominal tumors may cause renal hypoxia resulting in secondarily increased erythropoietin production and polycythemia. Whatever the exact mechanism, erythrocytosis is the most manageable of the ectopic hormone syndromes because of its association with benign conditions and resectable malignant disease and because phlebotomy is effective symptomatically, even in patients with poorly controlled malignancy.

ENDOCRINOLOGIC PRESENTATION

Ectopic hormone production can be divided into two categories: symptomatic and asymptomatic. With the advent of sensitive bioassays and radioimmunoassays for hormones, random study of cancer patients not clinically suspected of having ectopic hormone secretion often reveals elevated levels of hormone activity. There is a group of patients, however, whose primary clinical problem is related to symptoms caused by ectopic hormone secretion. Patients with these syndromes should be suspected of having occult malignancies so that valuable time is not lost before antineoplastic therapy is instituted.

Although derepression of the genome is a favored explanation for ectopic hormone secretion, inconsistencies in laboratory analyses initially appear to be incompatible with this hypothesis. The ectopic hormone found in the serum or the tumor may have biologic activity similar to the authentic hormone, but on radioimmunoassay it is found to be dissimilar. Amino acid sequencing has also demonstrated discrepancies between ectopic hormones and the parent polypeptide. If the mechanism of ectopic hormone production were only derepression, the ectopic hormones and the parent compound might be expected to be identical (Gordon and Roof, 1972).

Berson and Yalow (1971) have found by radioimmunoassay that large molecules consisting of complexes of the parent hormone circulate normally in small quantities, but that in some insulinomas, for example, the predominant ectopic hormone is the high molecular weight "big" insulin. The presence of these large molecules may explain some of the discrepancies in bioassays, radioimmunoassays, molecular weights, and amino acid sequences between ectopic and authentic hormones and, in addition, is compatible with genome derepression.

Ectopic Adrenocorticotropic Hormone

Logically one would expect patients with the adrenocorticotropic hormone (ACTH) syndrome to present clinically as Cushing's syndrome with the typical habitus of hyperadrenocorticism. This is not the case because adrenal hyperfunction must be present for comparatively long periods of time before this syndrome becames clinically apparent. Since 50% of patients with excess production of ACTH have the most virulent lung carcinoma (small cell carcinoma) as their underlying malignancy, they do not survive long enough to develop the characteristic phenotype. The other malignancies associated with ACTH secretion are pancreatic malignancy, including islet cell tumors and carcinoid (10%), thymic tumors (10%), neural crest tumors such as pheochromocytoma and neuroblastoma (5%), bronchial adenomas including carcinoid (2%), and medullary carcinoma of the thyroid (5%) (Amatruda and Upton, 1974).

Most of these patients present clinically with hypokalemic alkalosis and its associated weakness, glucose intolerance, or hyperpigmentation due to the concomitant secretion of melanocyte-stimulating hormone (MSH). Since most of the ectopic ACTH-secreting syndromes are associated with intrathoracic malignancy, an abnormal chest x-ray will alert the physician to the possibility of a hormone-producing malignancy. These patients should then have bronchoscopy and mediastinoscopy performed to establish a pathologic diagnosis.

In the less obvious cases a laboratory evaluation may help differentiate among adrenal hyperplasia of Cushing's disease, primary adrenocortical tumor, ACTH-producing pituitary tumor, ectopic ACTH production, and ectopic corticotropin-releasing hormone (CRH). This evaluation should include plasma ACTH and cortisol, serum potassium, and suppression of ACTH and cortisol secretion by high dose dexamethasone (2 mg orally every 6 hr for eight doses). As is seen in Table 1, Cushing's disease is associated with a minimally elevated ACTH level and rarely with hypokalemia, while ACTH and cortisol secretion can be suppressed by high dose dexamethasone. Primary adrenocortical tumors secrete cortisol which causes hypokalemia and suppresses ACTH secretion. Cortisol secretion by these tumors is not suppressible by dexamethasone. Pituitary adenomas secreting ACTH rarely are associated with hypokalemia and are not suppressible. The majority of ectopic ACTH-secreting tumors have high circulating ACTH levels resulting in high levels of nonsuppressible cortisol secretion which causes the clinically prominent hypokalemic alkalosis. Bronchial carcinoids may secrete CRH and small amounts of ACTH. These tumors are often suppressible by dexamethasone and are associated with hypokalemia (Odell, 1974).

Patients with ectopic ACTH secretion are best managed by control of the underlying malignancy. Since the majority have small cell carcinoma of the lung, specific radiotherapy or chemotherapy will be the best form of metabolic and neoplastic control. For those patients with less malignant disease the opportunity for long-term control is best with surgery. Medical control of the hyperadrenocorti-

Table 1. Differentiation of hyperadrenocortical disorders

Disease	Plasma cortisol	Plasma ACTH	Serum potassium	High dose dexamethasone suppression
Cushing's disease	↑	Normal, ↑	Normal	Yes
Adrenocortical tumors	↑	↓	↓	No
ACTH-producing pituitary adenomas	↑	↑	Normal	No
Ectopic ACTH	↑	↑↑	↓	No
Ectopic CRH	↑	↑	↓	Yes

cism may be achieved by metyrapone, o,p'DDD, or aminoglutethimide if the primary anti-neoplastic therapy is unsuccessful. Bilateral adrenalectomy should be considered only when the patient's long-term prognosis is relatively good.

Hypercalcemia

Patients presenting with weakness, gastrointestinal complaints, constipation, polyuria, polydipsia, drowsiness, confusion, and coma should be suspected of having hypercalcemia. It is important to remember that the cancer patient presenting with bizarre behavior may have hypercalcemia rather than metastatic brain disease.

Hypercalcemia in cancer patients may be caused by bone resorption associated with bony metastases and immobilization, ectopic secretion of parathyroid hormone, hyperparathyroidism, or iatrogenic hypervitaminosis D in patients with surgically induced hypoparathyroidism. The most common cause is bony resorption caused by immobolization of patients with bony metastases. Hypercalcemia associated with subclinical bony metastases is often difficult to distinguish clinically from ectopic hormone secretion. Since parathyroid hormone assays are not readily available in most clinical settings, evaluation for metastatic bone disease is often clinically helpful. Many patients with asymptomatic bony metastases with a normal bone survey may have either an abnormal bone scan or bone marrow biopsy. Immobilization of these patients may result in hypercalcemia.

The remaining small group of cancer patients without bony metastases may have the syndrome of ectopic parathyroid hormone secretion. Approximately 35% of the tumors producing parathyroid-like hormone are lung carcinomas with squamous cell histology being more frequent than the large cell anaplastic variety. Unlike many other syndromes associated with ectopic hormone secretion, small cell carcinoma of the lung is a relatively rare cause of parathyroid hormone secretion. Hypernephroma accounts for 25% of ectopic parathyroid hormone secretion while tumors of the ovary, endometrium, bladder, prostate, penis, esophagus, colon, and breast are less frequent (Odell, 1974).

Clinically, hypercalcemic cancer patients with hypophosphatemia are likely to have either hyperparathyroidism or ectopic secretion of parathyroid hormone while hyperphosphatemia is often associated with bony metastases. Breast carcinoma patients with metastatic bone disease may develop hypercalcemia after immobilization or after initiation of additive hormonal therapy. Since parathyroid hormone production is very rarely associated with breast carcinoma, hypercalcemic patients without bony metastases are more likely to have primary hyperparathyroidism than ectopic parathyroid secretion.

Cancer patients with hypercalcemia are best managed acutely by saline diuresis and diuretic administration and, if severely symptomatic, by mithramycin intravenously at a dose of 1 mg every other day. Thrombocytopenia may result if multiple doses of mithramycin are given. Prednisone may be effective, acute and chronically, particularly in patients with hematologic malignancy or breast cancer. Chronic control of hypercalcemia may be achieved by appropriate antineoplastic therapy, mobilization, oral inorganic phosphate administration, and occasionally intermittent mithramycin therapy (Muggia and Heinemann, 1970).

Inappropriate Antidiuretic Hormone Secretion

Hyponatremia in cancer patients is a particularly common problem. Dehydration due to vomiting, diarrhea, or diuretic therapy, as well as adrenocortical insufficiency caused by adrenalectomy or adrenal replacement by cancer, may cause a reduced intravascular volume, decreased glomerular filtration rate, and elevated blood urea nitrogen (BUN). As a compensatory mechanism, increased antidiuretic hormone (ADH) secretion results in water retention. If sodium deficiency is not also corrected, the patient becomes hyponatremic. These patients are best treated by hormonal replacement if Addisonian, as well as by careful rehydration and sodium replacement.

Other cancer patients, particularly those with small cell carcinoma of the lung, may present with hyponatremia, increased urinary sodium excretion, a normal BUN, and urine that is hyperosmolal as compared to plasma. These patients with the inappropriate ADH syndrome caused by the ectopic secretion of ADH by tumor are best managed primarily by specific anti-tumor therapy. The small cell carcinoma patients are best controlled by radiotherapy or, if metastatic, by chemotherapy. Water restriction is necessary when the syndrome is first diagnosed and may be chronically necessary if anti-tumor therapy is ineffective (Bartter, 1973).

Hypoglycemia

Tumors associated with hypoglycemia can be separated into two categories: the pancreatic islet cell insulinoma and the extrapancreatic tumors.

The insulinoma patients develop fasting hypoglycemia because of "big" and "little" insulin production by the tumor. Elevated levels of circulating insulin-like activity and immunoreactive insulin as well as insulin production by the tumor have helped to corroborate this hypothesis.

On the other hand, the extrapancreatic tumors associated with hypoglycemia are incompletely understood. Approximately 45% of these tumors are mesenchymal in origin. They are usually large retroperitoneal, peritoneal, or thoracic sarcomas. The other hypoglycemia-associated tumors include hepatomas (20%), gastrointestinal carcinomas (10%), adrenal tumors (9%), and lymphomas (5%) (Marks et al., 1974). Insulin-like activity, but not immunoreactive insulin, has been found in some of these tumors. Circulating "big" insulin may explain this apparent discrepancy. Not all hypoglycemia-associated tumors, however, have insulin-like activity.

Another possible mechanism of hypoglycemia is excessive glucose utilization by the tumors. Despite the logic of this theory, especially with large tumors, this has been hard to document. Differences in arteriovenous blood glucose values across tumors have been disappointingly small.

Inadequate glucose output by the liver in patients with hepatoma has also been suggested. At autopsy these patients may have significant volumes of normal liver despite extensive hepatic invasion by tumor. It has also been noted that patients, presumably with a small tumor burden, may present with hypoglycemia months before their hepatoma is diagnosed clinically.

It is also possible that extrapancreatic tumors may secrete an insulin-potentiating substance (Unger, 1966). At the present time, there is no universally accepted mechanism of hypoglycemia production for these extrapancreatic tumors. Surgical removal of these tumors can result in prolonged antineoplastic and metabolic control.

Ectopic Gonadotropin Secretion

Ectopic gonadotropins are most often secreted by trophoblastic disease in women, by teratomas and lung cancer in men, and by hepatoblastomas in young boys. Women present clinically with menstrual irregularities, men with gynecomastia, and boys with precocious puberty. Many of these patients do not secrete enough human chorionic gonadotropins to make pregnancy tests positive. It is therefore necessary to use more sensitive assays to detect the ectopic secretion of this hormone. These assays are also necessary for monitoring response to therapy (Odell, 1974).

Thyroid-stimulating Hormone

The relatively rare syndrome of thyroid-stimulating hormone production is associated with trophoblastic disease in the female and teratocarcinoma in the male. These patients characteristically have few symptoms or signs of hyperthyroidism. Clinically, tachycardia is common, but eye signs, thyroid enlargement, and tremor are not. Most patients excrete at least 100,000 I.U. per day of human chorionic gonadotropin. Their thyroid function tests may show elevated protein-bound iodine (PBI) and ^{131}I uptake values. Plasma and tumor thyroid-stimulating hormone values may be elevated by bioassay, but are normal by radioimmunoassay (Odell, 1974).

Growth Hormone

Growth hormone is rarely found to be elevated and, if elevated, is usually asymptomatic. One patient with ectopic secretion was found to have bronchogenic carcinoma and hypertrophic pulmonary osteoarthropathy (Steiner, Dahlback, and Waldenstrom, 1968).

Medullary Thyroid Carcinoma Syndromes

The medullary thyroid carcinoma (MTC) syndromes represent a multiple endocrine organ tumor syndrome which has several clinical variants. There are some families with a high incidence of pheochromocytomas and other families with an autosomal dominant inheritance of medullary thyroid carcinoma. Sporadically, there are patients with coexistent MTC and pheochromocytomas. The most intriguing variant is Sipple's syndrome, transmitted as an autosomal dominant with a high degree of penetrance, consisting of MTC, pheochromocytomas, parathyroid disease, and, in some instances, mucosal neuromas, marfanoid habitus, and megacolon.

MTC has characteristic dense calcification in both lobes of the thyroid on x-ray. Metastases in cervical nodes and liver may also contain radiographically visible calcification. On chest radiograph, metastases may be seen in the mediastinal and hilar nodes or as a characteristic interstitial multinodular pattern in the pulmonary parenchyma (Keiser et al., 1973).

These tumors characteristically secrete calcitonin, which during calcium infusion may be used to detect MTC in otherwise normal relatives of patients with this syndrome. Histaminase is also secreted by these tumors, but is found only in 50% of patients (Baylin et al., 1972). Elevated levels of calcitonin or histaminase after surgery are indicative of metastatic disease. Prostaglandins causing diarrhea, ACTH associated with Cushing's syndrome, as well as 3,4-dihydroxy-phenylalanine (dopa) decarboxylase and serotonin have also been found in association with MTC.

Patients with coexistent pheochromocytomas should undergo abdominal exploration before their neck dissection. At the time of the latter operation grossly abnormal parathyroid glands should be excised and a total thyroidectomy performed because of the associated parathyroid abnormalities and the bilaterality of the MTC.

GASTROINTESTINAL PRESENTATION

Various gastrointestinal syndromes associated with malignancy may be referred to the gastroenterologist for consultation. These include functioning islet cell tumors, the hereditary polyposis syndromes, and hepatomas with paraneoplastic manifestations.

Islet Cell Tumors

Zollinger-Ellison Syndrome   The Zollinger-Ellison syndrome (Zollinger and Ellison, 1955) is caused by "big" and/or "little" gastrin secretion by pancreatic islet cell tumors (Gregory and Tracy, 1972). Sixty percent of these tumors are malignant, 20% are multiple and benign, and 20% are single and benign. This diagnosis should be suspected in patients with recurrent gastrointestinal ulcers, particularly marginal ulcers after gastric resection, or persistent diarrhea. Elevated circulating gastrin levels are diagnostic of this syndrome, but are not available in most laboratories. Therefore gastric hypersecretion of greater than 1 liter and 100 meq of gastric acid during an overnight 12-hr fast provide indirect evidence for this diagnosis.

Recurrent ulcers are caused by gastric acid hypersecretion. The diarrhea results from the large volume of gastric acid secretions, impairment of absorption by acid-damaged intestinal mucosa, bile salt precipitation, and inactivity of pancreatic lipase at low pH. Since less than 25% of patients have surgically resectable islet cell tumors, the primary palliative form of therapy is total gastrectomy (Schein et al., 1973).

Glucagon-secreting Tumors   Glucagon-secreting islet cell tumors are very rare and have not been well studied. The few patients thought to have this syndrome have had diabetes and an associated dermatitis.

Islet Cell Insulinomas   Islet cell insulinomas secrete "big" and "little" insulin which cause fasting hypoglycemia. Because 80% of these tumors are single and benign, exploratory pancreatic surgery is often curative. Hypoglycemia in nonsurgical patients may be symptomatically managed by the administration of diazoxide. Anti-neoplastic chemotherapy with streptozotocin results in palliative improvement in approximately 50% of patients with islet cell cancer.

Diarrheogenic Islet Cell Tumors   The syndrome of watery diarrhea resulting in hypovolemia and hypokalemia with weakness and renal damage in the absence of gastric hypersecretion is thought to be caused by islet cell tumors producing a secretin-like hormone (Schein et al., 1973).

Hereditary Polyposis Syndromes

This group of cancer-associated syndromes, although not strictly paraneoplastic, represents a group of hereditary disorders often having extragastrointestinal manifestations, which, if recognized, may lead to the discovery and cure of asymptomatic malignancy (Stauffer, 1973).

Peutz-Jeghers Syndrome   This autosomal dominant syndrome is characterized by labial, buccal, and fingertip melanin-containing spots (Jeghers, McKusick, and Katz, 1949). All patients with these mucocutaneous stigmata have hamartomas of the small intestine, which rarely undergo malignant degeneration. There are, however, several case reports of periampullary adenocarcinoma (Achord and Proctor, 1963; MacDonald et al., 1967; Reid, 1965; Williams and Knudsen, 1965) as well as an increased incidence of theca cell ovarian tumors (Humphries, Sheppherd, and Peters, 1966). Surgery is necessary only if patients develop intussusception, obstruction, uncontrolled bleeding, or malignant degeneration.

Gardner's Syndrome   Patients presenting with bony and soft tissue tumors should be suspected of having the autosomal dominantly transmitted Gardner's syndrome (Gardner, 1962). These patients have colonic adenomatous polyps which usually undergo malignant transformation. They may also have adenomas of the stomach and small bowel. These patients should be followed closely for evidence of malignant degeneration particularly in the colon, but also in the small bowel (MacDonald et al., 1967; Schnur et al., 1973). Although prophylactic total colectomy or subtotal colectomy with ileorectal anastomosis may be lifesaving, this does not preclude malignant degeneration of small bowel polyps.

Familial Polyposis This syndrome is transmitted as an autosomal dominant without extragastrointestinal manifestations. It is important that family members of affected patients be evaluated because prophylactic colectomy for colonic polyposis before malignant degeneration occurs is lifesaving.

Hepatic Tumors

Both benign and malignant hepatic tumors are associated with a number of paraneoplastic syndromes. Adenomas of the liver have been associated with polycythemia. Hemangiomas have caused sequestration of platelets. Young boys presenting with precocious puberty are often found to have hepatoblastomas with elevated circulating levels of gonadotropins. Hepatomas are associated with hypoglycemia, polycythemia, and various tumor markers including α-fetoprotein, carcinoembryonic antigen, and variant alkaline phosphatase (Gluckman and Turner, 1974).

RHEUMATOLOGIC PRESENTATION

The acute onset of connective tissue disorders may signal the presence of an underlying malignancy while chronic connective tissue patients may develop malignancies in the sites of previous connective tissue activity.

Connective Tissue Disease with Underlying Malignancy

Dermatomyositis Dermatomyositis and variant myopathic-neuropathic syndromes are associated in 15 to 20% of cases with an underlying malignancy. Often the onset of the proximal myopathy is acute. Since most cases of dermatomyositis unassociated with malignancy occur before age 50, any patient over this age presenting with this syndrome should be evaluated for underlying malignancy (Bohan and Peter, 1975). Approximately 50% of this group will eventually develop cancer. These patients with underlying malignancy often do not have a pure dermatomyositis or polymyositis, but do have electromyographic evidence of neuropathy as well as myopathy. When these patients have their malignancy treated, the symptomatic relief from the connective tissue-related symptoms is often rewarding, whereas steroid therapy has been disappointing.

Hypertrophic Pulmonary Osteoarthropathy   Patients presenting with hand swelling, or arthritis of the wrists, knees, or ankles should be suspected of having hypertrophic pulmonary osteoarthropathy. This diagnosis is confirmed by radiographic demonstration of periosteal new bone formation along bone margins proximal to the involved joints. Clubbing of the fingers may be associated with this syndrome although it is more commonly not associated with osteoarthropathy. Most patients presenting with this syndrome have an associated intrathoracic malignancy, usually lung cancer. It has also been seen in patients with colon carcinoma and ulcerative colitis. Neurogenic and hormonal theories for this syndrome have been proposed, but have not clarified its pathogenesis (Holling, 1967). Palliative relief is obtained with control of the primary tumor, salicylates, and analgesics.

Amyloidosis   Amyloid joint involvement may present as a painless limitation of joint movement or as a painful arthritis of the hand due to amyloid infiltration of the carpal tunnel. Most of these patients have underlying immunoglobulin disorders such as multiple myeloma or Waldenstrom's macroglobulinemia. Besides symptomatic analgesia, the only helpful procedure has been decompression of the carpal tunnel (Wiernik, 1972).

Malignancy Developing in Areas of Previous Connective Tissue Disease

Patients with long-standing connective tissue disease may develop malignancy in areas of previous connective tissue activity. The most striking example is the development of bronchoalveolar tumors in patients with long-standing pulmonary fibrosis associated with scleroderma (Zatuchni, Campbell, and Zarafonetis, 1953; Weaver, Divertie, and Titus, 1967). Patients with discoid lupus may develop squamous cell carcinoma of the face and a few patients with documented systemic lupus erythematosus have developed lymphomas (Nilsen, Missal, and Condemi, 1967).

DERMATOLOGIC PRESENTATION

Certain dermatoses may cause the dermatologist to suspect an underlying malignancy. One group consists of dermatoses characteristically associated with malignancy. The second group resembles relatively common skin disorders, but because of atypical clinical behavior may cause the dermatologist to suspect an associated malignancy.

Syndromes Often Associated with Malignancy

Malignant Acanthosis Nigricans   Acanthosis nigricans is characterized by dark, hyperkeratotic areas in the body folds, particularly the axillae. Although this syndrome can be seen in children as a benign condition, the acute onset of this disorder in an adult almost always signals the presence of an internal adenocarcinoma.

Malignant Down   Patients with a sudden growth of facial and body hair should be evaluated for malignancy.

Acquired Pachydermoperiostosis   If a patient without a family history of pachydermoperiostosis presents with large extremities, particularly the hands, knees, and elbows, as well as generalized thickening of the skin of the scalp, forehead, upper lids, ears and lips, evaluation for bronchogenic carcinoma should be initiated.

Acquired Ichthyosis   Adults who develop ichthyosis often have underlying hematologic malignancy although other malignancies have been reported.

Plantar and Palmar Keratoses   Families with hyperkeratoses of the palms and soles have a high incidence of squamous cell carcinoma of the esophagus in later life. Interestingly, unaffected family members do not develop esophageal carcinoma.

Flushing   Episodic cutaneous flushes in patients with ileal carcinoid and the more prolonged and severe flushing associated with facial and periorbital edema in patients with bronchial carcinoids may be the presenting symptoms of patients with underlying carcinoid tumors.

Generalized Reticulohistiocytoma with Polyarthritis   Patients presenting with generalized reticulohistiocytoma, a rare syndrome characterized by pinkish cutaneous nodules and a destructive polyarthritis, may have underlying malignancy.

Erythema Gyratum Repens   Erythema gyratum repens, also a rare dermatologic syndrome, manifests itself as a knotty pine-appearing dermatosis of the trunk and extremities and is almost always associated with an underlying malignancy. The regressions and progressions of the underlying cancer are mirrored by the skin manifestations.

Syndromes Occasionally Associated with Malignancy

The following dermatologic syndromes are usually not associated with cancer, but in some instances, particularly if the clinical behavior of the dermatosis is atypical, may cause the dermatologist to suspect an underlying malignancy.

Hyperpigmentation   Hyperpigmentation may occur in patients with malignancies secreting ACTH and melanocyte-stimulating hormone (MSH). Patients with malignant melanoma may develop a characteristic generalized cutaneous melanin deposition.

Erythema Multiforme   Although this dermatosis is not usually associated with malignancy, it may be associated with cancer or may be triggered by radiation therapy.

Atypical Dermatitis Herpetiformis   Dermatitis herpetiformis is a bullous disease of young people that responds to sulfa drugs. However, in the older patient who does not respond to sulfa or sulfones, malignancy should be suspected.

Pemphigoid   Another bullous disease, pemphigoid is associated with antibodies to the basement membrane. In some instances it is associated with cancer.

Pruritis   Generalized itching may antedate an underlying malignancy by several years. Patients with diabetes and obstructive jaundice characteristically have pruritis, but some patients with malignancy have pruritis for unknown reasons. The pruritis of Hodgkin's disease, the leukemias, and mycosis fungoides is well known.

Urticaria   Urticaria is a relatively common dermatologic problem often associated with allergy. In some patients, however, it is a manifestation of cancer (Curth, 1971).

SUMMARY

The large number of paraneoplastic and cancer-associated syndromes preclude any extensive review in this brief discussion. In this presentation, cancer-associated syndromes are discussed using as a format clinical symptom complexes presenting to medical subspecialists in hematology, endocrinology, gastroenterology, rheumatology, and dermatology.

The clinically most common paraneoplastic syndrome presenting to the hematologist is erythrocytosis. Polycythemia vera, spurious polycythemia, and erythrocytosis secondary to diminished arterial oxygen saturation, abnormal hemoglobin structure, or ectopic erythropoietin secretion must be differentiated. Ectopic erythropoietin secretion is the most manageable of the ectopic hormonal syndromes because of its association with benign tumors and surgically controllable malignancy.

The endocrinologist must distinguish benign hormonal hyperfunction from ectopic hormonal secretion. Particular attention is paid to Cushing's syndrome, hypercalcemia, inappropriate ADH, hypoglycemia, and the medullary thyroid carcinoma syndrome.

The gastroenterologist may be asked to see patients with functioning islet cell tumors presenting as recurrent upper gastrointestinal ulcers and diarrhea (Zollinger-Ellison syndrome), diabetes (glucagon secretion), hypoglycemia (insulinoma), or severe diarrhea (secretin-like secretion). Patients with the hereditary Gardner's and familial polyposis syndromes, although few in number, should be diagnosed and followed closely because of the high incidence of colorectal adenocarcinoma.

Patients with occult malignancy may present initially to the rheumatologist with dermatomyositis, hypertrophic pulmonary osteoarthropathy, or amyloid involvement of the joints or carpal tunnel. Rheumatologic patients may also develop malignancy in the sites of previously active connective tissue disease.

The dermatologist recognizes specific dermatoses often associated with underlying malignancy and suspects malignancy in other patients having atypical variations of common dermatoses.

Although many of these syndromes are not common, the physician's knowledge of their association with cancer may result in early diagnosis and successful treatment of cancer. This knowledge can also clarify the nature of a patient's disability and may result in the use of effective symptomatic palliative measures, even in patients with far-advanced malignancy.

REFERENCES

Achord, J. L., and H. D. Proctor. 1963. Malignant degeneration and metastasis in Peutz-Jeghers syndrome. Arch. Intern. Med. 111:498–506.

Amatruda, T., and G. V. Upton. 1974. Hyperadrenocorticism and ACTH-releasing factor. Ann. N.Y. Acad. Sci. 230:168–180.

Bartter, F. C. 1973. The syndrome of inappropriate secretion of antidiuretic hormone. *In* Endocrine and Nonendocrine Hormone-producing Tumors, pp. 115–142. Yearbook Medical Publishers, Chicago.

Baylin, S., M. Beaven, L. Buja, and H. Keiser. 1972. Histaminase activity: A biochemical marker for medullary carcinoma of the thyroid. Amer. J. Med. 53:723–732.

Berson, S. A., and R. S. Yalow. 1971. Heterogeneity of peptide hormones in plasma as revealed by immunoassay. *In* Proceedings of XI Reunion of French-Speaking Endocrinologists, pp. 105–135. Masson et Cie, Paris.

Bohan, A., and J. Peter. 1975. Polymyositis and dermatomyositis. New Eng. J. Med. 292:344–347, 403–407.

Cramer, F., and W. Kimsey. 1952. The cerebellar hemangioblastomas. Review of 53 cases with special reference to cerebellar cysts and the association of polycythemia. Arch. Neurol. Psychiatr. 67:237–252.

Curth, H. O. 1971. Cutaneous manifestations associated with malignant internal disease. *In* T. B. Fitzpatrick, K. A. Arndt, W. H. Clark, A. Z. Eisen, E. J. Van Scott, and J. H. Vaughan (eds.), Dermatology in General Medicine, pp. 1561–1580. McGraw-Hill Book Co., New York.

Ebbe, S., B. Wittels, and W. Dameshek. 1962. Autoimmune thrombocytopenic purpora ("ITP" type) with chronic lymphocytic leukemia. Blood 19:23–35.

Fahey, R. J. 1951. Unusual leukocyte response in primary carcinoma of the lung. Cancer 4:930–935.

Gardner, E. J. 1962. Follow-up study of a family group exhibiting dominant inheritance for a syndrome including intestinal polyps, osteomas, fibromas and epidermal cysts. Amer. J. Hum. Genet. 16:376–390.

Gluckman, J., and M. Turner. 1974. Systemic manifestations of tumors of the small gut and liver. Ann. N.Y. Acad. Sci. 230:318–331.

Gordon, G. S., and B. S. Roof. 1972. "Humors for tumors": diagnostic potential of peptides. Ann. Intern. Med. 76:501–502.

Gregory, R. A., and H. J. Tracy. 1972. Isolation of two "big gastrins" from Zollinger Ellison tumor tissue. Lancet 3:797–799.

Hammond, D., and S. Winnick. 1974. Paraneoplastic erythrocytosis and ectopic erythropoietins. Ann. N.Y. Acad. Sci. 230:219–227.

Hertko, E. J. 1968. Polycythemia (erythrocytosis) associated with uterine fibroids. Case report with erythropoietic activity demonstrated in the tumor. Ann. Intern. Med. 68:1169.

Holling, H. E. 1967. Pulmonary hypertrophic osteoarthropathy. Ann. Intern. Med. 66:232–234.

Humphries, A. L., M. H. Sheppherd, and H. J. Peters. 1966. Peutz-Jeghers syndrome with colonic adenocarcinoma and ovarian tumor. JAMA 197:296–298.

Jeghers, H. J., V. A. McKusick, and K. H. Katz. 1949. Generalized intestinal polyposis and melanin spots of the oral mucosa, lips, and digits. New Eng. J. Med. 241:993–1005.

Keiser, H., M. Beaven, J. Doppman, S. Wells, and L. Buja. 1973. Sipple's Syndrome. Medullary thyroid carcinoma, pheochromocytoma and parathyroid disease. Ann. Intern. Med. 78:561–575.

Levin, J., and C. L. Conley. 1964. Thrombocytosis associated with malignant disease. Arch. Intern. Med. 114:497–500.

MacDonald, J. H., W. C. Davis, H. R. Crago, and A. D. Berk. 1967. Gardner's syndrome and periampullary malignancy. Amer. J. Surg. 113:425–430.

Marks, L., J. Steinke, S. Podolsky, and R. Egdahl. 1974. Hypoglycemia associated with neoplasia. Ann. N.Y. Acad. Sci. 230:147–160.

McFadzean, A. J. S., D. Todd, and S. C. Tso. 1967. Erythrocytosis associated with hepatocellular carcinoma. Blood 29:808–811.

Muggia, F., and H. Heinemann. 1970. Hypercalcemia associated with neoplastic disease. Ann. Intern. Med. 73:281–290.

Nilsen, L., M. Missal, and J. Condemi. 1967. Appearance of Hodgkin's Disease in patient with systemic lupus erythematosis. Cancer 20: 1930–1933.

Odell, W. D. 1974. Humoral manifestation of nonendocrine neoplasms— ectopic hormone production. In R. H. Williams (ed.), Textbook of Endocrinology, 5th Ed., pp. 1105–1115. W. B. Saunders Co., Philadelphia.

Reid, J. D. 1965. Duodenal carcinoma in the Peutz-Jeghers syndrome. Cancer 18:970–977.

Rosen, S. W., and B. Weintraub. 1975. Humours, tumors, and caveats. Ann. Intern. Med. 82:274–276.

Rosenbaum, D. L., G. W. Murphy, and S. N. Swisher. 1966. Hemodynamic studies of the portal circulation in myeloid metaplasia. Amer. J. Med. 41:360–368.

Schein, P., R. DeLellis, C. R. Kahn, P. Gordon, and A. Kraft. 1973. Islet cell tumors: Current concepts and management. Ann. Intern. Med. 79:239–257.

Schnur, P. L., E. David, P. W. Brown, O. H. Beahrs, W. H. ReMine, and E. G. Harrison. 1973. Adenocarcinoma of the duodenum and the Gardner syndrome. JAMA 223:1229–1232.

Stauffer, I. Q. 1973. Hereditable multiple polyposis syndromes of the gastrointestinal tract. In M. Sleisinger and J. Fordtran (eds.), Gastrointestinal Disease, Pathophysiology, Diagnosis, Management. W. B. Saunders Co., Philadelphia.

Steiner, H., O. Dahlback, and J. Waldenstrom. 1968. Ectopic growth hormone production and osteoarthopathy in carcinoma of the bronchus. Lancet 1:783–785.

Unger, R. H. 1966. The riddle of tumor hypoglycemia. Amer. J. Med. 40:325–329.

Waldmann, T. A., W. F. Rosse, and R. L. Swarm. 1968. The erythropoiesis-stimulating factors produced by tumors. Ann. N.Y. Acad. Sci. 149:509–515.

Weaver, A. L., N. B. Divertie, and J. Titus. 1967. The lung in scleroderma. Mayo Clin. Proc. 42:754–766.

Wiernik, P. H. 1972. Amyloid joint disease. Medicine 51:465–479.

Williams, J. P., and A. Knudsen. 1965. Peutz-Jeghers syndrome with metastatic duodenal carcinoma. Gut 6:179–184.

Zatuchni, J., W. Campbell, and C. Zarafonetis. 1953. Pulmonary fibrosis and terminal bronchiolar ("alveolar cell") carcinoma in scleroderma. Cancer 6:1147–1158.

Zollinger, R. M., and E. H. Ellison. 1955. Primary peptic ulceration of the jejunum associated with islet cell tumors of the pancreas. Ann. Surg. 142:709–728.

Concepts in Cancer Rehabilitation

Nathaniel H. Mayer, M.D.

"Rehabilitation" is fast becoming a major concept of cancer management in the 1970's. "Rehabilitation" as a recently developing aspect of cancer control programs may soon join in clinical partnership with the traditional big three: Surgery, Chemotherapy, and Radiotherapy. Indeed, after these latter treatment modalities are applied, the patient's need for rehabilitation may be even greater. But what is "rehabilitation"? Is it a faddish abstraction devised by health administrators to hound the harried clinician with yet another health directive? Is it an assault "team" of social working, physiotherapeutic, occupational psychologists poised to disrupt the sacred "oneness" of the doctor-patient relationship? Is it to be given intravenously when all else fails?

The ability of a person to function day by day is central to the theme of rehabilitation. It was once pointed to by Mary Switzer that physicians who are preoccupied with eradication of disease often forget that ". . . people live day by day and that the day's comfort is very important" (Rehabilitation of the Cancer Patient, 1972). Can the patient feed and bathe himself? Can he walk, talk, run a household, hold a job? Can the patient engage in adaptive, purposeful,

This work was supported by Contract NO1-CN-45126 from the National Cancer Institute of the Department of Health, Education, and Welfare.

goal-oriented behavior which he perceives to be necessary for his daily needs? The theme of cancer rehabilitation is the theme of quality survival—not how long a person lives (this is an index of our attack on disease) but how well he lives within the constraints of his disease. It is simple in a technical way to prescribe a Canadian hip disarticulation prosthesis for a 25-year-old housewife with fibrosarcoma of the thigh. It is more complicated to deal with the social and emotional consequences of this situation which decidedly influence efforts at physical restoration. Depression, loss of self-esteem, the ignominy of bodily mutilation, and the fear of a husband's rejection all will play a role in contouring the rehabilitation process and its eventual outcome for this patient. What of her children, and household responsibilities? What of her future schooling or vocational interests? What of the imposed financial burdens on the family unit? The physician bent on controlling disease shares the patient's uppermost concern for biologic survival; the rehabilitationist, on the other hand, concentrates on the restoration of function both for the patient and his family. The goal of rehabilitation services for the cancer patient is "to restore the patient to that point where he can function at his optimal level physically, socially, emotionally, and vocationally" (National Cancer Plan). The purpose of this paper is to describe a way of thinking about the needs of patients with cancer in functional terms. It is hoped that this approach will illustrate the major management concept behind rehabilitation which is to restore function.

A 59-year-old, right-handed, retired federal employee was admitted with complaints of recent dysphagia. He also had been having difficulty walking for 7 months and he complained of increasing tiredness during gait. A review of his medical records indicated that a diagnosis of squamous cell carcinoma of the hypopharynx had been made in the past and that cerebral metastases had been identified 7 months previously as the cause of his left-sided weakness. Pulmonary metastases had also been found. He was treated with radiotherapy, chemotherapy, and steroids during this time interval with apparent control of tumor activity and some improvement in symptomatology. The patient was living at home with his wife who had recently fractured her right wrist. He climbed stairs with difficulty and he was ambulatory with a cane in his right hand. However, he had fallen a number of times because his left knee "gave way." He continued to drive to the hospital for outpatient appointments by using his right-sided extremities. Examination revealed the presence of a left hemiparesis with marked proximal weakness of the scapular stabilizers, one fingerbreadth shoulder subluxation, but rather good distal extremity function including isolated hand and finger movement. The left lower extremity was largely synergy bound and, during gait, inadequate dorsiflexion made it difficult for him to clear the floor during swing phase, while stance phase revealed poor control and recurvatum at the knee. His cane was too long and he preferred to hold on to the wall or room furniture when he ambulated. There were no gross visual field deficits or major sensory or cognitive impairments, but he did have some word-finding difficulties as well as difficulty with lower extremity dressing. The patient was depressed by his physical impairments which did not seem to be improving over the previous months and he was particularly distressed by his new symptoms of dysphagia.

This case illustrates many aspects of rehabilitation concern. The patient's major complaints relate to problems of function: he has difficulty swallowing foods, he has difficulty walking, and he tires easily. His concerns are relevant to his daily functional needs and he would like treatment aimed at improving these functional impairments. It is interesting that hemiparesis had been present for 7 months with resulting gait disturbance yet no gait-training program had been considered in his management program. Perhaps it was felt that the patient's prognosis was so poor that it would not be "worth the effort." But let us consider what happened and what could have happened. The patient has survived at least 7 months after his hemiparesis, very likely because of intensive medical efforts (chemotherapy, radiotherapy, steroids, etc.). Though prognosis still remains poor, what survival time should we assign to this specific patient? How many more weeks or months of ambulation shall we predict for him? Should we allow him to continue to function as he has with an energy-consuming gait pattern (certainly contributing to his "tiredness"), run the risk of future falls (perhaps to fracture his hip?, perhaps to die of pulmonary embolization?) or shall we provide (and might we not have provided) a foot-ankle orthosis ("short leg brace") adjusted to stabilize the knee as well as to eliminate inadequate dorsiflexion at the ankle? May we not shorten the height of the cane so that it can be used more effectively as an assistive device? There are other issues of concern. Patients with cerebral metastases may have perceptual problems which interfere with function. How confident are we about this patient's ability to be a safe driver? He may physically be able to control the steering wheel with his right hand and press the gas with his right foot but are his perceptions of movement and visual-spatial relations intact? Extensive perceptual testing is indicated in this type of situation, particularly because the patient has insisted on driving to the hospital and his wife is unable to drive. Other difficulties that bear looking into are in the area of activities of daily living (lower extremity dressing difficulties) and speech pathology (subtle word-finding difficulties). What family stresses exist because of the husband's protracted medical problems? How much assistance can the wife provide to her husband in the face of her recent dominant extremity wrist fracture? If stair climbing is undesirable, can home facilities be modified such that living is accomplished on one floor level? Evaluation by psychosocial personnel is invaluable in defining these management issues which are often a complex blend of psychologic and practical stresses. This case emphasizes the need for identifying the functional problems of the patient with cancer as soon as they arise so that a program of rehabilitation can be devised pari passu with the program for cancer control. "It must be noted that the simple survival of patients treated for cancer is not tantamount to total recovery" (National Cancer Plan). When a patient is viewed from the perspective of his functional abilities rather than his disease process, management becomes more attuned to his rehabilitation needs and the quality of his remaining life.

A 63-year-old, right-handed, retired sales clerk was admitted to the hospital with a pathologic fracture of the distal left femur. The patient had undergone a right radical mastectomy 5 years previously for an infiltrating duct carcinoma. Axillary recurrence developed 1 year later and bowel obstruction requiring surgical decompression occurred 3 years later. During these years her disease had been managed with radiotherapy, chemotherapy, and hormonal therapy. Despite pain at the fracture site, the patient found that she could ambulate to the bathroom with the help of a cane in her left hand. She could not use a cane in her right hand because of the presence of marked lymphedema in the right upper extremity. The patient indicated that she first noticed some swelling in this extremity 2 years previously but that it had caused no functional difficulties. One month prior to admission, however, the arm "blew up" to the point where she had difficulty fitting her clothes, could not lift her "heavy arm," and had to rely on her left upper extremity for most of her daily activities. It was noted that in the previous months the patient had been returning to the outpatient clinic at more frequent intervals for follow-up care. Blood tests, particularly finger sticks, were being obtained more frequently and the patient recalls that they were often taken from the arm on the mastectomy side.

This case illustrates a number of dysfunctional consequences of breast cancer and its treatment. The occurrence of lymphedema in patients who have undergone axillary dissections has been variously reported in the literature and tends to be high, percentage-wise, in those series specifically looking at this question (Britton and Nelson, 1962; Healy, 1971). The relationship between lymphedema and loss of function in the upper extremity has not been looked at as carefully. Depending on duration, volume, and anatomical extent of lymphedema, patients will complain of arm heaviness (sometimes associated with pain in the shoulder-neck region because of traction on the supporting tissues of this area by the weight of the heavy arm); loss of range of motion at the shoulder, elbow, wrist, even fingers leading to impairment of reach, grasp, transport, power, and precision functions of the upper extremity; poor cosmetic appearance of the extremity as well as ill fitting, tight clothes. These consequences are as disastrous to the "domestic engineer" (housewife and homemaker) as they are to the career person outside the home. A major role in the sudden lymphedematous ballooning of an extremity has commonly been attributed to infection (Britton, 1959). Lesser causes have been occlusion of the axillary vein, occult recurrent neoplasm, and fibrosis of lymphatic channels after radiotherapy (Zeissler, Rose, and Nelson, 1972).

A carefully taken history will usually elicit episodes of minor trauma with skin breaks in the days or weeks before the patient seeks help. Patients who work in a kitchen are often subject to burns, cuts with a knife, and minor nailbed trauma. Patients who work in the garden without gloves are prone to being stuck by thorns or sharp instruments and insect bites. An occult offender which should receive greater attention is the venipuncture or finger stick which we subject our patients to when progression of disease necessitates frequent laboratory tests (as illustrated in the above case). Rarely do we specify the appropriate arm for obtaining blood samples. Treatment programs should emphasize preventive education for the patient in the immediate postsurgical period *before* development of lymphedema. A few sensible precautions at home, at work, and in the laboratory will help minimize the functional castastrophes that can result from this condition. If an infectious etiology can be identified as the likely factor in the development of lymphedema, appropriate antibiotics should be used. Subsequently, a pneumatic compression device should be applied in a monitored treatment program to milk the arm's fluid back into the systemic circulation (Stilwell, 1962). Pitting lymphedema seems most responsive to compression treatments whereas brawny long-standing edema has a much poorer prognosis for reduction. (However, I have had patients with the latter condition who have achieved significant improvement in range of motion of distal upper extremity joints which helped them functionally though cosmetically they remained unsatisfied). One cause of failure in regimens of pneumatic compression is a lack of adequate maintenance of arm girth by a diligent wrapping program with ace bandages after the pneumatic compression treatment. Many patients have told me that they had in the past applied elastic wrappings to their arms after a compression treatment—for 20 min q.i.d.! These wraps must be applied continuously to prevent re-accumulation of fluid as much as possible. Elevation of the extremity to take advantage of gravity flow should also be encouraged. Ultimately when serial measurements of arm girth appear to have plateaued, an elastic sleeve with a distal to proximal pressure gradient can be fitted. I also encourage isometric exercises of the lyphedematous extremity with the hand held higher than the elbow, elbow higher than shoulder in order to take advantage of muscle pumping action and gravity effect on tissue fluids. This may be accomplished more easily by having the patient exercise in the supine position, especially in the presence of lost range of motion at the shoulder. If motion has been impaired (and it usually is), a range of motion exercise program should accompany the lymphedema treatment program.

The crucial management concept for these patients is the restoration of upper extremity function and not merely the reduction of lymphedema. By attending to the patient's functional needs, the requisites of rehabilitation will have been served. Functional considerations need not be restricted to postoperative complications. For example, preoperative surgical planning is vital with respect to shoulder motion. A tight constricting scar pursuant to an unnecessarily high axillary incision may cause significant limitation of motion particularly if there is adherence of tissues to the underlying chest wall. In a similar way, attention to the functional consequences of breast amputation has been a concern of the Reach to Recovery program in the immediate postoperative period (American Cancer

Society). When called upon, the mastectomy volunteer presents information on preventing shoulder dysfunction as well as early prosthetic restoration. Some hospital programs have emphasized formation of mastectomy groups where physical, social and emotional consequences of a mastectomy are handled in a group setting. In addition, establishment of a couples group has been found to be helpful for marital as well as personal adjustments to a mastectomy (Schmid, Kiss, and Hibert, 1974).

Patients with metastatic involvement of bone without visceral involvement often live for long periods of time but they may have considerable dysfunction. These patients are prone to pathologic fractures as is illustrated in the case history cited above. Functional problems of such patients relate to their inability to bear weight on the fractured extremity and the clinician must adopt programs which will minimize or eliminate weight bearing on the extremity at risk. A program of graded physical therapy emphasizing the use of assistive devices to unload weight on a particular lower extremity is extremely helpful in keeping these patients mobile and out of bed. Many of these patients are prone to hypercalcemia which may be exacerbated by bedrest, thus compounding the clinician's management problems. When weight bearing becomes problematical in both lower extremities, a program of wheelchair independence can be undertaken. The physical therapist teaches the patient how to transfer from bed to chair using a low friction transfer board. Use of the upper extremities is important in this type of transfer. If pathologic fractures are present in the upper extremities as well, a device such as the Hoyer lift can be obtained. This device can be operated easily by one person (excluding the patient) and will allow the clinician to keep the patient from becoming bedridden upon discharge from the hospital. In the case illustration above, a "walking" cast was placed on the left lower extremity and the patient was trained to ambulate with a walker and partial weight bearing on that extremity prior to discharge from the hospital. In fact, pneumatic compression of the lymphedematous upper extremity reduced the swelling in the hand and wrist region sufficiently to allow her to grasp the walker during such ambulation.

A 54-year-old accountant underwent a right hemimandibulectomy and resection of the floor of the mouth, tongue, and submaxillary triangle for squamous cell carcinoma. A right radical neck dissection was performed 2 months later. Over the course of the next 16 months, the patient remained free of recurrence and metastatic disease. At this time, the patient complained of pain in the right shoulder and neck region, difficulty with arm raising, and problems with speech. Examination revealed weakness of the trapezius on the right resulting in poor scapula stabilization during abduction and elevation movements at the shoulder. The opened jaw deviated to the side of the hemimandibulectomy and the partially resected tongue coudl not touch the palate resulting in distortion of the tongue tip sounds "t," "d," and "n." The patient indicated that people at work had gotten used to his speech patterns but new clients initially had difficulty understanding him. The patient had grown a Van Dyke beard for cosmetic purposes.

Patients with cancer of the head and neck region may face a myriad of functional problems as a consequence of their disease process and its treatment. Functional deficits in speech, chewing, swallowing, salivary control, and taste, as well as severe cosmetic problems, are common. Section of the spinal accessory nerve results in marked trapezius weakness leading to a protracted painful shoulder with impaired scapular rotation and stabilization during functional activities. When a disease process forces a patient to literally "lose face," his vocational and social outlets may become constricted. Returning to a previously held job may be very unpleasant if other workers seek to avoid the facially disfigured patient. Patients with total laryngectomy have a major functional problem with communication (Lauder, 1971). The use of a magic slate or writing pad should be made available immediately after surgery. Training in the technique of esophageal speech (inhaled or injected air vibrates the walls of the esophagus to make sounds for speech) should be carried out preferably by a qualified speech therapist or a successful esophageal speaker usually available through local laryngectomy clubs. In addition to communication problems, there are many other functional problems which these patients face. For example, they cannot go swimming because of the permanent tracheal stoma and they must be careful when bathing or taking showers (shower collars are helpful). Programs of functional restoration for problems of orofacial disfigurement should include consideration of plastic reconstructive surgery, maxillofacial prosthodontics, and prosthetic replacement (Proceedings, Conference on Research Needs in Rehabilitation of Persons with Disabilities Resulting from Cancer, 1965; Neoplasm of Head and Neck, 1974). An obturator appropriately fabricated to cover a palatal defect can be invaluable in improving speech and swallowing functions. In the case illustration above, compensation for restricted tongue motion was achieved by constructing a thickened upper denture in such a manner as to facilitate contact between the tongue tip and the palate. Speech intelligibility improved dramatically. An exercise program in occupational therapy coupled with an elastic shoulder harness alleviated the painful traction syndrome on the side of the radical neck dissection. Patients attempt to hide disfigurement in many ways, such as the growth of a beard to mask distorted facial anatomy. Self-imposed social ostracism is another means of "hiding" disfigurement. Timely psychologic intervention may be helpful for the patient and his family in adjusting to this difficult situation. Supportive and skillful nursing practice, particularly emphasizing the patient's self-care management of his stoma and nasogastric tube feedings, plays the key role in early rehabilitation of these patients in the immediate postsurgical period.

A 48-year-old barber had the removal of a malignant melanoma from the dorsum of the left foot 6 years ago. One year later he underwent a left groin dissection followed subsequently by immunotherapy. Two years later, recurrence in the left calf region resulted in an above knee amputation. The patient was taught proper stump hygiene, strengthening exercises, and stump wrapping with ace bandages. A plaster pylon (temporary prosthesis) was fabricated for gait training and stump shrinkage. When the stump size appeared to have stabilized, a definitive prosthesis was prescribed. This consisted of a total contact socket with pelvic belt suspension, a hydraulic knee, and a SACH (solid ankle cushion heel) foot. The patient was trained on ramps, curbs, and stairs with his prosthesis and returned to work on a part-time basis. An application for sponsorship of the prosthetic training program was rejected by the Bureau of Vocational Rehabilitation because the patient's financial assets exceeded the legal limit for such sponsorship. One year has gone by and the patient remains free of metastases. His stump has continued to shrink and he will require a new prosthetic socket. He is currently working full time.

The functional goals for this patient were quite clear when he was first seen: he wanted a prosthesis to be able to walk and to return to work. Limb amputation secondary to malignancy occurs most commonly because of bone tumors and many feel that a prosthesis should be fitted at the earliest possible date provided the stump is in suitable condition and metastases are not present (Leavitt, 1972). However, there may be many good functional reasons to provide a prosthesis or a much less expensive sturdy pylon for patients who already have metastases. The presence of metastatic disease is not necessarily a contraindication to prosthetic prescription (Shea, 1972). The key consideration (aside from physical feasibility) should be the patient's need of a prosthesis, both functionally and psychologically.

The prosthetic program for a cancer amputee is similar to that of any amputee who has lost a limb from other causes such as accident or peripheral vascular disease. Ideally, these patients should be seen preoperatively by the rehabilitation team to let him know that his amputation is not the end point of medical care but the beginning of a functional restoration program. Information on social, financial, and vocational considerations can begin to be collected because it will have important implications in determining functional goals for the patient. Early upper extremity strengthening exercises and instruction in crutch walking may be particularly helpful to the patient who will be undergoing a hip disarticulation or a hemipelvectomy procedure. In the postoperative period, goals of stump healing and shaping are adopted as well as gait training with a pylon. For the cancer amputee, this program may be affected by whether or not the patient will be undergoing chemotherapy or radiotherapy. The patient may develop side effects such as nausea and vomiting which may usurp his strength and motivation for a rigorous training program. Fluctuations in the size of the stump may also be particularly troublesome while the patient undergoes chemotherapy. Knowledge of prognosis and future treatment plans by the medical oncology team is important for prescription of prosthetic components for the definitive prosthesis. If frequent stump size fluctuations are to be anticipated, a prosthesis with suction suspension will not be desirable. Similarly, the decision to fit a radiation-treated stump with suction socket suspension or with pelvic joint and belt may be difficult. The level of amputation has a definite bearing on training and prosthetic considerations. For example, the hip disarticulation patient has an intact ischium which provides a solid weight-bearing surface allowing good prosthetic stability. The patient with a hemipelvectomy, on the other hand, has no ischium and must carry weight on soft tissues which provide relatively poor stability. Both of these patients must have good flexibility in the lumbrosacral spine because flexion of the prosthetic hip joint is accomplished by performing a posterior pelvic tilt which swings the prosthesis forward. This contrasts with the above knee amputee who uses his intact hip flexors to advance the prosthesis forward. Prosthetic devices are also available for the upper extremity amputee. Given the prostheses commonly available, clinical experience has taught that a cable-controlled hook is the terminal device which is most functional (though not cosmetic) for the patient. On the other hand, the prosthesis for a forequarter amputation permits little or no function and is chiefly cosmetic. Most amputees request prostheses for function and many would sacrifice appearance for the sake of increased functional capabilities. At the present time, however, external power and control of upper extremity prostheses are still an active area for research and development, particularly with respect to high level amputations.

Every state in the union has a Division or Bureau of Vocational Rehabilitation and their vocational counseling service can be invaluable for patients with physical impairments who have vocational potential. They can be instrumental in sponsorship of rehabilitation and vocational training programs for appropriately referred patients, though until recently their involvement with cancer patients has been limited. With improving survival times and better cancer control, it should be anticipated that more patients with cancer would benefit from vocational guidance and services.

There are many rehabilitation problems which we have not touched on, e.g., rehabilitation needs of the colostomy patient or the patient with spinal cord metastasis (Katona, 1967; Dietz, 1969; Krusen, Kottke, and Ellwood, 1971; Lenneberg, 1972). Emphasis on functional considerations continues to be the hallmark of rehabilitation management in these areas as well. To rehabilitate is to restore function. When patient problems are viewed from the perspective of function, management becomes more responsive to patient needs. If we can orient ourselves to this approach, we will have come a long way towards achieving quality survival for the patient with cancer.

REFERENCES

American Cancer Society. Reach to Recovery Program.
Britton, R. C. 1959. Management of peripheral edema, including lymphedema of the arm after radical mastectomy. Cleve. Clin. Q. 26(2):53.
Britton, R. C., and P. A. Nelson. 1962. Causes and treatment of postmastectomy lymphedema of the arm. JAMA 180(2):95.
Dietz, J. H., Jr. 1969. Rehabilitation of the cancer patient. Med. Clin. North Amer. 53(3):607–624.
Healy, J. E. 1971. Role of rehabilitation medicine in the care of the patient with breast cancer. Cancer 28:1656 ff.

Katona, E. A. 1967. Learning colostomy control. Amer. J. Nurs. 67(3).

Krusen, F., F. Kottke, and P. Ellwood (eds.). 1971. Handbook of Physical Medicine and Rehabilitation. 2nd Ed. W. B. Saunders, Philadelphia.

Lauder, E. 1971. 3rd Ed. Self-Help for the Laryngectomee.

Leavitt, L. A. 1972. Rehabilitation problems of the cancer patient. *In* Rehabilitation of the Cancer Patient. Year Book Medical Publishers, Inc., Chicago.

Lenneberg, E. S. 1972. Rehabilitation needs of patients with colostomy. *In* Rehabilitation of the Cancer Patient. Year Book Medical Publishers, Inc., Chicago.

National Cancer Plan. Cancer Program Objective 7. U.S. Dept. Health, Education and Welfare, National Institutes of Health, National Cancer Institute. p. 2–10.

Neoplasm of Head and Neck. 1974. Year Book Medical Publishers, Inc., Chicago.

Proceedings, Conference on Research Needs in Rehabilitation of Persons with Disabilities Resulting from Cancer. 1965. U.S. Dept. of Health, Education and Welfare, Vocational Rehabilitation Administration, and The Institute of Physical Medicine and Rehabilitation, New York University Medical Center.

Rehabilitation of the Cancer Patient. 1972. Year Book Medical Publishers, Inc., Chicago. p. 13.

Schmid, W. L., M. Kiss, and L. Hibert. 1974. The team approach to rehabilitation after mastectomy. AORN J. 19(4):821–836.

Shea, J. D. 1972. Amputation, rehabilitation, and tumors of the extremities. *In* Rehabilitation of the Cancer Patient. Year Book Medical Publishers, Inc., Chicago.

Stilwell, G. 1962. The physiatric management of postoperative lymphedema. Med. Clin. North Amer. 46(4):1051 ff.

Zeissler, R. H., G. B. Rose, and P. A. Nelson. 1972. Postmastectomy lymphedema: late results of treatment in 385 patients. Arch. Phys. Med. Rehabil. 53:159 ff.

Psychosocial Support Systems in Cancer

Melvin J. Krant, M.D.

A change in an individual's customary status is a challenge to the homeostatic adjustment to his environment, and such change can be cause for celebration, or anxiety or despair. When the essential integrity of an individual is disrupted through a disease process, great strains are placed upon him. The individual struggles to maintain a hold on himself and to correct the imbalance (change) as effectively as possibly in order to gain back the sense of stability previously defining him. Such struggle utilizes many psychologic operations, which can be looked on as coping mechanisms, or defense mechanisms, or any similar nomenclature, but which signify that the individual is doing something to maintain a sense of balance. At times such doings are maladaptive, in the sense that they interfere with what most health professionals agree upon as appropriate behavior. The woman who feels a lump in her breast and delays going to a physician is clearly behaving "maladaptively." She may deny to herself that she has felt the lump and may refuse to place her hand, or another's hand, anywhere in the vicinity of the indicting lump. She may argue with herself that it will go away, and she may anxiously examine herself for many weeks, imploring the "lump" to vanish, and finding reason to believe that it has indeed become smaller (temporarily). She may declare its "innocence" because of absence of pain or tenderness. Or, she may run immediately to the phone and request an appointment with her physician. We obviously call the latter behavior adaptional, or appropriate.

Any disruption to the usual stability of an individual is disturbing, but when thoughts or threats of cancer are encased in the disruption, the emotional result is invariably catastrophic. The threatened individual invariably experiences the shocking reality of vulnerability, of essential instability, of customarily out-of-mind potential mortality. More than that, such a catastrophic disruption is threatening to all who are caught in its glowering web, be it family, friends, employers, colleagues, or physicians. Few physicians are totally comfortable with the diagnosis of cancer. If the lesion is potentially fatal, a physician is often caught in disconcerting feelings of helplessness. If the lesion is curable but at the price of body mutilation, he may be so caught up in the attempts at the cure that he refuses to see, or cannot grasp, the consequences of his therapy.

I would like to address myself to two examples of clinical importance, in order to explore the "existential" nature of the despair from the patient's viewpoint. I will do so with an eye to enhancing an empathic grasp of these problems, delineated as psychosocial problems, but conceived of as existential, or living-one's-life problem, so that an appreciation of what can be offered may be suggested. There are three essential themes:

1. Human beings find meaning in their lives through interactions with others (family, friends, society) and with symbols (home, God, country, cause, jobs).

2. Body integrity is essential in working through such interactions. Loss of body integrity, through threat of disease or through treatment, disrupts a person's established interactive patterns. A readaptation to life has to be made, and this requires appropriate mourning for what has been lost.

3. Communication, verbal and nonverbal, is the essential commodity to establishing one's place and influence in the human interacting system, and in assisting readaptations to occur.

The two examples to be dealt with are early, curable cancer, in the form of breast cancer, and late-stage, terminal cancer, in the form of breast or bronchogenic cancer. The first example focuses on the problems associated with the meaning of cancer, even in its early stages, as well as the price paid for cure, namely, mutilation. The second example focuses on the chronicity of cancer, and the learning process of dying. Although important, no attempt has been made here to analyze factors associated with delay in seeking, advising, or accepting appropriate therapy.

The woman who has a "discovered" lump in her breast has two major stresses to deal with. The first is the question of cancer; the second is the need for hospitalization, surgery, and breast amputation. Our present approach to her frequently forces both stresses into a simultaneous mold; namely, she is asked to undergo a diagnostic biopsy and an amputation of the breast at the same time. Surgeons argue about efficiency and the preferability of one anesthesia exposure. An awareness of double, simultaneous, overwhelming stress would argue that a biopsy should first, and separately, be performed, and cancer verified or disproved. Only with that knowledge and subsequent attempted psychologic integration of the meaning of cancer should amputation follow. There is little experimental human data that dictate a one-stage operative procedure in the name of cancer control. It may well be that many, if not most, women would benefit from a two-stage procedure, so that they can face each stress singly and be helped to cope with each in turn. There is a need to absorb the fact that cancer exists and that the breast may then be sacrificed for the sake of cure. A patient can probably deal with the meaning of mastectomy more effectively when that is the operation to be done, rather than with the surgical procedure scheduled as one of uncertainty. I say probably because researched data are very limited in this regard. Conversations with a number of women postmastectomy, as well as with healthy women, lead me to believe that a hope (or fantasy) that the lump will not be cancer is the primary preoperative concern, and that mastectomy itself cannot really be dealt with when the certainty of cancer was doubted. There are probably many women who could not tolerate a two-stage procedure—that is, who would rather have it all over at once. Such women may have severe anesthetic and surgical phobias and feel defenseless and helpless in facing surgery. They may have severe cancer fear and could not wait for a second procedure. Certainly, discussion of such concerns with patients presurgery can elicit potential fears. If not verbalized directly by the patient, they are suggested by marked upset, restlessness, and sleeplessness in the days immediately prior to surgery. A person who possesses such incapacitating fears needs to verbalize them. I suggest that all people have a fear of anesthesia and surgery, as well as a fear of pain. Most of us do all right with a bit of assurance. Phobic individuals need much more help. At any rate, a two-step (double operation) approach to cancer diagnosis, and then to mastectomy, could help many women begin an appropriate grieving for a lost body part allowable in the name of cancer control and cure. But appropriate research is most needed.

The postoperative patient must deal with two phenomena, namely, cancer and mutilation, and must deal with these simultaneously. The diagnosis of cancer, and the mutilating mastectomy, are not time-limited events; they are long-range, ongoing concerns. Unfortunately, there is a scarcity of researched existential data on long-term follow-up of cancer-cured mastectomy patients. In one of the few physician-written articles on the subject Dr. Clinton Ervin (1973), a surgeon, commences his report by referring to three post-mastectomy suicides, and how these deaths forced him to realize that women may not simply be cured of their cancers—they may be wholly overwhelmed by the combined event of cancer, scarring, and a sense of self-repugnance. In discussing an additional 12 cases, he states that these women saw themselves as mutilated, repulsive, diseased, and, with all that, in the grasp of a disease which they felt could only end in a lingering, lonely, painful death.

Women are concerned with their external images, and frequently believe that men and women are staring at them and see right through their clothes. This may lead to social withdrawal, and at-home hostility, rage, and depression. Bard and Sutherland (1955) examine the problem of the painful fantasies involved in relating to people and to a hostile environment without an intact and acceptable body. Even if not depressed, postmastectomy women often harbor a conviction that a "deformed" or "disfigured" person is held in low esteem by the community at large, and that she can expect only pity, revulsion, intolerance, or some equally disturbing reaction from people in general. Mastectomy women may also see themselves as "vulnerable," now that the prior image of the inviolable body has been aborted, to general illness, general calamity, and life problems that they will not be able to deal with because of their permanent body (self) wound.

Many women see themeslves as the "strong" one in the family—the person on whom everybody else leans, the fortress that comforts and supports. The combination of mastectomy and cancer may strip them of that image of strength. For some the fear of becoming a burden instead of being strong and independent can be overwhelming. For others, their claim to legitimate dependency on a strong male who will protect them is diminished because of having less to offer in the bargain. Sexual attractiveness, as well as sexual "completeness," is invested in breast appearance. It should therefore hardly be surprising that anger and resentment, followed by guilt and depression, can haunt a woman long after mastectomy and erode her marriage, family life, or love relationships severely.

On top of these reactions is the ever present fear of death from cancer. "Was it worth it?" is a sentiment recorded, expressing both doubt and resentment at the physician for doing this to her, when she must die anyway from cancer. Husbands may harbor the same feelings of doubt. Dependent women may harbor resentment against their husbands for "allowing" cancer and mutilation to occur. Communication patterns in the family are often severely disrupted (Quint, 1965). Discussions of feelings, of fears, of "unacceptability," of concerns with spreading cancer, and of ever-haunting implication of dying and death, are usually avoided. Women may seek assurances from physicians that each and every ache or pain is not cancer, that all cancer was removed, and that the mutilation was "worth it," but such reassurances can seldom be forthcoming. Fear of the loss of the opposite breast is a frequent concern. Husbands want to go on with living, and often become confused by their wive's depression, reticence, resentment, nervousness, or irritating behaviors. Men frequently infantilize their wives, but after a while grow resentful that, after all they've done, things aren't back to normal. And of course, if a marriage has been borderline, or if a man is invested primarily in his wife's body, and not the person, or if he harbors neurotic feelings about deformity, illness, or weakness, he may find himself acting abusively or derisively.

Jeanne Quint (1964) has pointed out that homecoming after mastectomy may be a time of great nervousness, exhaustion, and feelings of anxiety. Some improvement may follow after 6 or 8 weeks at home, especially as the incision heals, and a prosthesis begins to be successfully used. Quint warns that in the 4th to 5th month after an operation, signs of depression return, and that many experience doubts about their future and an incapacity to "get-on" with life's activities. Her studies indicate that even 1 year after mastectomy, women reported feeling alone and lonely, finding death-talk necessary but depressing, and afraid to talk to their families about concerns for the future. These women were very aware of stories of other women with breast cancer who died, or who suffered from medical treatment, and felt that they just couldn't trust their physicians.

Betty Harker (1972), a social worker who had a long bout with breast cancer before dying, points out that the cancer patient tries to suppress her bitterness, or her angry sentiments, because of the fear of driving much needed people away. However, Harker points out that the patient is often driven to express her anger and then feels guilty about so doing, and consequently withdraws into silence and avoidance of meaningful communication. The patient often doesn't know how to open up conversation, and neither do family members or friends; the result is an augmented level of disagreeable tension.

Mastectomy procedures may cause long-lasting pain, or strange sensations over the chest. Often this pain interferes with simple daily hygiene functions such as washing, and a helpless anger can prevail. In many cultures, a high value is placed on not showing or talking of pain, otherwise one is labeled a "complainer." Patients from such cultures need permission from physicians and family to discuss their experience of pain, rather than always showing a "good face." Otherwise they must live with pain secretly and resentfully (Harker, 1972).

Psychosocial interventions are therefore directed at preventing or alleviating the disastrous consequences of cancer and mutilation. There are, in general, two broad concepts. They should be seen as mutually supportive, but are often operationally excluding. The first concept, and the one most popularized, can be called the positive approach. The idea is to get the patient actively rehabilitated through exercises, prosthesis, arm massages, etc. The Reach to Recovery program seems in their vein, namely, the visit of a postmastectomy recovered patient utilized to hasten reintegration into society.

An additional, and often needed, concept is that of mourning and reintegration. What is implied is a long-term process of support, which acknowledges that the patient and family will need time to adjust, that they may slip back into self-pitying and depressive days, and that they may need reassurance and encouragement to verbalize for a year or longer.

The physician is at the heart of such interventions. His willingness to grasp empathetically the existential issues at stake and to arrange for continued long-term interaction with the patient is critical. If he realizes that a mastectomy patient may be in for long-term emotional disarray, collaborative efforts with social workers, psychiatrists, ministers, and other counseling forces can deal with these issues on an ongoing basis.

Essential recommendations for such psychosocial approaches, for physician and a collaborative team, would be as follows:

1. Establish early a trusting relationship which encourages individual verbalizations of fears and concerns prior to surgery.
2. Help patient and family sort out the separate concerns for cancer and mastectomy.
3. Help patient begin appropriate mourning for the lost body image before surgery, and help with discussion of fear and concerns of the "self," and not just of the surgery.
4. Inform patient as to potential postmastectomy concerns, and help patient understand that such reactions are understandable and that the concerned group will be "there" to share and discuss possible anguish and life uncertainty. The team should reach out to patient.
5. Share all major therapeutic steps with patient and significant others.
6. Stay scrupulously honest about medical findings and their meaning, without imposing uncertain meanings.
7. Explore husband's reactions to wounds, scars, deformities, etc. Help him verbalize his rage, fear, frustrations, etc., separately from wife.
8. Recognize need for constant reassurance that the right steps were taken. Help patient discuss other "cases" that have progressed or died.
9. Provide an outlet for patient's bitterness or feelings of resentment.

Interventions of this kind are not one-time events, nor, as indicated, are they time limited. Interventions of the mourning-reintegration type may require months to even years before harmonious recovery is seen. Do not wait for the patient to come in complaining. Intervention of this nature should be intertwined with rehabilitation tasks, and with breast reconstruction plastic surgery where appropriate.

The existential problems of the fatally ill cancer patient, especially towards the end of his life, are essentially similar, except that they are organized around sets of physical as well as living-while-dying problems. First, it is undeniably true that when severe pain exists, little else exists in the conscious and unconscious world of the patient and his family. The patient is overwhelmed, and the family is pathetically helpless and at times furious. Every effort must be extended to relieve relentless pain. But two issues should always be considered in such an address: 1) anxiety can augment and distort pain, and anxiety needs to be considered, explored, and verbalized; and 2) patients may distrust and reject the narcotizing effect of pain medication and should be allowed to control such disturbing effects by modifying, changing, or refusing drugs.

When pain and other disabling physical phenomena do not overwhelm, then a patient should be helped to live his life and to die, in a fashion that promises his sense of unique personhood, his sense of control of his destiny within the limitations and framework imposed upon him by illness and nonindependence, and his desires to influence ongoing life events after his death. Being ill, especially chronically ill and fatally ill, obviously creates an intense alteration of the previously existing self—the strong, capable, independent, self-sufficient, lovable, purposive, immortal self. People deal with altered self-image by comparing this image to a past image and an idealized image. Coping forces and defensive forces appear organized to give both meaning to, and to protect against, the implication of the alteration.

For a person to truly understand this alteration is to enjoin a new identity. To have this new identity, one must know what is happening to him, and how he should see it. A person does not need intricate details; he really needs simply statements and symbols. He may deny the knowledge, and may attempt to behave as if his identity is unchanged. Or of even more difficulty for him, a patient may sense that others, such as family, are aware of information about him and are keeping it from him. Such states of awareness are troublesome and result in dissonance between patient, family, and health caregivers. Altered states of identity are hard enough to bear without feelings of resentment that one is being victimized through forced, but not trusting, dependency. A person cannot feel in control and purposive if he feels victimized, and he cannot accept a new and difficult identity if he is threatened with the loss of a much needed identity that was employed to "protect" him against a hostile environment.

When a fatal illness afflicts a person with a strong ego who has the capacity to grasp real events as real and to perceive and conceptualize the meaning of such events, then the problems of communication are greatly simplified. The sharing of knowledge, facilitation of appropriate expression of feelings, and encouragement of personal grieving for what has been changed and lost through illness, enhance a sense of control in the decisions affecting his life in the present and in the future. When fatal illness afflicts individuals who have a lessened ego ability to trust, to grasp and conceptualize the real meaning of events, or who are persistently threatened by the universe they inhabit, communication problems may be enormous. It is with such individuals that extraordinary degrees of denial, rage, or withdrawal are seen. Such individuals can become extremely clinging, dependent and impotent, or can act murderously and self-destructively. Such patients become extremely difficult management problems. They often need people to act out against, such as family or staff. Patients who may appear sweet, calm, and accepting to staff may be raging and resentful to their families. Such patients can make a medical staff and nursing staff get furious at their families. Staunchly independent folks can become tyrants to a medical staff, or their inconsolable bitterness may be too much for a doctor or nurse to take.

Psychosocial interventions by a trained staff should be directed at a patient, family, and medical staff. The latter group is particularly important to work with, for physicians, nurse, social workers, and other health care individuals have considerable interactive problems with patients, families, and each other. When a staff member identifies with a patient, or feels a sense of impotence in dealing with a relentless problem, or is under attack by an angered family member accusing malfeasance, incompetence, or plain stupidity, staff tend either to withdraw, find fault with each other, or respond sullenly and with their counter-rage. Unnecessary procedures may be ordered, extra medications given, or other inappropriate actions taken. Few of us are trained to be objectively, equinimitably, but empathetically concerned. Our own egos are too often at risk.

Essentially, one should look for four major areas of anxiety in terminal patients and their families. These anxieties, potential or actual, should be explored in words. They express, at least in part, the necessary adaptive steps that a patient and family must each endure for a reasonably healthy adaptation to the phenomena of dying and reintegration mourning. Healthy, by the way, does not mean happy or peaceful. Sadness, depression, and anger are all healthy reactions. First is the question of excessive denial which can lead to damaging and maladaptive behaviors in family or patient or in medical decisions. A person with a life expectancy of 2 or 3 months who decides to sell his business in order to reinvest in a long-term, marginal scheme, is cause for concern. Such individuals also tend to postpone or avoid other important decisions. They confuse family and staff, who are made uncomfortable by the denial stance. In certain borderline personalities, denial may be the only way to coping with terminality, and it would be foolish to disjoint such defenses. An appropriate intervention would be to help the family, or the staff, tolerate such denial.

Second, a sense of alienation should be explored. Alienation is the feeling of being out of harmony with the universal nature of things or with a moral order where goodness is appreciated and badness punished. One feels that there is an "injustice"—it's unfair. It can be expressed as "Why is this happening to me when that worthless bum down the street who never did anything for anybody just goes right on drinking?" Alienation implies rage, impotence, futility, and, of course, guilt, punishment, and, thusly, depression, self-pity, and a sharp drop in self-worth. One feels unloved, unloveable, and a burden. Role changes are implied with their distressing shift in values; independence turning into dependence changes the order of things— mothers are only mothers when they are mothering.

Feelings of alienation sensitize an individual's interpretation of other people's behaviors. Feelings and concerns of abandonment become aroused. This is especially true if there is concern as to trust and dependence, and if there are bitterness and resentment against fate. Bitterness drives people away; many individuals need permission and a feeling of trust and safety in order to express their bitterness. Absence of "safety" results in withdrawal, depression, poor communication, and actual and felt abandonment.

And last, interacting with alienation and abandonment is an anxiety of depersonalization. To be no longer a person, to be thought of only as the third person, to feel objectified, is to be devitalized—in other words, to see oneself as dead and annihilated. Annihilation implies a wiping out of all traces, an attitude of "no one will miss me, no one will know that I was here, no one will mourn me." There is a sense of the immortal in many of us; it can be expressed in terms of resurrection and of heaven-hell interface, but also in children, monuments, nature. Different cultural groups express it in their unique manner. There is a dread of annihilation and depersonalization. Psychosocial intervention must explore this. When the "I" changes to a third person—"They do terrible things to people here"—one should be one the lookout. Annihilation is nonimmortality—it is anger, projected rage at the cosmos for "meaningless" existence.

What is meant then by interventions is a program directed at exploring these anxieties through verbalization and behaviors in order to relieve the sense of suffering inherent therein. Help is offered to an individual to feel that his existence is meaningful and that he has permission to grieve for himself, to express his bitterness, to grasp understandingly his true identities, and to integrate his dying with his past, present, and future. Such efforts require working with families as well as with patients in order to resolve conflicts, clarify information, dispel fantasies, encourage adaptations through mourning, and offer an alliance in the postdeath period. Ongoing work with families after a death is frequently productive in facilitating expressions of mourning, answering lingering doubts and questions, and helping a family to accept and integrate their new identities. Such ongoing postdeath interventions may be required for many months and should be interlocked with community efforts to help people into new roles, such as widowhood or fatherlessness.

REFERENCES

Bard, M., and A. Sutherland. 1955. Psychological impact of cancer and its treatment. IV. Adaptation to radical mastectomy. Cancer 8:656–672.

Erwin, C. V. 1973. Psychological adjustment to mastectomy. *In* Medical Aspects of Human Sexuality. Vol. 7, pp. 42–65.

Harker, B. L. 1972. Cancer and communication problems. A personal experience. Psychiatry Med. 3:163–171.

Quint, J. 1965. Institutionalized practices of information control. Psychiatry 28:119–132.

Quint, J. 1964. Mastectomy: Symbol of cure, or warning sign. G. P. 29: 119–124.

Emotional and Personality Characteristics of Cancer Patients

Claus Bahne Bahnson, Ph.D.

Observations concerning psychologic aspects of cancer go all the way back to Galen (200 A.D.), who stated that melancholy women more often developed breast cancer than did sanguine women, and have reappeared in the literature during the 18th and 19th centuries. Guy (1759) wrote that malignancies occur in women with "hysteric and nervous complaints" and are peculiar to "the dull, heavy, phlegmatic, and melancholic," especially those who have met with "disasters in life, and occasion much trouble and grief." Walshe (1846) wrote frankly that "moral emotions ('mental misery, sudden reverses of fortune, habitual gloominess') produce defective innervation . . . which in its turn causes the formation of carcinoma." Amussat (1854), similarly, wrote that "the influence of grief appears to me to be . . . the most common cause of cancer." Between 1870 and 1890, there appeared a surge of "psychosomatic" statements about cancer by Paget (1870), Snow (1883, 1891), Parker (1885), Cutter (1887), Hughes (1887), and others, all referring in one terminology

This paper was delivered at the American College of Physicians' Course 3 on "Recent Developments in Medical Oncology," May 14, 1975, as part of session "The Patient with Cancer."

or the other to the influence of loss and bereavement, grief, or melancholy on the development of cancer. Meyer (1931) and Hoffman (1925) followed up with similar statements. Elida Evans (1926) reported on 100 cases of cancer which had been evaluated through intensive psychotherapy. She found that her patients had lost or had disrupted a major emotional relationship prior to the development of the disease. Evans thus was one of the first to express a dynamic formulation of cancer. Foque (1931), in Paris, pointed toward "the role of sad emotions as activating and secondary causes in . . . certain human cancers" and observed in many of his patients "great crises, grave depressive afflictions, profound mourning, and all the sad emotions which have prolonged repercussions . . ."

Psychology and psychoanalysis have sponsored two main approaches to cancer: one related to loss and depression as an antecedent to cancer, the other to a particular personality configuration characterized by denial and repression as well as strong internalized control and commitment to social norms. In recent years two or three groups, in particular, have brought the loss-depression hypothesis to the fore once again. Greene and associates (1954, 1956, 1966) and Schmale and Iker (1964, 1966) in a series of studies evaluated personality factors in patients with lymphomas and leukemias, and uterine malignancies, respectively, and found repeatedly that severe loss or separation, with concomitant depression, helplessness, and hopelessness, is a characteristic antecedent to the development of both of these types of malignancies. Greene, together with different collaborators, included a series of both male and female patients with reticuloendothelial diseases and consistently reported that separation from a significant person or the loss of a major goal, with ensuing depression, was the key factor gleaned from carefully analyzed clinical and test studies of these patient groups. Later, Greene and Swisher (1969) reported a study of monozygotic twin pairs discordant for leukemia, and showed again how the unfortunate twin who was subject to individual frustration or loss developed leukemia, whereas the more fortunate twin did not. Schmale and Iker (1966) used a predictive technique, selecting from a group of women at higher risk (Papanicolaou III smears) those who might develop cervical cancer, based on a recent history of loss and hopelessness. The predictions were correct beyond the 0.02 level of significance. Independent of the Rochester group, LeShan and co-workers (1956, 1960, 1966), after working clinically with more than 500 cancer patients, reached a similar conclusion. LeShan emphasized that serious and incapacitating depletion and depression (or as he prefers to call it: "despair," in the sense of Kierkegaard) earmarked these patients who were experiencing insoluble life situations prior to the onset of cancer. He also emphasized that some of the chronic personality aspects of cancer patients-to-be are: fragile or nonexisting affective objective relationships and a basic bleak hopelessness about ever achieving any real feeling or true meaning of life.

LeShan and Worthington (1956) studied cancer patients and controls by means of a personal history test developed by Worthington. They found that: 1) cancer patients had suffered a loss of an important relationship before the diagnosis of cancer; 2) cancer patients had no ability to express hostile feelings; and 3) cancer patients showed tension over the death of a parent, usually an event which had occurred many years previously. Their findings support the observation by several other workers that strong unresolved tensions concerning parental figures are characteristic of cancer patients.

Other researchers who have emphasized the importance of depression are: Kowal (1955), who stated that there is a loss of a significant figure or loss of a life goal, resulting in hopelessness, despair, and passive surrender, prior to the onset of cancer; and Meerloo (1954), who stated that all of his patients had severe depressions or other psychopathology prior to clinical onset. Neumann (1959) observed that 80% of her cancer patients had suffered the loss of a significant person within 1 or 2 years before onset of symptoms, and Stevenson (1964) suggested "that brain states signifying profound alarm or despondency, particularly in a medium of aging hormones, are connected with tumour formation . . ."

Brown, Katz, and Kaufman (1961) compared cancer patients, individuals coming to a Cancer Detection Center, and psychiatric out-patients, to each other by means of a drawing technique: the House-Tree-Person Test. Cancer patients and patients coming to the Cancer Detection Center differed from psychiatric out-patients and a control group of student nurses by presenting a personality pattern of "infantile oral-sadistic and anal-sadistic impulses, disturbed sexual identification, egocentricity and emotional immaturity, guilt feelings concerning hostile and sexual impulses, and defective interpersonal relationships." Oo (1965) emphasized the dysphoric flavor of these patients' interviews, as well as their TAT and Rorschach responses, and indicated that they appeared bleak and lacking of emotional expression. Sugar and Watkins (1961) found that patients with breast cancer, compared to those with benign lesions, were more depressed and showed marked emotional disturbances.

Hagnell (1966), within the parameters of a prospective population study of 2,550 persons in Sweden, found that female cancer patients, compared to controls, more often were "substable" in the terminology of Sjöbring's personality classifications, 10 or more years prior to the onset of disease. This "substable" personality type is characterized by being warm and hearty rather than cool, concrete rather than abstract, interested in people rather than in ideas, and tending to be a social extrovert rather than an introvert. This substable group has many characteristics in common with Bleuler's "syntonic," Kretschmer's "cyclothymic," Sheldon's "viscerotonic," and Eysenck's "extrovert" characteristics. An analysis was made of the relation of the incidence of cancer to body build and no relationship was found. That the "substable," or extrovert, personality predicts cancer is supported by a study by Coppen and Metcalfe (1963) who made a study of 50 women with cancer in London and found that these patients were significantly more extroverted compared with the controls without cancer. Kissen and Eysenck (1962) similarly found greater extroversion, using Eysenck's method, in cancer patients compared to control patients.

Goldfarb, Driesen, and Cole (1967) reviewed recent literature on the psychology of cancer and summarized the personality characteristics as follows: 1) maternal dominance, 2) immature sexual adjustment, 3) inability to express hostility, 4) inability to accept loss of a significant object, 5) pre-neoplastic feelings of hopelessness, helplessness, and despair. He also pointed out that free fatty acid levels are abnormally high in patients with rapidly growing malignancies and that this is also characteristic of depressed patients. He indicated that cancer patients and depressed patients share psychodynamic characteristics as well as some biochemical features.

Farberow et al. (1964) studied suicide among general medical and surgical hospital patients and reported that cancer patients account for a disproportionate amount of suicide deaths among hospital patients with serious diseases. He stated that cancer patients were more distressed by their illness, showed indications of severe emotional disturbance in a majority of cases, and had special problems with their family lives.

We shall now review the other main approach to psychologic factors in cancer, dealing with repression, denial, poor emotional outlet, and lack of self-communication. It should be said at once that several of those workers who have emphasized depression and loss also have reported striking observations of denial and "blandness" in their patients. Although a survey of the literature indicates that these observations "creep into" nearly all reports, the fact still remains that only a few groups have emphasized these long term psycho-dynamic aspects of the patients' personalities. Kissen and his co-workers in Glasgow (1962, 1963, 1964, 1965, 1966a, 1966b, 1966c, 1967) have pursued this particular approach over the last decades, starting with clinical observations and later moving into objective research, making use of the Maudsley Personality Inventory (MPI), developed by Eysenck, in order to validate on a quantitative and statistical basis their clinical impressions. Using well validated scales such as the Extraversion-Intraversion and Neuroticism Scales of the MPI, Kissen's group found that cancer patients have marked diffi-culty with emotional discharge and tend to be quite inhibited and repressive subjects when compared with control patients with other serious diseases of similar sites.

The Gengerelli Symposium (Gengerelli and Kirkner, 1954), which was one of the first publications signaling a renewed interest in the psychologic aspects of cancer, contains several contributions relating to ego defenses as well as to other aspects of personality and psychopathology. Blumberg, West, and Ellis reported MMPI findings from cancer versus control patients, and described the cancer patients as defensive, anxious, over-controlled subjects with no abil-ity to release tension through motor or verbal discharge or any kind of "acting out." Their MMPI and Rorschach results suggested that cancer patients with fast developing disease are more defensive and over-controlled than patients with slowly developing disease. The rapidly progressing cancer patients also showed lack of ability to de-crease anxiety, and presented a polite, apologetic, almost painful acquiescence. This was contrasted with the more expressive, and some-times bizarre, personalities of those who responded well to therapy with long remissions and long survival. The authors' impression is that the very development of cancer in man might conceivably result from the physiologic effect of long continued inner stress, which has remained unresolved by either outward action or successful adapta-tion. It seems to them that human cancer could represent, at least in many instances, a "non-adaptation syndrome." Also Klopfer, in the Gengerelli Symposium, related ego defense and ego strength to the differential development of fast and slow growing cancers. Using a theoretical model with two axes, 1) investment in ego defense and 2) impairment of reality testing, Klopfer found that fast growing cancers correlated significantly with high investment, and slow growing cancers with low investment, in ego defenses. Also, cancer appeared with decreasing incidence as impairment of reality testing increased. Perrin and Pierce (1959) emphasized that cancer develops slower in less inhibited individuals and faster in strongly inhibited individuals. Cobb (1952) stressed that all cancer patients regard emotional involvement as dangerous, and that they withdraw and encapsulate themselves due to fear of rejection and misfortune. West, in the 1954 Gengerelli Symposium, described the cancer patient with the poorest prognosis as a defensive, repressive person, with great need for appearing "good" and acceptable to others. Tarlau and Smalheiser (1951) also emphasized constriction and repression, deduced from Rorschach records of cancer patients, to be a particular feature of this condition. Reznikoff (1955), in his study of psychologic factors in breast cancer, stressed the appearance of rigidity and repression in his patients side by side with a basic discontent with their sex role. Valadares (1967) reports on the basis of a study of 163 cancer patients that inhibition of drive leads to biologic regression, masochism, self-destructive tendencies, and cancer.

This author and his co-workers have pursued the study of ego defenses using questionnaire methods, Rorschach assessments, drawing, TAT stories, adjective checklists of mood (conscious and preconscious), and clinical interviews. The results are reported in a number of publications (1964a, 1964b, 1965a, 1965b, 1966a, 1966b, 1967a, 1967b, 1969a, 1969b, 1970) and can be summarized as presenting general support and confirmation of the hypothesis that cancer patients, compared to other patient populations and to normal samples, make heavy use of denial and repression, have lost communication with their own covert needs and wishes, but present a realistic and pleasant interpersonal attitude although they live a constricted and bleak life. In a study making use of the Roe Parent-Child Relationship Questionnaire (1966) and introducing three control groups, our cancer patients were found to remember their parents as being noninvolved, cold, and nearly nonexistent in their early emotional lives. We concluded that the rigid defensiveness and lack of internal communication in cancer patients may be related to early interactions with parents, not allowing the patients (children) to develop affective communications with the parents, and thus impairing affective expression, depriving them of the experience of having stable object relationships.

Cutler (1954), working with terminal cancer patients, described them as individuals who fail to express themselves and who repress hostility. Often, the patient is an overly "good" person, expressing self-pity. Jacobs (1954), similarly, remarked on the pronounced self-destructive forces and rigid armoring of the cancer victim. Thus, an extensive literature exists relating depression, intolerable psychologic conflict, and a repressive personality pattern to the onset of clinical cancer.

RESULTS FROM RECENT STUDY OF CANCER PATIENTS

The results from one of this author's studies of the psychosocial profile of cancer patients are discussed below. In the SECON Health Study,[1] including heart, cancer, and other seriously ill patients as well as a normal stratified control population, we developed scales on the basis of a questionnaire, by item-analyzing a priori selected items pertaining logically to selected theoretical dimensions. Items were rejected until a reasonable approximation to uni-dimensionality was achieved, and the scales were then run against four nosologic groups: myocardial infarction (MI), cancer (CA), mixed sick controls (S), and normal controls (N). High and low socioeconomic status (SES) and age groups were stratified throughout.

Three-way analyses of variance, including nosologic group, age, and SES, were carried out with these subject groups. Four different anxiety scales, each measuring a different aspect of the anxiety complex, all revealed that the cancer group rated lowest and the MI group high, or highest. On the scale of "Psychic Anxiety" (Table 1) cancer patients rated lowest at a probability level of <0.01, whereas the other patient groups (MI and mixed sick) rated highest, with the normal control group at an intermediate level. The fact that cancer and the other sick groups, exposed to similar upsetting hospital procedures, fall in opposite ends of the distribution suggests that we

[1]The SECON study (principal investigators: Dr. Walter I. Wardwell and Dr. Claus B. Bahnson) was supported in part by Grant HE 07522 from the National Heart Institute.

Table 1. Means of scaled scores for "psychic anxiety"
(SES × nosologic group)[a]

SES	MI	S	N	CA	SES	F	p
High	174.5	221.4	175.3	120.6	174.2		
Medium	201.0	185.3	164.6	102.0	177.3	4.98	<0.01
Low	225.0	211.5	202.2	211.8	212.0		
Nosologic group	197.9	200.8	176.5	154.4		4.05	<0.01

[a]Conclusions: 1) CA < N < MI, S; 2) SES: Low > Medium, High; 3) med CA < all other groups.

here deal with a true and not a spurious difference in personality characteristics. Exactly the same sequence was obtained for the scale "Autonomic Indicators of Anxiety" (Table 2), $p < 0.05$. The cancer group also fell lowest on the scales of "Somatic Anxiety" and "Phobic Anxiety," with the MI group holding higher ratings, although the differences here did not attain statistical significance. On the two anxiety scales, obtaining significance, then, the cancer group fell lowest, indicating that they exhibit fewer anxiety symptoms, and also report less awareness of feelings of anxiety, whereas the MI group rated high on these anxiety measures.

Two scales pertain to a person's general proneness to suffer from minor somatic symptoms: "Somatization" and "Self-Image: Bodily Strength." On the scale of "Somatization" (Table 3), the cancer group again fell lowest, $p < 0.02$, and young subjects reported more somatic symptoms than old, $p < 0.01$. The MI group again rated high.

Consistent with this finding, the cancer group also fell highest on the scale "Self-Image: Bodily Strength" (Table 4), $p < 0.01$,

Table 2. Means of scaled scores for "autonomic indication of anxiety"
(age × nosologic group)[a]

Age	MI	S	N	CA	Age	F	p
35–54	94.8	100.0	73.4	70.6	85.6	13.26	<0.01
55–64	69.2	70.8	61.3	49.2	64.2		
Nosologic group	83.8	88.5	68.4	59.6		3.72	<0.05

[a]Conclusions: 1) CA < N < S < MI; 2) young > old; 3) old CA < all other groups.

Table 3. Means of scaled scores for "somatization"
(age × nosologic group)[a]

Age	MI	S	N	CA	Age	F	p
35–54	50.3	52.7	44.3	43.0	47.9		
55–64	45.5	42.8	42.8	33.0	42.5	8.09	<0.01
Nosologic group	48.2	48.8	43.7	37.9		3.75	<0.02

[a]Conclusions: 1) CA < N < MI, S; 2) young > old; 3) old CA < all other groups.

again a very significant result because the three comparison groups here did not differ much from each other. This scale measures a person's perception of his own physical health and resiliency. Although variance by SES did not obtain significance, interestingly the high SES cancer subjects, in particular, perceived themselves as healthier and possessing more bodily strength than their high SES controls. The perception of physical strength thus has little to do with actual disease, and, instead, reflects personality organization and defense.

In order to evaluate the stress hypothesis, pertinent scales for stress variables were run for the four groups. On the scales "Recent Stress" (Table 5) and "Stress at Work" (Table 6), the cancer group rated lowest and the MI group highest, ($p < 0.01$). On "Recent Stress," old cancer subjects, in particular, rated lower than all other groups. For "Stress at Work," young, and high and middle SES, cancer patients rated lower than all other groups. In contrast, cancer patients rated highest and MI patients lowest ($p < 0.10$) on "Stress

Table 4. Means of scaled scores for "self-image, bodily strength"
(SES × nosologic group)[a]

SES	MI	S	N	CA	SES	F	p
High	145.8	135.6	143.3	170.0	145.9		
Medium	139.0	142.4	143.8	139.9	141.7	1.56	n.s.
Low	130.7	1320.	139.1	154.1	136.9		
Nosologic group	139.3	137.2	142.6	154.6		4.22	<0.01

[a]Conclusions: 1) CA > N, MI, S; 2) high CA > all other groups.

Table 5. Means of scaled scores for "recent stress"
(age × nosologic group)[a]

Age	MI	S	N	CA	Age	F	p
35–54	7.2	6.3	6.6	5.1	6.6	8.59	<0.01
55–64	6.0	5.0	6.1	3.6	5.5		
Nosologic group	6.7	5.8	6.4	4.4		5.07	<0.01

[a]Conclusions: 1) CA < S < N < MI; 2) young > old; 3) old CA < S < N < MI.

in the Family of Orientation" (Table 7), reflecting the quality of relationships to parents during childhood, and conflict between or separation of the parents. Thus, the effects of an early life stress seem to operate in cancer patients, whereas MI patients suffer from recent stress and conflict with authority.

On two scales, "Behavior Pattern A" (Table 8) and "Perception of External Control" (Table 9), both reflecting the feeling of being pushed or controlled by external demands, cancer patients clearly fall

Table 6. Means of scaled scores for "stress at work"[a]

Nosologic group	MI	S	N	CA	X̄	F	p
	14.9	14.4	14.5	12.9			
Age 35–54	15.5	14.9	14.8	12.0	14.8	1.58	n.s.
Age 55–64	14.0	13.5	14.1	13.8	13.9		
SES							
High	14.7	16.3	15.1	11.9	14.8		
Medium	15.3	13.8	14.0	12.1	14.3	0.88	n.s.
Low	14.3	14.4	14.3	14.1	14.3		
Nosologic group	14.9	14.4	14.5	12.9		7.46	<0.01

[a]Conclusions: 1) CA < MI, S, N; 2) young, high, and medium SES, CA < all other groups.

Interactions: F   p
A × N   5.67   < 0.01
SES × N   3.06   < 0.01

Table 7. Means of scaled scores for "stress in family orientation" (SES ×
nosologic group)[a]

SES	MI	S	N	CA	SES	F	p
High	348.5	278.5	344.8	390.1	344.1		
Medium	281.4	280.3	292.0	351.1	289.6	2.26	<0.10
Low	298.0	368.3	276.3	324.6	317.6		
Nosologic group	306.2	316.8	307.6	350.9		2.51	<0.10

[a]Conclusions: 1) CA > S > N, MI; 2) high > low > medium; 3) high
CA > all other groups.

lowest ($p<0.01$). These scales bring out the differential personality
and perception of life conditions of myocardial infarction and cancer
patients, both representing a position expected on theoretical grounds.

In order to assess social commitment and conformity variables,
three revelant scales were run in this personality area: "Commitment
to Social Norms," "Religiosity," and "Alienation" (Tables 10 to 12).
As predicted, cancer patients fell highest on "Commitment" (Table

Table 8. Means of scaled scores for "Pattern A"[a]

		MI	S	N	CA	X̄	F	p
		54.7	47.2	51.0	41.3			
Age	35–54	58.0	50.0	52.2	44.8	53.0	12.66	<0.001
	55–64	48.6	43.0	48.3	38.0	46.2		
SES								
High		54.7	62.5	56.2	38.7	54.7		
Medium		55.4	44.0	47.0	36.8	48.5	3.37	<0.01
Low		49.9	46.1	48.1	46.0	47.6		
Nosologic group		54.0	47.2	51.0	41.3		8.58	<0.005

[a]Conclusions: 1) CA < S < N < MI; 2) young > old; 3) SES: high >
medium, low; 4) medium, high SES CA < all other groups; 5) old CA < all
other groups.

Interaction:	F	p
SES × N	3.37	< 0.01

Table 9. Means of scaled scores for "internal versus external control: perception of outer world (degree of external control)" (age × nosologic group)[a]

Age	MI	S	N	CA	Age	F	p
35–54	5.9	5.3	5.7	4.4	5.6		
55–64	5.7	5.4	5.3	5.5	5.5		
Nosologic group	5.8	5.4	5.5	5.0		4.52	<0.01

[a]Conclusions: 1) CA < S, N < MI; 2) young CA < all other groups.
Interaction: F   p
A × N   3.93   < 0.01

10), with MI patients falling lowest ($p<0.01$). A similar trend was observed for "Religiosity" (Table 11).

Our "Alienation" scale[2] is a second order scale, constructed by combining seven item scales: "Commitment," "Paranoid Mistrust," "Paranoid Sensitivity," "Social Desirability," "Estrangement from Others," and two scales referring to "External Control," one measuring the perception of the outer world, the other a person's awareness of adapting self to environment. On this combined scale (Table 12), cancers fell significantly lower than the three other groups, which did not differ much from each other ($p<0.05$). As indicated by the two significant interactions, age × nosologic group, and SES × nosologic group, young, and high and medium SES cancer patients rated lower

Table 10. Means of scaled scores for "commitment to social norms" (SES × nosologic group)[a]

SES	MI	S	N	CA	SES	F	p
High	429.7	479.0	489.0	515.3	470.7		
Medium	475.7	458.9	462.2	566.8	471.8	3.76	<0.05
Low	428.8	450.7	433.0	477.1	444.0		
Nosologic group	450.9	458.0	465.6	510.8		4.71	<0.01

[a]Conclusions: 1) CA > N, S, MI; 2) SES: high, medium > low; 3) medium SES CA > all other groups.

---

[2]Like the other scales, this scale was constructed together with Dr. Walter I. Wardwell on the basis of the SECON study data pool.

Table 11. Means of scaled scores for "religiosity"
(age × nosologic group)[a]

Age	MI	S	N	CA	Age	F	p
35–54	72.0	72.9	76.3	91.1	75.4		
55–64	77.4	76.9	82.6	77.1	79.2		n.s.
Nosologic group	74.3	74.5	78.9	83.9		2.34	<0.10

[a]Conclusions: 1) CA > N > S, MI; 2) young CA > all other groups.

Interaction:	F	p
A × N	2.85	< 0.05

Table 12. Means of scaled scores for "alienation"[a]

	MI	S	N	CA	X̄	F	p
	6.6	6.5	6.6	6.0			
Age 35–54	7.0	6.4	6.7	5.6	6.6		
Age 55–64	6.2	6.8	6.3	6.5	6.4	0.13	n.s.
SES							
High	6.4	6.2	6.0	4.7	6.0		
Medium	6.4	6.5	6.6	4.9	6.4	13.32	<0.01
Low	7.6	6.7	7.4	7.7	7.3		
Nosologic group	6.6	6.5	6.6	6.0		2.96	<0.05

[a]Conclusions: 1) CA < S, N, MI; 2) low SES > medium > high; 3) young, high SES CA < all other groups.

Interactions:	F	p
A × N	2.76	< 0.05
SES × N	2.13	< 0.05

than all other groups; whereas, young heart patients rated higher than all other groups.

MEDIATING PSYCHOPHYSIOLOGIC MECHANISMS

In a quest to understand how the psychophysiologic pathways between personality, emotions, and cancer may have developed, several researchers have studied how neurologic, endocrinologic, and immunologic processes are modified by, or modify, psychologic processes.

Studies, particularly by the Russian experimentalists Kavetsky et al. (1966 and 1969) and Balitsky, Kapshuk, and Tsapenko (1969), have addressed themselves to the relationship between CNS changes and malignancies. Kavetsky has shown that lesions of the paraventricular and ventromedial nuclei of the hypothalamus lead to regression of adenomatosis in thyroid tumors. Balitsky, studying changes in bioelectric activity of the cerebral cortex in animals with grafted tumors, observed that bioelectrical activities in the cortex changed and that the frequency of afferent impulsation of involved nerves declined. Here, then, are hard-nosed empirical data pertinent to our broader schema. Rakoff (1962, 1963, 1966) emphasized the important role of the hypothalamic-pituitary system in carcinogenesis and indicated that two alternate pathways of transmittal from the hypothalamus to the target tissues may be operating. One leads via the endocrine glands through hyperfunction to carcinogenesis and the other, more directly, triggers carcinogenesis through neuroendocrine mechanisms and biomechanical changes.

Different workers have emphasized different aspects of the transmittal from the CNS to the target tissues. Kissen and Rao (1969) find that cancer patients compared to control patients show less initial adrenergic response at the time of admission to the hospital, but otherwise retain higher and more fluctuating levels. Cardon and Mueller (1966) concluded that the elevated free fatty acid levels in cancer patients may be related to adrenergic preponderance. Corson (1966) suggested on the basis of his experimental research with dogs that "unstable" animals exhibiting a predominance of adrenergic factors may be more prone to develop tumors. In a later paper (1969), Corson suggested that lack of extinction of visceral responses to stress in dogs, which occurs in animals exhibiting nonadaptive reactions to change in the external situation, may be related to chronic visceral disturbance in these dogs and, possibly, to carcinogenesis. Seymour Levine (1961), who studied the effects of early handling of rats, concluded that one of the reasons that handled rats resist implanted tumors better than nonhandled rats was that their adrenal cortical response was more vigorous, although briefer. Stein's work (Stein, Schiavi, and Luparello, 1969) is of particular importance because it relates hypothalamic changes (lesions) to immune processes by way of modification of circulating antibodies as well as of neuroendocrine and ANS intervening processes. Katz et al. (1969), in an important study of corticoid and androgenic steroids in women with breast cancer, found that the corticoid-androgenic ratio predicted prognosis in cancer of the breast, with high corticoid outputs related to poor prognosis, and low relative corticoid outputs predicting a good prognosis. His group also was able to obtain an impressive correlation (0.56, $p<0.01$) between breakdown of ego defenses and hydrocortisone production in the patients. These findings support those of the workers mentioned above, but raise an important question since elevated rates in their study were associated with a breakdown of defenses, and low rates with hope, faith, control, and denial. In order to relate these findings to the denial hypothesis, it will be imperative to define more clearly in future studies exactly what is meant by defensive failure. The exact defensive mechanisms must be outlined and measured. Moore (1964) clearly demonstrated the importance of hormonal activity when showing that virus alone is hardly carcinogenic, whereas, in combination with hormonal stimulation, it appears highly carcinogenic. Marmorston et al. (1966) compared hormone metabolites in malignant and nonmalignant tumors and found significant differences. Multivariate analyses of such hormones as estrone, 17-ketosteroids, Porter-Silber Chromogen, and the beta part of 17-ketosteroids, all discriminated significantly between the two tumor types. Marmorston et al. (1965a, 1965b, 1965c) showed that estrogen, androsterone, dehydroepiandrosterone, 17-ketogenic steroids, 17-hydroxycorticosteroids, and other hormone metabolites were diminished in cancer patients, when compared with nonmalignant and healthy control patients. She also showed that every cancer type has its own profile of changed hormone production, so that such a profile may serve as a predictor.

Turning now to the immune reactions, reference will be made only to a few basic points. In our psychosomatic model of complementarity, emotional decompensation could well be likened to immunologic failure, in the sense that both processes refer to diminished control, organization, integration, and capacity for resistance and defense. Soloman and Moos (1964) have suggested that stress may reduce the antibody response, and that adult immunologic responsivity may be a function of early infantile experiences. These hypotheses find support in the studies of Ader and Friedman (1964), showing that early life experiences and environmental manipulations modify responses to injected Walker-256 carcinoma, by Ader and Friedman's finding (1965) that rats prematurely separated from their mothers have greater mortality rates from implanted tumors, and Newton's results (1964) that rats handled and petted early in life resist Walker carcinoma 256 longer than rats raised in isolation and without handling.

Weiss (1969) finds that native or acquired immunologic disability often precedes the onset of neoplasia and has suggested several mechanisms by which psychogenic stimuli may affect host-tumor interactions via the immunologic apparatus. Rasmussen (1969) directs himself to the intricate effects of stress on both immunologic and anaphylactic responses, pointing out that stress may stimulate as well as deplete immunologic defensive reactions. Kidd (1961) and Sommers (1958) have approached the immune problem from a slightly different point of view, suggesting that latent cancer cells often are present in body tissues without developing further, and that the sudden proliferation of such cancer cells may be a function of the breakdown of the immune resistance at a particular time. Southam and Siegel (1966) in their careful experiments have gone far to show that immune reactions definitely influence the course of cancer, paying special attention to autoimmune processes. Bennette (1965), in addition to his psychobiologic theorizing and interest in immunologic relationships, emphasizes the role of DNA as a carrier of information and suggests that immunologic reactions may interfere or interact with the distribution of the information code carried along by the DNA molecules for the purpose of identification.

POSTSCRIPT

This brief survey has carried us from the level of broad and abstract psychosocial thinking to the concrete and precise areas of endocrinology and immunology. The frames are different, but the psychologic and immunologic considerations show many conceptual similarities. They both have to do with relationships to self, on the psychologic or somatic levels; with exhaustion and breakdown of defensive systems; and, probably, with dual control systems governing each area. There is a peculiar isomorphism between the psychologic self-alienation and narcissism and the biologic self-propagation and inhibition of immune reactions, which should allow for a theoretical reformulation on a higher level of abstraction, including both levels of psychobiologic processing. Early life experience, self-relationships and self-image, hormonal reactions, autoimmune processes, and the mechanisms of RNA communication, all may have to be considered within a single global theory as multifaceted expressions of the total psychobiologic process. Although we are not this far as yet, there seems to be no doubt that such a theoretical development is the next necessary step which will enable us to conceive of, and not only describe, the malignant process as a total life development, encompassing data which today still are understood as reflecting independent, and at most interactive, phenomena. This monistic construct implies a leap away from the disciplinary segregation characterizing cancer research today, but will be worthwhile, since it will allow for integration and mutual stimulation of all participating disciplines.

REFERENCES

Ader, R., and S. B. Friedman. 1964. Social factors affecting emotionality and resistance to disease in animals. IV. Differential housing, emotionality, and Walker-256 carcinoma in the rat. Psychol. Rep. 15:535–541.

Ader, R., and S. B. Friedman. 1965. Social factors affecting emotionality and resistance to disease in animals. V. Early separation from the mother and response to a transplanted tumor in the rat. Psychosom. Med. 27:119–122.

Amussat, J. Z. 1854. Quelques Reflexions sur la Curabilite du Cancer. E. Thunot et Cie., Paris.

Bahnson, C. B., and M. B. Bahnson. 1964a. Denial and repression of primitive impulses and of disturbing emotions in patients with malignant neoplasms. In D. M. Kissen and L. L. LeShan (eds.), Psychosomatic Aspects of Neoplastic Disease, pp. 42–62. Pitman, London.

Bahnson, C. B., and M. B. Bahnson. 1964b. Cancer as an alternative to psychosis: A theoretical model of somatic and psychological regression. In D. M. Kissen and L. L. LeShan (eds.), Psychosomatic Aspects of Neoplastic Disease, pp. 184–202. Pitman, London.

Bahnson, C. B., and M. B. Bahnson. 1965a. Ego defensive functioning in cancer patients: The utilization of denial and projection as measured by self-attributed and projected mood and emotion. Paper presented at the Fourth International Conference on Psychosomatic Aspects of Neoplastic Disease, Turin, Italy.

Bahnson, C. B., and M. B. Bahnson. 1965b. Psychodynamics of cancer. Paper presented at the Fourth International Conference on Psychosomatic Aspects of Neoplastic Disease, Turin, Italy.

Bahnson, C. B., and D. M. Kissen (eds.). 1966a. Psychophysiological aspects of cancer. Ann. N.Y. Acad. Sci. 125(3):1028–1055.

Bahnson, C. B., and M. B. Bahnson. 1966b. Role of the ego defenses: denial and repression in the etiology of malignant neoplasm. Ann. N.Y. Acad. Sci. 125(3):827–845.

Bahnson, C. B. 1967a. Psychological aspects of cancer. Paper presented at the International Congress for Psychosomatic Medicine and Hypnosis, Kyoto, Japan, July.

Bahnson, C. B. 1967b. Psychodynamische Prozesse und Persönlichkeitsfaktoren bei Krebskranken. *Prophylaxe*. Internat. J. of Prophylactic Med. Soc. Hyg. 6(2):17–26.

Bahnson, C. B. 1969a. Psychophysiological complementarity in malignancies: Past work and future vistas. Ann. N.Y. Acad. Sci. 164(2): 319–334.

Bahnson, C. B. 1970. Basic epistemological considerations regarding psychosomatic processes and their application to current psychophysiological cancer research. Int. J. Psychobiol. 1:57–69.

Bahnson, M. B., and C. B. Bahnson. 1969b. Ego defenses in cancer patients. Ann. N.Y. Acad. Sci. 164(2):546–559.

Balitsky, K. P., A. P. Kapshuk, and V. F. Tsapenko. 1969. Some electrophysiological peculiarities of the nervous system in malignant growth. Ann. N.Y. Acad. Sci. 164(2):520–525.

Bennette, J. G. 1965. Immunological mechanisms in possible mediators of psychosomatic competence in relation to chemical, viral and physical carcinogenic changes. Paper presented at the Fourth International Conference on Psychosomatic Aspects of Neoplastic Disease, Torino, Italy, June.

Blumberg, E. M., P. M. West, and F. W. Ellis. 1954. A possible relationship between psychosomatic factors and human cancer. Psych. Med. 16:277–286.

Brown, F., H. Katz, and M. K. Kaufman. 1961. The patient under study for cancer: A personality evaluation. Psychosom. Med. 23(2):166–171.

Cardon, P. V., Jr., and P. S. Mueller. 1966. A possible mechanism: Psychogenic fat mobilization. Psychophysiologic aspects of cancer. Ann. N.Y. Acad. Sci. 125(3):924–927.

Cobb, B. 1952. A socio-psychological study of the cancer patient. Unpublished doctoral dissertation. University of Texas, Austin, Texas.

Coppen, A. J., and M. Metcalfe, 1963. Cancer and extraversion. Brit. Med. J. 5348:18–19.

Corson, S. A. 1966. Neuroendocrine and behavioral response patterns to psychologic stress and the problem of the target tissue in cerebrovisceral pathology. Ann. N.Y. Acad. Sci. 125(3):890–915.

Corson, S. A. 1969. Discussion. Physiologic responses to avoidable and unavoidable psychologic stress in relation to genetic differences. Ann. N.Y. Acad. Sci. 164(2):526–534.

Cutler, M. 1954. Behavioral characteristics of 40 women with cancer of the breast. *In* J. A. Gengerelli and F. J. Kirkner (eds.), The Psychological Variables in Human Cancer. University of California Press, Berkeley.

Cutter, E. 1887. Diet on cancer. Albany Med. Ann., July and August.

Evans, E. 1926. A Psychological Study of Cancer. Dodd, Mead, New York.

Farberow, N. L., E. S. Shneidman, and C. V. Leonard. 1964. Suicide among general medical and surgical hospital patients with malignant neoplasms. New Physician, January.

Foque, E. 1931. Le problem du cancer dans ses aspects psychiques. Gaz. Hop., Paris, 104:827–833.

Gengerelli, J. A., and F. J. Kirkner (eds.). 1954. The Psychological Variables in Human Cancer: A Symposium. University of California Press, Berkeley.

Goldfarb, C., J. Driesen, and D. Cole. 1967. Psychophysiologic aspects of malignancy. Amer. J. Psychiatry 123:1545–1552.

Greene, W. A. 1954. Psychological factors and reticuloendothelial disease. I. Preliminary observations of a group of males with lymphomas and leukemias. Psychosom. Med. 16:220–230.

Greene, W. A., L. E. Young, and S. N. Swisher. 1956. Psychological factors and reticuloendothelial disease. II. Observations on a group of women with lymphomas and leukemias. Psychosom. Med. 18:282–303.

Greene, W. A. 1966. The psychosocial setting of the development of leukemia and lymphoma. Ann. N.Y. Acad. Sci. 125(3):794–801.

Greene, W. A., and S. N. Swisher. 1969. Psychological and somatic variables associated with the development and course of monozygotic twins discordant for leukemia. Ann. N. Y. Acad. Sci. 164:394–408.

Guy, R. 1759. A Essay on Scirrhous Tumours and Cancers. W. Owen, London.

Hagnell, O. 1966. The premorbid personality of persons who develop cancer in a total population investigated in 1947 and 1957. Ann. N.Y. Acad. Sci. 125(3):846–855.

Hoffman, F. C. 1925. Some Cancer Facts and Fallacies. Newark.

Hughes, C. H. 1887. The relations of nervous depression to the development of cancer. St. Louis Med. Surg. J., May.

Jacobs, J. S. L. 1954. Cancer: Host-resistance and host-acquiescence. *In* J. A. Gengerelli and F. S. Kirkner (eds.), The Psychological Variables in Human Cancer. University of California Press, Berkeley.

Katz, J. L., T. Gallagher, E. Hellman, E. J. Sachar, and H. Weiner. 1969. Psychoendocrine considerations in cancer of the breast. Ann. N. Y. Acad. Sci. 164(2):509–516.

Kavetsky, R. E., N. M. Turkevich, and K. P. Balitsky. 1966. On the psychophysiological mechanism of the organism's resistance to tumor growth. Ann. N.Y. Acad. Sci. 125(3):933–945.

Kavetsky, R. E., N. M. Turkevich, R. M. Akimova, I. K. Khayetsky, and Y. D. Matveichuk. 1969. Induced carcinogenesis under various influences on the hypothalamus. Ann. N.Y. Acad. Sci. 164(2):517–519.

Kidd, J. G. 1961. Does the host react against his own cancer cells? Cancer Res. 21:1170.

Kissen, D. M., and H. J. Eysenck. 1962. Personality in male lung cancer patients. J. Psychosom. Res. 6:123.

Kissen, D. M. 1963. Personality characteristics in males conducive to lung cancer. Brit. J. Med. Psychol. 36:27–36.

Kissen, D. M. 1964. Lung cancer, inhalation, and personality. *In* D. M. Kissen and L. L. LeShan (eds.), Psychosomatic Aspects of Neoplastic Disease, pp. 3–11. Pitman, London.

Kissen, D. M. 1965. Possible contribution of the psychosomatic approach to prevention of lung cancer. Med. Officer 114:343–345.

Kissen, D. M. 1966a. The significance of personality in lung cancer in men. Ann. N.Y. Acad. Sci. 125(3):820–826.

Kissen, D. M. 1966b. The value of a psychosomatic approach to cancer. Ann. N.Y. Acad. Sci. 125(3):777–779.

Kissen, D. M. 1966c. Psychological factors, personality and prevention in lung cancer. Med. Officer 116:135–138.

Kissen, D. M. 1967. Psychosocial factors, personality and lung cancer in men aged 55–64. Brit. J. Med. Psychol. 40:29–43.

Kissen, D. M., and L. G. S. Rao. Steroid excretion patterns and personality in lung cancer. Ann. N.Y. Acad. Sci. 164(2):476–482.

Klopfer, B. A. 1954. Results of psychological testing in cancer. *In* J. A. Gengerelli and F. J. Kirkner (eds.), The Psychological Variables in Human Cancer. Univ. of California Press, Berkeley and Los Angeles, California.

Kowal, S. J. 1955. Emotions as a cause of cancer: Eighteenth and nineteenth century contributions. Psychoanal. Rev. 42:217–227.

LeShan, L., and R. E. Worthington. 1956. Some recurrent life history patterns observed in patients with malignant disease. J. Ment. Dis. 124:460–465.

LeShan, L., and M. Reznikoff. 1960. A psychological factor apparently associated with neoplastic disease. J. Abnorm. Soc. Psychol. 60:439–440.

LeShan, L. 1966. An emotional life-history pattern associated with neoplastic disease. Ann. N.Y. Acad. Sci. 125(3):780–793.

Levine, S. 1961. Plasma-free corticosteroid response to electric shock in rats stimulated in infancy. Science 135:795–796.

Marmorston, J., H. W. Gierson, S. M. Myers, and E. Stern. 1965a. Urinary excretion of neutral 17-ketosteroids and pregnanediol by patients with lung cancer and emphysema. Amer. Rev. Respir. Dis. 92:404–416.

Marmorston, J., L. J. Lombardo, S. M. Myers, H. W. Gierson, and E. Stern. 1965b. Urinary excretion of neutral 17-ketosteroids and pregnanediol by patients with prostatic cancer and benign prostatic hypertrophy. J. Urol. 93:276–286.

Marmorston, J., L. G. Crowley, S. M. Myers, E. Stern, and C. E. Hopkins. 1965c. Urinary excretion of neutral 17-ketosteroids and pregnanediol by patients with breast cancer and benign breast disease. Amer. J. Obstet. Gynec. 92:447–459.

Marmorston, J. 1966. Urinary hormone metabolite levels in patients with cancer of the breast, prostate and lung. Ann. N.Y. Acad. Sci. 125(3):959–973.

Marmorston, J., P. J. Geller, and J. M. Weiner. 1969. Pretreatment urinary hormone patterns and survival in patients with breast cancer or lung cancer. Ann. N.Y. Acad. Sci. 164(2):483–493.

Meerloo, J. A. M. 1954. Psychologic implications of cancer. Geriatrics 9:154–156.

Meyer, W. 1931. Cancer. P. B. Hoeber. New York.

Moore, D. H., and M. J. Lyons. 1964. The role of viruses in breast cancer causation. Presented at the Fifth National Cancer Conference, Philadelphia, September.

Neumann, C. 1959. Psychische Besonoerheiten bei krebspatientinneiu (Psychic peculiarities of female cancer patients). Z. Psychosom. Med. 5:91–101.

Newton, G. 1964. Early experience and resistance to tumor growth. In D. M. Kissen and L. LeShan (eds.), Psychosomatic Aspects of Neoplastic Disease. J. B. Lippincott Company, Philadelphia.

Oo, M. 1965. Personality examinations of cancer patients. Presented at the Fourth International Conference on Psychosomatic Aspects of Neoplastic Disease, Turin, Italy, June.

Paget, Sir J. 1870. Surgical Pathology, 3rd Ed. Longmans, Green, and Co. London.

Parker, W. 1885. Cancer, a study of three-hundred and ninety-seven cases of cancer of the female breast. G. P. Putnam's Sons, New York.

Perrin, G. M., and J. R. Pierce. 1959. Psychosomatic aspects of cancer: A review. Psychosom. Med. 21:397–421.

Rakoff, A. E. 1962. Polycystic disease of the ovaries: Its relationship to the Stein-Leventhal Syndrome and other endocrine dysfunctions. J. Germantown Hosp. 3:25–35.

Rakoff, A. E. 1963. Hormonal patterns in psychogenic amenorrhea and anovulation. Adv. Neuroendocrinol. 14:460–510.

Rakoff, A. E. 1966. In panel. Retrospects and prospects. Ann. N.Y. Acad. Sci. 125:1029–1031.

Rasmussen, A. J., Jr. 1969. Emotions and immunity. Ann. N.Y. Acad. Sci. 164(2):458–462.

Reznikoff, M. 1955. Psychological factors in breast cancer: A preliminary study of some personality trends in patients with cancer of the breast. Psychosom. Med. 17:96–108.

Schmale, A. H. Jr., and H. P. Iker. 1964. The affect of hopelessness in the development of cancer. I. The prediction of uterine cervical cancer in women with atypical cytology. Psychosom. Med. 26:634–635.

Schmale, A. H. Jr., and H. P. Iker. 1966. The psychological setting of uterine cervical cancer. Ann. N.Y. Acad. Sci. 125(3):807–813.

Snow, H. 1883. Clinical Notes on Cancer. J. & A. Churchill, London.

Snow, H. 1891. The Proclivity of Women to Cancerous Diseases. J. & A. Churchill, London.

Soloman, G., and Moos, R. H. 1964. Emotions, immunity and disease. Arch. Gen. Psychiatry 2:657–674.

Sommers, S. C. 1958. Host factors in fatal human lung cancer. AMA Arch. Pathol. 65:104–111.

Southam, C., and A. H. Siegel. 1966. Serum levels of second component of complement in cancer patients. J. Immunol. 97:3.

Stein, M., R. Schiavi, and T. J. Luparello. 1969. The hypothalamus and immune process. Ann. N.Y. Acad. Sci. 164(2):464–472.

Stevenson, D. L. 1964. Evolution and the neurobiogenesis of neoplasia. *In* D. M. Kissen and L. L. Shan (eds.), Psychosomatic Aspects of Neoplastic Disease. Pitman, London.

Sugar, M., and C. Watkins. 1961. Some observations about patients with a breast mass. Cancer 14:979–988.

Tarlau, M., and I. Smalheiser. 1951. Personality patterns in patients with malignant tumors of the breast and cervix: An exploratory study. Psychosom. Med. 13:117–121.

Valadares, E. A. 1967. Psychological features in E.N.T. oncology: Preliminary notes. Semana Medica Vol. 9, No. 443, November.

Walshe, W. H. 1846. Nature and Treatment of Cancer. Taylor and Walton, London.

Weiss, D. W. 1969. Immunological parameters of the host-parasite relationship in neoplasia. Ann. N.Y. Acad. Sci. 164(2):431–448.

Index